WE 810 BUN

WE 810 BUN

Clinical Challenges
in Orthopaedics:
The Shoulder

Clinical Challenges in Orthopaedics: The Shoulder

Edited by

Timothy D. Bunker

Consultant Orthopaedic Surgeon,
Princess Elizabeth Orthopaedic Hospital, Wonford Road, Exeter, UK

Peter J. Schranz

Consultant Orthopaedic Surgeon,
Princess Elizabeth Orthopaedic Hospital, Wonford Road, Exeter, UK

I S I S
MEDICAL
MEDIA

Oxford

© 1998 by Isis Medical Media Ltd.
59 St Aldates
Oxford OX1 1ST, UK

First published 1998

British Library Cataloguing in Publication Data.
A catalogue record for this title is available from
the British Library

ISBN 1 899066 74 8

Bunker, T (Tim)
Clinical Challenges in Orthopaedics: The Shoulder
Timothy D. Bunker and Peter J. Schranz

Always refer to the manufacturer's Prescribing
Information before prescribing drugs cited in this book.

Typeset by
Creative Associates, 115 Magdalen Road, Oxford OX4 1RS, UK

Printed and bound in Hong Kong

Distributed in USA by
Mosby-Year Book Inc., 11830 Westline Industrial Drive
St. Louis Mo. 63146, USA

Distributed in the rest of the world by
Oxford University Press,
Saxon Way West, Corby, Northamptonshire,
NN18 9ES, UK

Contents

List of contributors

Timothy D. Bunker MCh(Orth) BSc MB BS FRCS FRCSEd
Consultant Orthopaedic Surgeon, Princess Elizabeth Orthopaedic Hospital, Wonford Road, Exeter, EX2 4UE, UK

J. Kiss MD
Senior Lecturer in Orthopaedic Surgery (former Shoulder Fellow to Professor Wallace), Department of Orthopaedics, Semmelweis University of Medicine, Budapest XI, Karolina ut 27, 1113 Hungary

D.J. Ogilvie-Harris BSc Hons MB ChB MSc FRCSC
Associate Professor, University of Toronto; Orthopaedic Surgeon, 1-032 Edith Cavell Wing, The Toronto Hospital, Western Division, 399 Bathurst Street, Toronto, M5T 2S8, Canada

E. Sarrosa MD FPCS FPOA
The Toronto Hospital, Western Division, 399 Bathurst Street, Toronto, M5T 2S8, Canada

Peter J. Schranz LRCP MRCS FRCSEd FRCSEdOrth
Consultant Orthopaedic Surgeon, Princess Elizabeth Orthopaedic Hospital, Wonford Road, Exeter, EX2 4UE, UK

W.A. Wallace MBBS FRCSEd
Professor of Orthopaedic Surgery, Department of Orthopaedic and Accident Surgery, University of Nottingham, Queen's Medical Centre, Nottingham, NG7 2UH, UK

Clive D. Warren-Smith BSc MBBS FRCS
Consultant Orthopaedic Surgeon, The Alexandra Hospital, Mill Lane, Cheadle, Cheshire, SK8 2PX, UK

Preface

Why is there a need for yet another book on the shoulder? This book is one of a series which will cover the whole extent of orthopaedic surgery. It tackles a set of challenging topics on the shoulder; some such as recurrent anterior dislocation have now yielded their secrets so that we can treat them in a rational and scientific manner, while others such as frozen shoulder are beginning to yield their secrets and some such as cuff arthropathy remain unsolved. Every chapter is richly illustrated, with full colour photographs, X-rays and line diagrams.

The book is aimed primarily at orthopaedic surgeons approaching their final examinations. It is not a didactic book, but more a challenging one which will stimulate the reader to think beyond the standard texts. We hope that it will catch also the imagination of surgeons who are committed to the field of shoulder surgery since it is forged from the very latest research and written by experts in the field. However, it is not a series of disconnected essays, as are so many 'up-to-date' texts, for the contributors are held together by a common heritage. They share the same background in that they were trained under the tutelage of Professor Angus Wallace in his shoulder unit in Nottingham. The exception is Professor Ogilvie-Harris and his associate Dr Sarrosa, for surgery in the UK has a conservative streak and has fallen behind North America in the field of arthroscopic surgery.

The book starts with a chapter on taking a history and examining a patient with a disordered shoulder. To date this area has been poorly covered in books on the shoulder, most treating clinical skills with contempt and concentrating on high-tech investigations. The British school has always been strong on clinical symptoms and signs and we hope that this is conveyed in this highly illustrated chapter. The second chapter discusses investigations, including MRI. Professor Ogilvie-Harris tackles the present state of arthroscopic surgery around the shoulder, including subacromial decompression, frozen shoulder and repair of both the cuff and dislocations. Next comes a scientific investigation of impingement and cuff tears and an introduction to all the tricks of the trade used by shoulder surgeons to extricate themselves, and their patients, from difficult situations. Dislocation follows, with one chapter on traumatic dislocation and the second by Professor Wallace on the multidisciplinary approach to atraumatic dislocation. Mr Bunker discusses the exciting advances which have occurred recently in the understanding of the pathology of frozen shoulder and its treatment. Chapter nine discusses how new understanding of shoulder morphology has led to the development of the third generation shoulder replacements. Chapters ten and eleven get to grips with those awkward areas, the acromioclavicular and sternoclavicular joints. Four chapters on difficult fracture problems follow: two- and three-part fractures, four-part fractures, the clavicle and fractures of the glenoid. Finally we wind up our tour of shoulder challenges with a thorough analysis of neurological problems, the 'icing on the cake' for the shoulder surgeon.

We would like to acknowledge our publishers, *Isis Medical Media Limited*, who have helped us so much with the design of the book. We would like to thank the medical illustration department at the Royal Devon and Exeter Hospital for all their assistance with the illustrations. Finally we thank our wives, Sue and Ann, for their tolerance during the writing of this book.

T. Bunker and P. Schranz
Princess Elizabeth Orthopaedic Hospital, Exeter
December, 1997

CHAPTER 1

The art of diagnosis in the mystery shoulder

T. Bunker

Introduction

'The shoulder is the most rewarding joint in the whole body. It possesses the salient merits of honesty and curability. When movement is limited or painful the significance regularly implies what on anatomical grounds it ought' (Cyriax).

Unfortunately, in the minds of many surgeons, the shoulder, lying buried under the cloak of deltoid, remains a joint shrouded in mystery, difficult to diagnose and difficult to treat. For three-quarters of this century the shoulder was the forgotten joint. Whilst the bulk of orthopaedic surgeons worked on hip and knee replacements, and on spinal and trauma instrumentation, the shoulder was ignored. Over the earlier decades of this century pioneers, such as Codman, DePalma and Neer, made significant inroads into the mysterious realm of the shoulder. However, in the last two decades, our understanding of the shoulder has developed at breathtaking speed. In the field of diagnosis, arthroscopy and magnetic resonance imaging (MRI) have cast new light on the physiology and pathology of the shoulder. Advances in soft-tissue surgery, in particular arthroscopic surgery, suture-anchor techniques and laser surgery, have decreased the morbidity and improved the outcome of surgery to the shoulder. Third generation modular prostheses have revolutionized the results of shoulder replacement. Additionally, primary-care physicians and public-health officials have awoken to the fact that 10% of the population have one or more episodes of shoulder pain at some point in their lives, and 5% of all primary-care consultations are for shoulder problems. Against such a background this book will help to unveil the enigmas of

the shoulder for the surgeon who has the ambition to learn more about this fascinating and rewarding joint.

In fact the shoulder is no different from any other joint and, although every shoulder presents as a diagnostic challenge, the great majority can be correctly diagnosed with a carefully taken history and a structured examination.

Despite the most meticulous history and examination, a minority of shoulder problems will remain a mystery. Fortunately, we now have a range of diagnostic facilities at our disposal: blood tests, plain radiographs, arthrography, ultrasound, MRI, computerized tomography (CT) scanning, shoulder arthroscopy, bursoscopy, neurophysiological testing, surgical exploration and histopathology.

Four golden rules should always be observed when making a diagnosis for patients presenting with a shoulder problem: (1) *never take for granted the diagnosis of the referring physician*. Remember that the referring physician may have very little understanding of shoulder pathology, he may be a generalist or a specialist from another discipline such as a spinal surgeon. Respect the referring physician; he may well be more knowledgeable than you in other disciplines, but has recognized his limitations in shoulder surgery and hence has referred the patient to you.

The referral of a frozen shoulder is the classic trap. Many primary-care physicians, and even some orthopaedic surgeons, think that any painful stiff shoulder is a frozen shoulder. Of 150 patients referred to Dr Wiley (1991) as a frozen shoulder, only 37 truly had the condition. So respect the referring physician, but confirm his or her diagnosis; (2) *never jump to conclusions*. If the patient says that their arm goes dead, it does not necessarily mean that they have 'dead arm syndrome' (shoulder subluxation). Record it and note it, for the patient is usually right, but don't jump to a diagnosis and blot everything else out of mind.

Always wait until the history has been completely taken and a full examination performed before making the diagnosis. Diagnosis is like solving a jigsaw puzzle, the puzzle is not solved when the four corners have been found, but only when the last piece has been put in place.

Recently a patient was referred to me who said that he went to his doctor with a painful shoulder. The doctor asked him, whilst he was still fully dressed, to raise his arm. The patient raised his arm to shoulder height, but could raise it no further. The doctor made a diagnosis of a frozen shoulder, indicated the need for a manipulation and implied that this course of action would lead to the patient's recovery. The doctor was incorrect in all three assumptions; the patient in fact had a rotator-cuff tear, did not need a manipulation (but had two) and failed to recover. It was also inexcusable for the doctor not to have undressed and examined the patient properly. There is no better example of the disaster of jumping to conclusions, or thinking the jigsaw puzzle is solved when the four corners alone have been exposed; (3) *leave enough time for each patient*. After spinal disorders the shoulder is probably the most difficult joint to diagnose accurately.

Most shoulder problems are soft-tissue disorders, such as impingement, cuff tears, contractures and dislocations, hence they are not revealed on radiographs. At least 20 minutes should be booked for a new patient, and 15 for an old patient. Also, leave enough time for injection studies; (4) *listen to the patient*. The patient is nearly always right. Let the patient tell their story, prompt but don't lead, give them time, inspire confidence, draw them out.

This chapter will describe a structured clinical assessment based upon the recommendations of the American Shoulder and Elbow Surgeons (ASES) research committee (Richards *et al.*, 1994) (Fig. 1.1).The next chapter will look at the role of investigations in diagnosing the mystery shoulder.

Method of referral

In the US and some parts of Europe the patient may self-refer. In this case prior information is scant. However, in the UK, and increasingly in the USA, the patient will

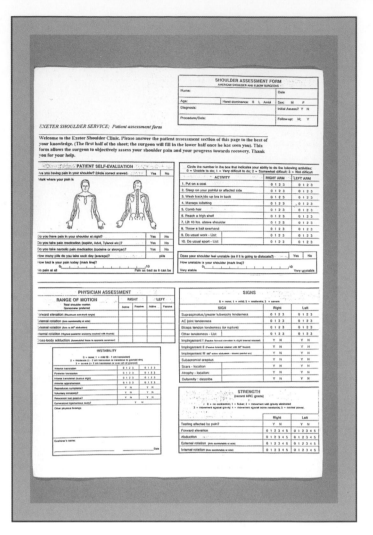

Figure 1.1 – *The American Shoulder and Elbow Surgeons assessment form. This consists of a patient self-assessment form, which assesses pain, function and instability. It also contains a proforma for the examination, filled in by the examining surgeon, which assesses clinical examination, range of movement, impingement signs, instability signs and strength.*

have been referred by a primary-care physician or orthopaedic colleague. Surgeons usually build up a referral base and learn that some colleagues are immensely talented and others mediocre at best. The former will give tremendous help in their letter of referral, the latter scant detail.

The ideal referral letter (Table 1.1) will detail the problem, be it pain, loss of function, deformity, instability or weakness. It will detail in which shoulder the problem lies, when and how the problem started, what treatment has been given so far and how it has helped. It will also detail the clinical findings made at the time of referral.

Table 1.1 – The contents of an ideal referral letter.	

- The problem   Pain; loss of function; deformity; weakness; instability
- Which shoulder
- Onset   When and how?
- Treatment   What and how effective?
- Relevant findings
- The patient   Pen portrait
- The family
- Employment
- Home circumstances
- Past history   Medical and surgical
- Drugs

As important, the letter will give a history of the patient themselves, their family background, employment and home circumstances, which will allow you to probe into these areas with greater ease.

Finally the referral letter will give details of the previous medical and surgical history and the medication that the patient is currently on. It is surprising how patients will forget important medical events, let alone what medication they are taking. How often do we have the patient (usually a man) deny that he has ever had a day's illness in his life, only to have his wife inform us that he had a myocardial infarct 3 months ago!

Patient self-evaluation

While the patient is waiting to be seen he or she is asked by the clinic receptionist to fill in the ASES self-evaluation form. The self-evaluation form has three parts, relating to experience of pain, activities of daily living and instability. Questions on the form relating to pain include: 'do you have pain?', 'where is the pain?', 'do you have night pain?', 'do you take pain medication?', 'do you take narcotic pain medication?', 'how many pills do you take every day?' There is also a visual analogue score to complete.

There are 10 daily-living activities listed, each of which is measured on a 4-point ordinal score (from 0 to 3, where 0 = unable to do; 1 = very difficult to do; 2 = somewhat difficult; 3 = not difficult). The 10 activities are: put on a coat; sleep on affected side; wash back/do up bra; manage toilet; comb hair; reach a high shelf; lift 10 lbs above shoulder height; throw a ball overhead; do usual work (list); do usual sport (list).

The final self-evaluation question asks if the shoulder feels unstable and if so the patient is asked to indicate the degree of instability on a visual analogue score.

The self-evaluation form allows objective scoring of pain (out of 10) and activities (out of 30). It is a permanent record which can be retrieved for research purposes, and since it has been agreed by the ASES, it allows comparisons between clinics. The ASES shoulder score can be calculated from it using the formula $([10-VAS] \times 5) + (5/3 \times ADL)$ which gives a score out of 100.

The proforma also shows that your clinic means business and gives the patient something to think about whilst they wait to see you. Once the patient has filled in the self-evaluation form it is time for patient and surgeon to meet.

Initial impressions

It was Sherlock Holmes who said 'Observe, my dear Watson, don't just look'. The physician's observations should start as soon as he meets the patients. How old do they look? How do they hold the shoulder? How does their neck move during the interview? How do they dress? How do they shake hands? Are they depressed, angry, confrontational? Do they have an obvious medical condition that could affect their shoulder? Are there any scars visible which may have a bearing on the shoulder? The rationale behind this approach is as follows: (a) *How old is the patient?* Bearing in mind the importance of not jumping to conclusions when making a diagnosis, there are two aphorisms worth remembering. Firstly 'All patients under the age of 40 have instability' and secondly 'grey hair equals cuff tear'. (Fig. 1.2). Age has a bearing on the disease, the quality of tissue that needs to be repaired and the rehabilitation potential of the patient; (b) *How does the patient hold the shoulder?* Is the patient being protective of the shoulder? Is the shoulder moving freely during the interview? Is there disparity of movement from interview to examination? Finally, beware of the patient who attends the clinic wearing a sling, either they have a devastating problem, or they are amplifying their pain;

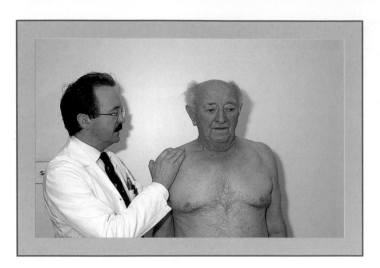

Figure 1.2 – *'Grey hair equals cuff tear'. Rotator-cuff tears are associated with ageing.*

rheumatoid, the Heberden's nodes of the polyosteoarthritic, the skin burns of the syringomyelic. The author has seen all of these in his shoulder clinic; (h) *Does the patient have surgical scars of relevance?* The initial observations are made before the patient undresses so only the skin of the face, neck and hands will be apparent until later. However, the scar in the posterior triangle of the neck, from a bottle fight, or a poorly trained surgeon, which has divided the spinal accessory nerve may well have a bearing upon shoulder function.

These initial observations only take seconds, whilst the surgeon is introducing himself and shaking the hand of the patient, and thanking them for filling in the self-assesment form. Now it is time to start taking a history.

Taking the history

The shoulder patient will usually present because of pain, loss of function, stiffness, weakness or instability. All of these symptoms are indicative of potential problems, so the first question should be 'Your doctor has asked me to see you because of your shoulder, what is the trouble?'

Pain

The commonest presentation is pain. Ask the patient where they get the pain. Observe how they answer. True shoulder pain is difficult to pinpoint and the patient will take the palm of the other hand and rub it over the deltoid (Fig. 1.3) to explain where the pain is. This is called the 'palm sign'. Contrast this with acromioclavicular joint pain which is quite specific, for here the patient will take the index finger of the opposite hand and point to the acromioclavicular joint (Fig. 1.4). This is called the 'finger sign'. Check the patient's consistency by noting where the patient has drawn the site of the pain on the ASES form. True shoulder pain must be differentiated from referred pain. The key to this is in the radiation of the pain. Where does the pain go? True shoulder pain radiates down to the insertion of the deltoid; if severe it will radiate down to the elbow and on to the radial side of the forearm, sometimes to the radial side of the wrist, exceptionally to the thenar emminence, but never to the fingers.

the outcome is going to be poor either way; (c) *How does the patient move their neck?* Shoulder pain can be referred, commonly from the neck. Watch the neck throughout the interview before the patient is aware of your covert observation; (d) *How does the patient dress?* Patients with shoulder pain have difficulty dressing. In particular they have difficulty putting clothing over their heads. Many people in the shoulder clinic will have button-up shirts or dresses, and will wear cardigans and not pullovers. Observe how they dress and undress. Don't let your clinic nurse help them. Use every opportunity to observe their shoulder function; (e) *How does the patient shake hands?* The shoulder-shrug of the patient with a massive rotator-cuff tear is pathognomonic for, unable to reach, he is forced to leave the elbow at the side and shrug the whole forequarter to shake hands; (f) *Is the patient depressed, angry, or confrontational?* The psychological attitude of the patient is important to their prognosis. The patient with night pain may have been worn down by the torture of sleep deprivation, over many months, and may be radically improved by shoulder surgery. The angry patient may have litigation ongoing against an employer and will not get better until the lawyers have cleared the field. The confrontational patient may never be content, so try to avoid surgery in these patients; (g) *Does the patient have overt medical problems?* Secondary arthritis is common in the shoulder. Watch out for the prognathic jaw and big hands of the acromegalic, the pitted fingernails of the psoriatic, the swollen proximal interphalangeal (PIP) joints of the

If the pain radiates to the fingers look elsewhere for the site of the pain, usually the cervical spine. Thoracic-

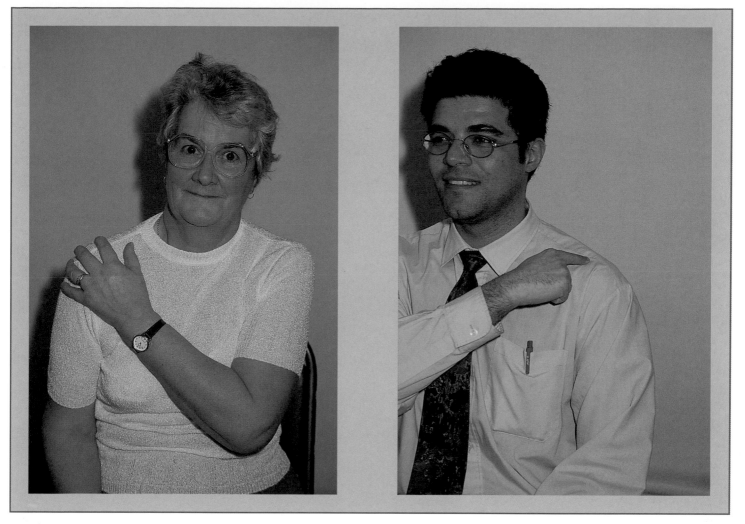

Figure 1.3 – *The palm sign of true shoulder pain. The patient rubs the affected shoulder to show the vague distribution of the pain.*

Figure 1.4 – *The finger sign of acromioclavicular joint pain. Acromioclavicular joint pain is quite specific and the patient will point directly to the joint as the source of their pain.*

outlet pain usually radiates to the ulnar side of the hand and arm (C8 and T1), sometimes even to the chest wall (T2). Beware of subluxation which can cause a heavy feeling in the fingers, or a dead feeling, but this is different from pain.

Patients with true shoulder pain may get aching or fatiguing in the trapezius. This is because they are protecting the glenohumeral joint and rotator cuff by overusing scapulothoracic movement. This fatigues the scapular muscles.

Acromioclavicular pain may radiate to the neck, or be felt anywhere in the epaulette region (that region supplied by the C4 nerve root).

Sternoclavicular joint pain classically radiates along the course of the clavicle.

Beware of those rare cases of visceral referred pain, angina to left shoulder and gall bladder to right scapula. These are exceedingly rare.

Once again refer to the drawing on the ASES self-assessment form, and add your own annotations as necessary.

When did the pain start?

How did the pain start? Was the onset insidious or violent? If there was an accident, either sporting, at work or in the home, how did it happen? What position was the arm in? How violent was it? Did the pain come on immediately? Was there a hiatus in the pain, did it become worse that evening (typical with a rotator-cuff tear)? If there was an injury how was it managed? Did the patient go to hospital? Were radiographs taken, and if so what did they show? How was the injury managed? To what degree did it recover and in what time frame? Is litigation pending?

How bad is the pain?

The ASES form asks four questions of the patient to assess the severity of pain. These relate to (1) the presence of night pain, (2) the need for medication, (3) the need for narcotic medication, and (4) how many pills are needed per day. Finally, the patient is asked to fill in a visual-analogue scale of pain severity. Often the patient will need to be led through these questions again by the physician, with annotations as necessary. Beware of patients who say they are in continual agony. Beware of stoics. Be ready to listen to the patient's partner; some patients will overplay their pain, some will underplay it. It was Codman who said he would much rather listen to the spouse's description of the severity of the pain, because they always described it with more honesty!

What is the pain like?

This is always a difficult question for the patient to answer. Most patients describe their pain as more of an ache. However, there is one characteristic pain — the crescendo pain — like a severe toothache, which builds up rapidly to reach an intolerable level, that can only mean one thing, acute calcific tendonitis. Vasomotor pain of thoracic-outlet syndrome may be recalled as 'icy water trickling down the arm'. Referred pain from the neck often has a 'burning' nature.

What movement exacerbates the pain?

Pain on movement is usually termed the painful arc (Fig. 1.5). Classically, the painful arc is due to rotator-cuff pathology, it starts at 70° of elevation and eases at about 140°. The high painful arc which starts at 140° and becomes worse when the arm is elevated further is often associated with acromioclavicular joint disorders. Both rotator-cuff pathology and acromioclavicular disorders may be combined, the pain starts at 70° and does not let up until the end point of movement is reached — this is the combined painful arc.

The painful arc may be worse in abduction rather than elevation. Pain may be exacerbated by passive internal rotation of the arm at 90° of elevation.

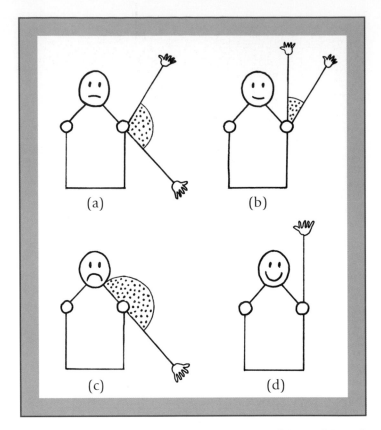

Figure 1.5 – *The painful arcs. (a) Classic painful arc, (b) High painful arc of acromioclavicular joint disease, (c) Combined painful arc, (d) Normal.*

Some patients will state that there is a particular pain brought on with a hitch or catch when the arm, which is held at 90° of abduction, is rotated actively; some physicians will say this is associated with a partial thickness top-surface tear of the rotator cuff.

Acromioclavicular joint pain may be exacerbated by cross body adduction, and also by full internal rotation with the hand up behind the back (the wrestling 'half Nelson' position). Acromioclavicular joint pain is increased by compression of the joint surfaces, for instance when doing a press-up.

The pain of dislocation may be brought on by bringing the arm up into the position of apprehension (90° of abduction and full external rotation) (Fig. 1.6), or the cocking position of throwing.

Rotator cuff pain occurs when reaching. This is classically the case, so ask the patient about typical reaching positions, lifting a coffee pot, lifting a cup, changing gear with a stick-shift gearchange, putting the ignition-key in the car, using a computer keyboard, dressing, reaching up to a shelf, holding out a newspaper. Some patients will even have changed their

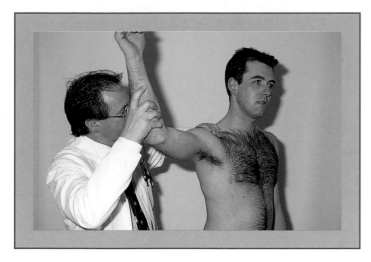

Figure 1.6 – *The position of apprehension. The arm is abducted 90° and fully externally rotated.*

newspaper, from full size to tabloid to avoid this fatiguing, reaching ache. Many of these activities will be covered again when the 'activity' section of the ASES form is run through with the patient.

Pain at rest should alert the attention of the surgeon; this is how metastases and sepsis present.

Other exacerbating features

Night pain is typical of true shoulder pain. The patient may have difficulty in getting to sleep, may awaken early, may awaken during the night, or may adopt a particular sleeping position in an attempt to avoid the pain.

The pain may be made worse by lifting or carrying. Patients with frozen shoulder often register severe pain if the arm is jerked.

What treatment has the patient had?

How much did it help? If the patient had an injection did it relieve the pain and, if so, for how long? Was it relieved for the duration of the local anaesthetic? Was there no relief? Where was the injection sited? Have they had physiotherapy? What form of physiotherapy, was it ultrasound, interferential, hands-on manipulation, Theraband exercises, deep frictions? Which of these modalities helped and which made the pain worse? Has the patient had fringe management, osteopathy, chiropractics, acupuncture, aromatherapy? The answers to these questions can be of vital importance. Moreover, if you have failed to discover that the patient has already had physiotherapy, and that it made the pain worse, and then suggest that physiotherapy is the best treatment for

them, the patient's confidence in you as a shoulder specialist will be sorely tested!

Loss of function

The patient's main complaint may be loss of function. This may be quite specific such as not being able to play overhead shots at tennis, or it may be quite general. The ASES self-assessment form is extremely helpful in that it covers most functions and allows further dialogue to flesh out the details. The form covers eight activities, plus work and sport. Be careful as sometimes patients will fill in the form as a mirror-image of what it should be.

Putting on a coat. Many patients with shoulder pain will have great difficulty in dressing. In particular, they have difficulty putting on a coat and have to put the injured arm in first. They may even have to ask a partner to help them dress.

Sleeping on the painful side. This is commonly painful. The next two activities are a function of restriction of internal rotation. *Washing the back/doing up bra at back*, is a function which requires quite a good range of internal rotation. Less internal rotation is required for managing toilet/wiping the bottom, but is such a prime social responsibility that it needs noting.

Combing the hair, is a function of elevation and external rotation, but is also inseparable from hand dominance. If the non-dominant hand is affected ask how the patients manage to wash their hair.

The next three questions relate to activities that are a function of reaching overhead. The first is *reaching a high shelf*, the second *lifting 10 lbs overhead* which requires strength as well, and the third is throwing a ball which requires elevation, strength and dexterity.

Work. The type of work undertaken by the patient is ascertained and the activities involved in such work are listed. This allows the surgeon to look into environmental causes of pain in the shoulder, and allows him to obtain a description of the workplace and what the patient actually does and needs to do. Overhead workers, such as carpenters and electricians, often suffer from impingement pain.

Sports. Ask which sports the patient plays, how often and at what level? Ask whether the patient can still participate, and if not why not? The self-assessment form allows the surgeon to elaborate on areas where the patient is disabled.

Instability

The patient will usually volunteer that the shoulder 'Goes out'. The instability may have started with a traumatic episode. In this case it is important to document when this happened. Exactly how did it happen? How much force was involved, minimal or great? Did the shoulder reduce spontaneously? Was it put in by a friend, first aider, or paramedic? Did the patient have to go to hospital? If so which hospital? Was a radiograph taken? What type of anaesthetic was needed to reduce the dislocation? Which way did it come out, front or back? How many times has it gone out since ? How much force was required to put it out the second and subsequent times? How many times has it gone out altogether? Does the shoulder give trouble between episodes of dislocation? Does it feel vulnerable? Is it protected? What can the patient not do, because of the worry of it coming out again?

The shoulder may have become unstable without a clear-cut episode of trauma. This story should ring alarm bells. Patients who dislocate without trauma are 'born loose' and are consequently far more difficult to treat. Again ask how often the shoulder comes out? What position is the arm in when it dislocates? Does the shoulder seem to come out forward, backwards or downwards, or a combination of these? How does the shoulder trouble the patient between episodes of dislocation? How vulnerable does the patient feel? How restricted are they at home, at work and at sports?

The final group of instability patients are those who present with subluxation. These are a difficult group to diagnose and often fall into the 'mystery shoulder group'. The patient may complain that the arm feels heavy, or dead. They may complain of neurological symptoms in the forearm and hand. The differential diagnosis includes referred neurological irritation arising from the neck or the thoracic outlet. This type of mystery shoulder will often need investigation. Examination under anaesthetic and arthroscopy of the shoulder become vital tools to the investigating surgeon.

Stiffness, weakness, deformity and noises, may be the chief complaints of your patient. These are all revealed during the examination and we will deal with each as we run through the shoulder examination.

By this stage the surgeon should have a fair idea of what is wrong with the patient and their shoulder. At this point it is useful to move on to the general history and to ask the four key questions on previous medical history, previous surgical history, drug history and allergies.

The general medical history may be very relevant, for instance frozen shoulder is common in patients with diabetes. Remember to keep an open mind, just because a patient has diabetes it does not necessarily mean that they have frozen shoulder, just as, if they have sickle cell disease, it does not necessarily follow that they have avascular necrosis of the humeral head, again the fact that they are on dialysis does not necessarily mean that they have an amyloid deposit in the coraco-acromial ligament causing impingement; but the association should flash instantly through your mind.

The clinical examination

Introduction

The examination will follow the standard pattern of look, feel, move, strain and investigate.

Observation

Clearly the patient must be unclothed for the examination. Ladies should keep their bra on for the sake of propriety and decorum. However, all other clothing above the belt must be taken off, including vests. Watch the patient undress because this is enlightening. Can the elbow leave the side? Can the patient reach? How protective of the shoulder are they? How clumsy are they with buttons? Have they developed reverse dominance?

Deformity

Look at the patient from the front, side and back. The patient may actually present with a main complaint of deformity (Fig. 1.7). This may appear trivial, such as the male model who presented with an acromioclavicular dislocation, but this actually deprived him of his livelihood of modelling shirts for mail-order catalogues; or the body-builder who presented with a partial tear of pectoralis major, which to him was a disaster as it ruled him out of winning any further major body building contests. On the other hand the patient may present with a major deformity caused by a congenital anomaly such as congenital pseudarthrosis of the clavicle, Sprengel's shoulder, Erb's palsy or Poland's anomaly.

Observe the attitude of the shoulder. In particular look at the sternoclavicular and acromioclavicular joints. Are they swollen? Are they misplaced? Look for asymmetry between the shoulders. Look at the humeral head in relation to the scapula — does it appear

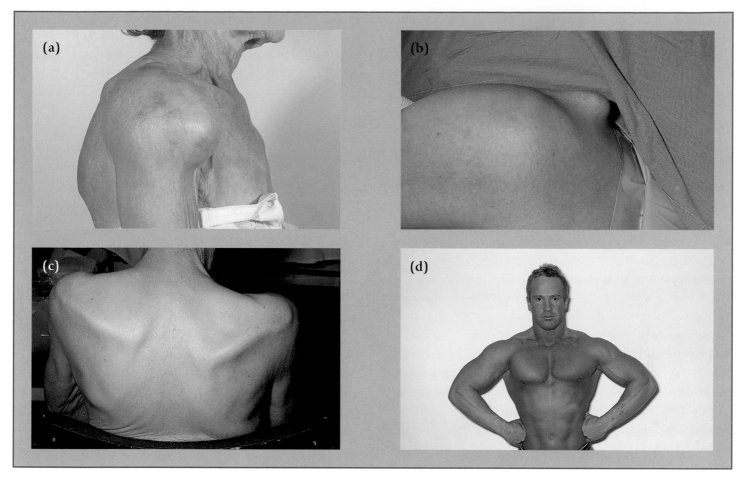

Figure 1.7 – *Deformity. (a) Swollen shoulder, (b) Wasting of infraspinatus and supraspinatus (old cuff tear), (c) Dislocated acromio-clavicular joint, (d) Pectoralis major rupture, on the right.*

medialized? Is it elevated? Does it appear abnormally prominent either anteriorly or posteriorly?

Atrophy

Atrophy may be caused by disuse, a partial or complete tear of the muscle, or by neurological disease. Note not only the presence of wasting, but also the degree of wasting. For instance a mild degree of wasting of infraspinatus may be caused by disuse or impingement, whereas marked wasting is more likely to follow a tear of infraspinatus or suprascapular nerve entrapment. Mild wasting of deltoid may signify disuse, whereas severe wasting may mean there is a palsy of the axillary nerve. Is there any winging of the scapula?

Look for hypertrophy as well as atrophy. The classic is the 'Popeye' muscle with a torn long-head of biceps (Fig. 1.8). The 'Superman' appearance of fascioscapulohumeral dystrophy, where the deltoid appears hypertrophied compared to the wasted arm and scapular muscles, is a good

example. Muscle spasm may mimic hypertrophy such as the trapezius spasm of the patient with a cervical disc prolapse.

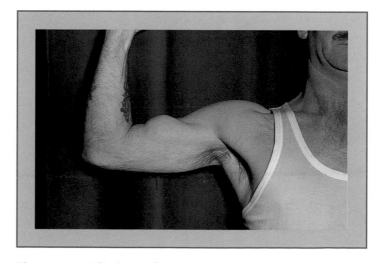

Figure 1.8 – *The 'Popeye' muscle caused by a rupture of the long head of biceps tendon.*

Scars

Scars are vital evidence and so should be noted. If the scar is wide, cross hatched and perpendicular to Langer's lines then it is likely that the surgery underneath will be just as inept. The scar is the signature of the surgeon (Fig. 1.9). Alternatively, if the scar is in the skin crease but widened then the patient may have a hypermobility syndrome and a lax shoulder.

Physical examination

Having circled the patient and carefully observed the shoulder, a physical examination should be made. Always examine the asymptomatic shoulder first and then turn to the symptomatic side. Identify the landmarks — the posterior angle of the acromion, the spine of the scapula, the clavicle, the acromioclavicular joint, and the coracoid process.

First just run the hand over the shoulder. Is the skin normal to touch? Is it hot? Is it extra sensitive? Feel the sternoclavicular joint. Is it swollen? Is it abnormally mobile? Is it tender? Feel the acromioclavicular joint. Is it swollen, hypermobile or tender? Feel the greater tuberosity, the key area where cuff tears originate (Fig. 1.10). Is the tuberosity tender? Can you feel the sulcus of a tear or the emminence of osteophyte on the tuberosity beyond a tear? Is there an abnormally prominent anterior acromion or an abnormal spike of bone in the insertion of the coraco-acromial ligament? Feel the muscles, in particular supraspinatus and infraspinatus, feel how wasted they are. Biceps tendon is very difficult to feel, unless the patient is cachectic. Run the hand

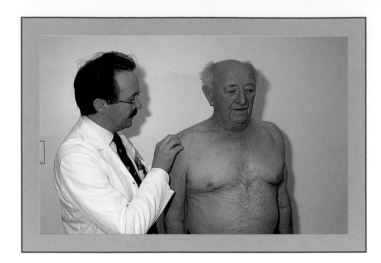

Figure 1.10 – *Palpating the greater tuberosity.*

down the arm. Look at the hand. See if there is any wasting of the interossei, any evidence of Dupuytren's disease, any nail pitting or clubbing.

Note any areas of tenderness on the ASES form, along with the degree of tenderness. Note that the worse the tenderness the higher they score, exactly the opposite of the scoring for activity.

Movement of the joint

The joint must be moved in three different ways. First actively by the patient (Fig. 1.11). Look at the rhythm of the movement, the ratio of scapular movement to glenohumeral movement, comparing side to side, particularly as the arm comes back down from full elevation, because this is when a protective pattern of

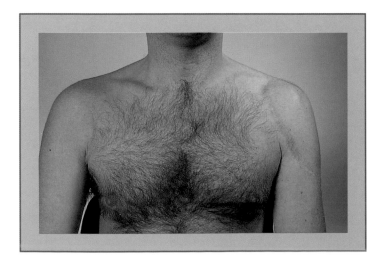

Figure 1.9 – *A wide scar on the left shoulder and a skin-crease scar on the right shoulder.*

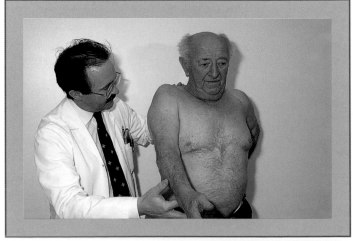

Figure 1.11 – *Active elevation. The surgeon watches the patient's eyes as the arm traverses the painful arc of movement.*

movement (reversed scapular rhythm) is most noticeable. Active movement will be affected by pain and weakness. Next the joint must be moved passively by the surgeon. If the range of passive movement is greater than that of active movement, it confirms that either weakness or pain is limiting the active movement. However, if the passive movement is restricted as much as the active movement this implies either a contracture of the capsule, joint disease, such as arthritis, or locked dislocation. Finally the joint should be moved against resistance to assess muscle strength.

The range of motion is assessed actively and then passively. Forward elevation is measured as combined glenohumeral and scapulothoracic motion. The maximum arm trunk angle is recorded. Differentiating glenohumeral from scapulothoracic movement is not consistent (according to the research committee of the ASES), but it is useful to place your examining hand over the top of the scapula to give some feel as to the rhythm and pattern of movement as well as to feel for crepitus, and to grade that crepitus.

During passive elevation, record the presence of impingement, the degree of pain and wincing, the amount of resistance and spasm, as the arm comes up into the painful arc (Fig. 1.12). The ASES proforma has three boxes to record impingement. I is passive forward elevation in slight internal rotation. II is passive internal rotation with the arm in 90° of elevation, which is slightly more sensitive. III is the classic painful arc at 90° of active abduction, which is less sensitive.

External rotation is measured both actively (Fig. 1.13) and passively (Fig. 1.14), with the elbow held comfortably to the side, using the forearm as the pointer of a goniometer. Restriction of passive external rotation can only mean one of three things: (1) that the patient has a frozen shoulder, (2) arthritis, or (3) locked posterior dislocation. External rotation can also be tested with the arm at 90° of abduction.

Internal rotation is measured using the functional method of the highest vertebral level touched by the extended thumb (Figs 1.15 and 1.16). The normal position reached by the thumb is the bottom of the scapula — T7. Levels above this mean that there is excessive movement in the joint, suggesting instability, levels below this suggest either stiffness or pain. End-point pain on internal rotation is typical of impingement.

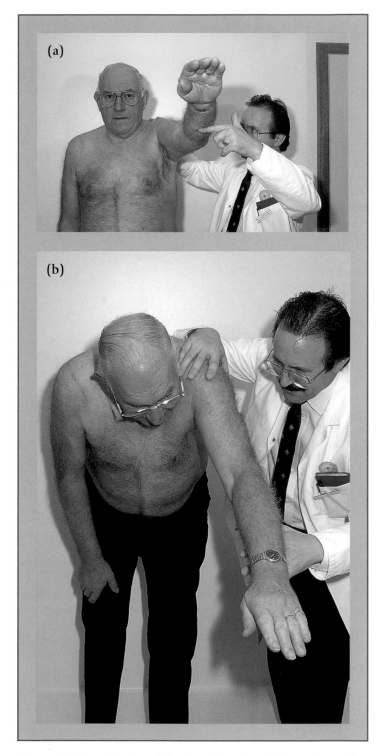

Figure 1.12 – *Passive elevation. Standing (a), and stooping (b). In rotator cuff disease the patient is able to relieve impingement pain by stooping.*

Beware of the patient who has elbow disease because this method of measuring internal rotation depends upon having normal and symmetric elbow movement, thus its use is invalid in rheumatoid or generalized arthritis.

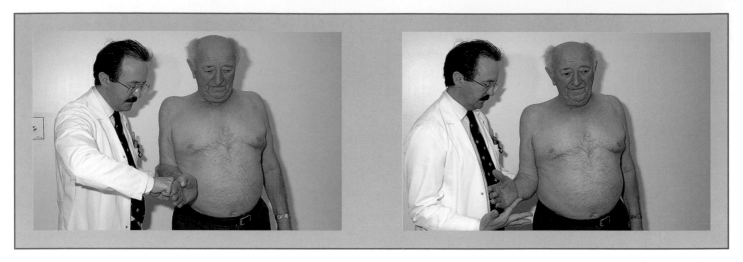

Figure 1.13 – *Active external rotation. This tests infraspinatus, the anterior capsule and pain.*

Figure 1.14 – *Passive external rotation. This tests if the anterior capsule is contracted.*

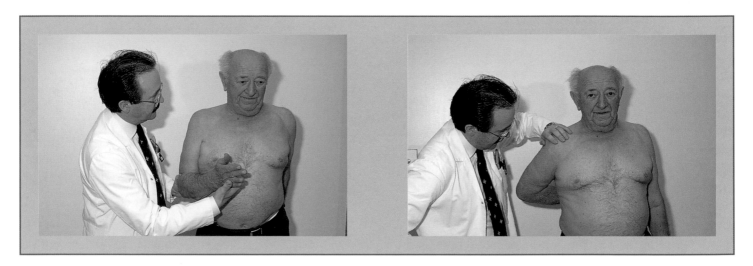

Figure 1.15 – *Active internal rotation. This tests subscapularis, the posterior capsule and pain.*

Figure 1.16 – *Passive internal rotation. This tests if the posterior capsule is tight.*

Finally we measure cross-body adduction both actively and passively.

Crepitus

Some patients may actually present with the complaint that 'the shoulder makes noises'. These noises are important, but all too often neglected. Ask what type of noise it is? Where does it come from? Is it from the glenohumeral joint, the acromioclavicular joint, or from the cuff? Is it the clunk of relocation? Is it the click of a labral tear? Is it the squeaking stiction-friction of arthritis? Is it the washerboard rattle of snapping scapula? Is it the crepitus of a rotator-cuff tear? If so, is it the soft crepitus of a partial-thickness tear or the harsh crepitus of a full-thickness tear?

Feel the shoulder as the patient reproduces the noise. Take every opportunity to tune your hand in to noises in the shoulder.

Strength

Strength is recorded according to the Medical Research Council (MRC) grade 0 = no contracture; 1 = flicker; 2 = movement with gravity eliminated; 3 = movement against gravity; 4 = movement against some resistance; 5 = normal strength. If the strength is impaired the surgeon should make a judgement as to whether this weakness is caused by pain inhibition alone, or by true weakness of the muscle.

Forward elevation tests anterior deltoid and also tests the integrity of the cuff to stabilize the fulcrum of the shoulder. Watch to see if the humeral head rises forwards and upwards on initiation of elevation.

Abduction tests both supraspinatus and deltoid, each of which contribute to about 50% of the torque of abduction (Fig. 1.17). If you need to test supraspinatus in a more isolated fashion then resisted abduction should be tested at 90° of abduction, with the arm internally rotated. This is called 'Jobe's test'.

External rotation tests infraspinatus and teres minor (Fig. 1.18).

Internal rotation is taken as a test of subscapularis (Fig. 1.19), but is actually a much more composite movement powered by latissimus dorsi, teres major, and even pectoralis major.

Instability testing

The apprehension test

This is the classic test for anterior instability. This test can be performed with the patient either sitting or standing. To test the right arm the examiner stands to the right and just behind the patient. The examiner bends the patient's elbow to 90° and holds the elbow in his/her right hand. The examiner places his/her hand over the patient's shoulder with the thumb on the back of the humeral head. The affected arm is fully externally rotated at 45°, then at 90° and finally at 135°. As the arm is externally rotated the patient realizes that the shoulder is about to 'slip out'. At this point the patient winces and involuntarily resists any further movement (Fig. 1.20).

The crank test

This is a continuation of the apprehension test. If the patient does not wince at full external rotation then

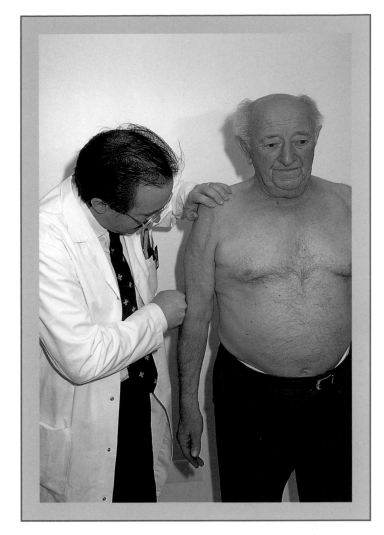

Figure 1.17 – *Abduction test for supraspinatus. Resisted active abduction.*

overpressure is applied, or the shoulder is cranked out. Again the end-point is apprehension (Fig. 1.21)

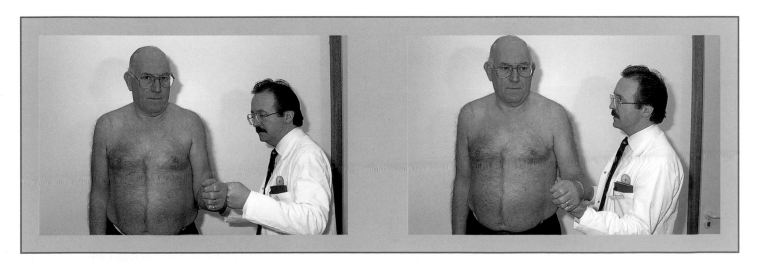

Figure 1.18 – *External rotation tests infraspinatus.*

Figure 1.19 – *Resisted internal rotation tests subscapularis.*

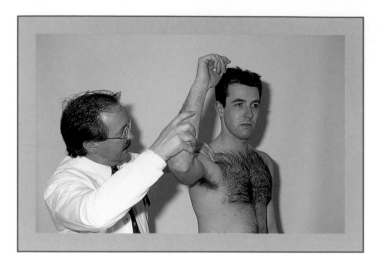

Figure 1.20 – *The apprehension test. The patient is brought into the position of apprehension and shows evidence of muscle spasm, wincing and wariness.*

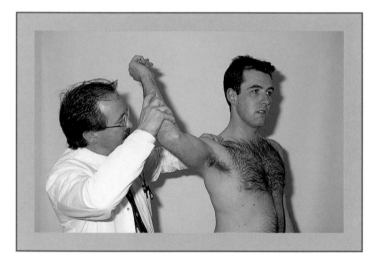

Figure 1.21 – *The crank test. With the patient in the position of apprehension the arm is cranked, gently, into even more external rotation. The patient becomes agitated.*

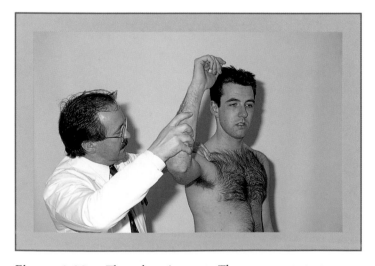

Figure 1.22 – *The relocation test. The surgeon puts pressure upon the anterior humeral head, pushing it back into joint.*

The relocation test

This is the third part of the apprehension test. When the patient starts to feel the joint slipping out the examiner presses backwards on the humeral head, thereby relocating it. The patient's wince disappears and the muscles relax, the patient once again becomes comfortable with the examination (Fig. 1.22).

The anterior drawer test

This test is analogous to the anterior drawer test of the knee. The test was first described by Gerber and Ganz (1984) and their description of the test is very precise, but has been incorrectly copied into major textbooks.

This test must be performed with the patient supine, it can not be performed with the patient sitting or standing as this makes the test unreliable. The shoulder

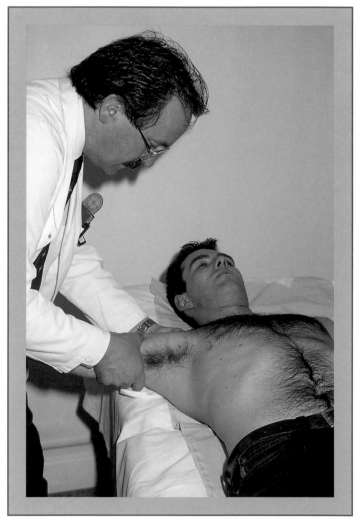

Figure 1.23 – *The anterior drawer test. The patient must be supine. The surgeon stands and supports the weight of the arm in his axilla. The arm is widely abducted and, in this position, the surgeon assesses the amount of abnormal anterior translation.*

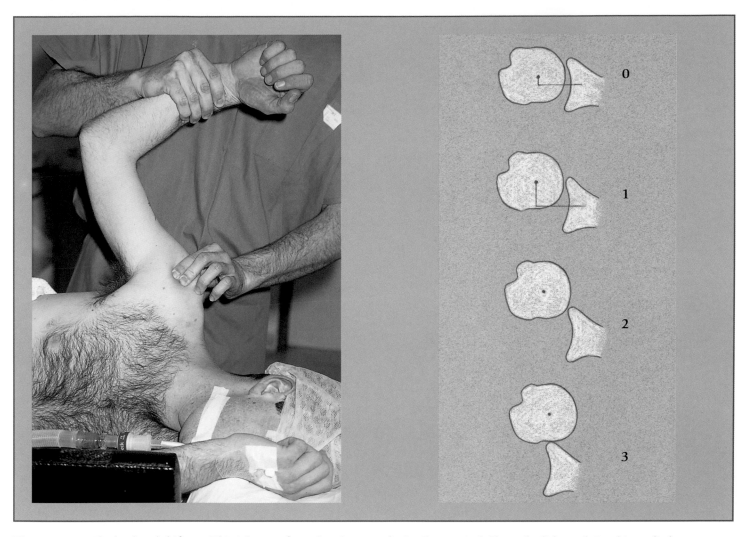

Figure 1.24 – *The load and shift test. This is best performed under anaesthetic. The arm is deliberately dislocated. Load is applied to compress the head against the glenoid and then the joint is relocated with a 'clunk'. The degree of instability is graded 0 (normal) to 3 (dislocated).*

is held in 80–120° of abduction, 10° of forward flexion and neutral rotation. To examine the right arm the patient's wrist is gripped in the surgeon's axilla, and the elbow held by the examiner's right hand. The examiner's left hand stabilizes the scapula. With the patient fully relaxed, the humerus is drawn forwards and back with a force comparable to that in the Lachman test.

The key elements to this test are that the patient is supine, the arm abducted and the patient relaxed (Fig. 1.23).

Some major textbooks suggest that the test be performed with the patient seated and with no abduction. In this position subscapularis protects the front of the shoulder and the test is unreliable.

The load and shift test

This test can be performed in the clinic but caution must be exercised as it can provoke a true dislocation. There are recorded episodes of such a dislocation being irreducible, and the patient requiring a general anaesthetic for reduction! This is a provocative test, being the shoulder equivalent of the Barlow and Ortolani test of the hip, or the pivot shift in the knee. Every opportunity should be taken to practise this test on the anaesthetized patient prior to every surgical repair (Fig. 1.24).

The patient is positioned supine or semirecumbent. For the right shoulder the surgeon stands at the side of the couch and stabilizes the scapula with his/her left hand. The patient's elbow is flexed and held in the surgeon's right hand. The shoulder is then abducted to 100° and externally rotated to just below the apprehension threshold. Pressure is then applied to the arm compressing the joint surfaces (as in the pivot shift). With the shoulder loaded the humeral head is shifted forwards, the surgeon taking the attitude that he/she is going to dislocate the shoulder! The resulting shift is graded. Grade 0 is normal; Grade 1 is anterior translation to the edge of the glenoid; Grade 2 is subluxation over the front of the glenoid, easily reduced; Grade 3 is the full clunk of dislocation, and the clunk of relocation.

Having completed the tests for anterior instability the surgeon must see if there is an element of inferior, posterior or generalized laxity.

Sulcus sign

The clinical diagnosis of inferior instability is made by gentle downward traction on the relaxed upper arm (Neer & Foster, 1980). This produces a sulcus between the lateral acromion and the humeral head. The test is conducted with the patient upright. The sulcus sign is the hallmark of multidirectional instability (Fig. 1.25).

Posterior jerk test

Tests for posterior instability are poorly covered in the literature. The key to posterior subluxation and

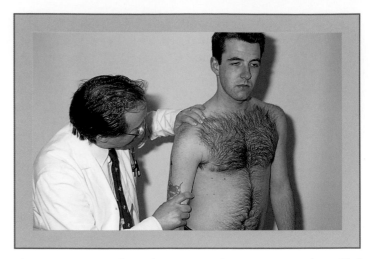

Figure 1.25 – *The sulcus sign. The arm is gently pulled downwards to see whether a sulcus appears between the humeral head and the acromion.*

dislocation is that it occurs with the arm in internal rotation that is then elevated in the plane of flexion and not in the plane of abduction (Fig. 1.26).

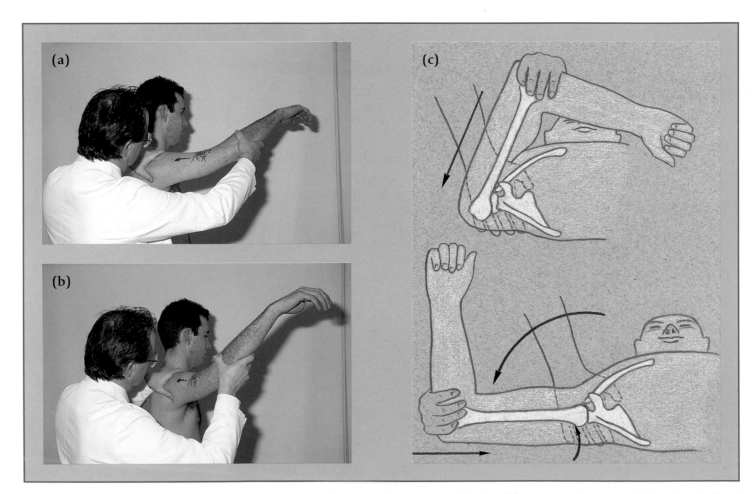

Figure 1.26 – *The posterior jerk test. The arm is elevated in internal rotation and slight adduction. At about 30° of elevation the head dislocates posteriorly (a). The arm is then brought into the plane of abduction and the head is felt to reduce with a jerk (b).*

To test the right arm the surgeon stands behind and to the right of the patient. The surgeon's hand is placed over the scapula with the thumb on the back of the humeral head. This is very important because it is the surgeon's thumb that detects the subtle posterior translation in subluxation. The surgeon takes the patient's elbow in his/her right hand and fully internally rotates the humerus. The shoulder is then slowly elevated in the plane of flexion and slight adduction. Almost immediately (30° of flexion) the humeral head is felt to sublux and then to dislocate. Often the patient is not aware of the subluxation, but may be aware of full dislocation. The arm is further elevated to 100°, at this point the arm is moved from the plane of flexion to the plane of abduction and the humeral head relocates with a jerk, the patient experiences brief pain and then relief from pain.

Once again every sentence of this description must be followed precisely. If the test is performed in neutral or external rotation the patient will not dislocate. If the test is conducted in the plane of abduction and not the plane of flexion the patient will not dislocate.

The posterior drawer test

The patient must be supine. To examine the right shoulder the surgeon stands level with the shoulder (Gerber & Ganz, 1984). The patient's elbow is flexed to 120° and supported by the surgeon's right hand. The shoulder is held abducted by 80–120° and slightly flexed. The surgeon places his/her left hand over the shoulder with the fingers on the scapular spine and the thumb just lateral to, but still in contact with, the coracoid process. (Fig. 1.27).

The shoulder is internally rotated and flexed to 80°, and at the same time the thumb of the left hand presses back upon the humeral head. The amount of posterior displacement of the head, relative to the coracoid and the spine of the scapula, can be felt and graded.

Generalized joint laxity

The patient must be examined for generalized laxity. Generalized laxity is graded 0–9. Points are scored for wrist flexion (thumb to forearm), finger extension (little finger and wrist extend so that the little finger is parallel with the forearm), recurvatum at elbow and recurvatum at knee. Both sides are tested giving a potential score of 8. Finally spinal flexion, so that the patient can place the palms of the hand on the ground, scores the ninth point.

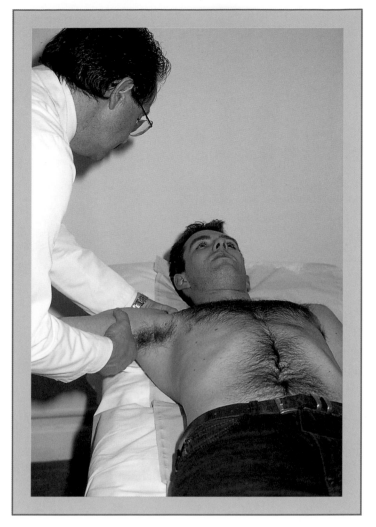

Figure 1.27 – *The posterior drawer test. This is similar in all respects to the anterior drawer test except that abnormal posterior translation is assessed.*

Shoulder laxity may be isolated and is characterized by excessive movement, external rotation to 95°, internal rotation to a T5 vertebral level and a positive 'orang-utan' sign (Fig. 1.28).

Finally a word of caution about applying these tests to children and adolescents. Emery (1991), using the drawer tests, found positive results in 57% of boys and 48% of girls, all of whom had asymptomatic shoulders.

Neurological testing

Neurological disorders may present to the shoulder surgeon with pain (usually referred), weakness or paralysis (often causing deformity), loss of function and even instability (for instance after polio).

The history and examination should determine firstly whether this is an upper motor-neurone lesion, or a lower motor-neurone lesion; secondly whether the lesion is

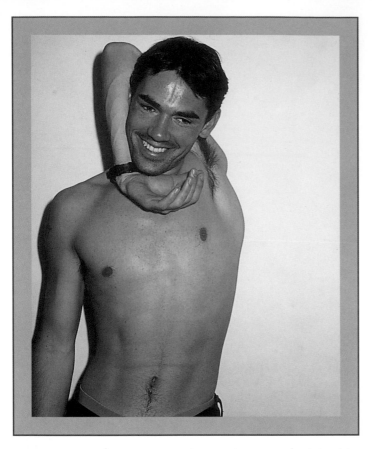

Figure 1.28 – *The 'orang-utan' sign. This is a test of shoulder laxity. The patient has the ability to fold the arm over their head and tickle their ipsilateral ear.*

diffuse or discrete; and thirdly whether the lesion is complete or incomplete, recoverable or irrecoverable.

Both upper and lower motor-neurone lesions will present with weakness. Upper motor-neurone lesions rarely present in the shoulder service, the commonest lesions being 'Stroke shoulder', cerebral palsy and demyelinating disease. These usually present late, as a contracted shoulder, and the diagnosis is not difficult because the patient has weakness, spasticity and brisk tendon reflexes.

Lower motor-neurone lesions will commonly present in the shoulder clinic. The key findings in lower motor-neurone lesions are weakness, fasciculation, muscle wasting, hypotonia and diminished tendon reflexes.

Identifying whether a lesion is discrete or diffuse depends upon a careful neurological examination, allied to a thorough knowledge of the nerve pathways in the upper limb.

Lower motor-neurone lesions may originate from the spinal cord and roots (the commonest being syringomyelia, cervical spondylosis, polio, neuralgic amyotrophy); from the brachial plexus (the commonest

being obstetric palsy, traumatic brachial plexus palsy, thoracic-outlet syndrome); and lesions of the peripheral nerves (commonly the axillary nerve, the musculocutaneous nerve, the suprascapular nerve, the long thoracic nerve, and the spinal accessory nerve). These nerves may be damaged by trauma, compression neuropathy, and toxic and metabolic polyneuropathies.

In the shoulder clinic the surgeon does not have the time to do a complete muscle mapping, and should this be needed (for instance in traumatic brachial plexus lesions) it should be delegated to a neurophysiotherapist. The shoulder surgeon takes a limited number of key muscles and examines each for bulk, tone, strength, reflexes and coordination. Each of these muscles should be familiar to the surgeon in terms of their nerve supply and root value.

In the time allotted in the clinic a favoured selection of muscles are: shoulder shrug (trapezius, spinal accessory nerve, cranial nerve XI); abduction (deltoid, axillary nerve, C5, deltoid jerk); external rotation (infraspinatus, suprascapular nerve, C5); internal rotation (subscapularis, nerves to subscapularis, C5); elbow flexion (biceps, musculocutaneous nerve, C5,6, biceps jerk); elbow extension (triceps , radial nerve, mainly C7, triceps jerk); wrist extension (extensor carpi radialis brevis (ECRB), extensor carpi radialis longus (ECRL), radial nerve, C6); power grip (flexor digitorum profundus (FDP), median nerve, C8, finger jerk); metacarpophalangeal (MCP) joint abduction (interossei, ulnar nerve, T1). It should be noted that there is some root overlap, for instance triceps is actually supplied by C6,7 and 8, but for the sake of simplicity the main root value only is expressed above.

Sensation can be tested for light touch, joint position sense, vibration, pain and temperature, but with the constraints of time imposed by the shoulder clinic the shoulder surgeon usually only has enough time to examine for light touch. Only if a condition such as syringomyelia is suspected should the whole gamut of sensory techniques be employed, and sometimes it is more helpful to request a neurological opinion.

A useful quick sensory exam can be performed by testing light touch in the following areas; acromioclavicular joint, epaulette region (supraclavicular nerves, C4); deltoid insertion (axillary nerve, C5); radial border of forearm (musculocutaneous nerve, C5,6); thenar emminence and volar-aspect index finger (median nerve, C6); extensor-aspect middle finger (radial nerve, C7); hypothenar emminence (ulnar nerve, C8); ulnar border of forearm (medial cutaneous nerve of forearm, T1).

Neurological examination is incomplete without looking for abnormalities of the sympathetic nervous system, Horner's syndrome, skin mottling or discolouration, lack of or excessive sweating.

If the neurological pattern is diffuse and the clinical symptoms are suggestive of a thoracic-outlet syndrome (TOS) (diffuse aching or throbbing in the arm, radiating down the ulnar border to the little finger, or sometimes the chest wall, worse with carrying and overhead activities, sometimes with vascular mottling) then the specific tests for TOS should be carried out.

Roos' test

This is the best objective test for TOS. The test is carried out by abducting both arms and shoulders to 90° and asking the patient to open and close their hands slowly but forceably for a period of 3 minutes (Fig. 1.29). The test is sometimes called the overhead exercise test, and most patients with TOS will not be able to perform the test for anything like 3 minutes on the affected side.

The military brace test

The patient stands with the hands comfortably to his/her sides. The surgeon places a stethoscope over the supraclavicular fossa and feels the radial pulse with the other hand. The patient is then asked to forceably brace the shoulders backwards and downwards as though a soldier on parade (Fig. 1.30). The test is positive if the pulse fades or a bruit appears.

Adson's test

Although this eponymous test was one of the first for TOS it is not as accurate as Roos' test or the 'military brace test'. Adson called this his 'vascular test'. The patient sits comfortably, with the surgeon palpating the radial pulse. The patient is then asked to take a deep breath, as in Valsalva's manoeuvre, and to turn the neck to the affected side with the chin thrust upwards (Fig. 1.31). The test is positive if the pulse fades.

Injection studies

Injection studies are part of the routine clinical examination for the shoulder and provide confirmation

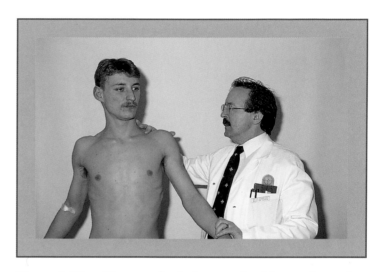

Figure 1.30 – *The costoclavicular test. In this test the patient braces their shoulders backwards whilst the surgeon feels their pulse and listens for turbulent flow (a bruit) in the subclavian vessels.*

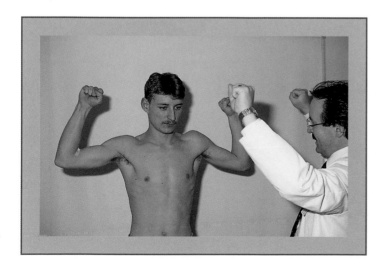

Figure 1.29 – *Roos' test. This is termed the overhead exercise test. The patient holds both arms in the air and then forcefully squeezes and releases the hand. This causes claudication of the arm in patients with vascular thoracic outlet syndrome.*

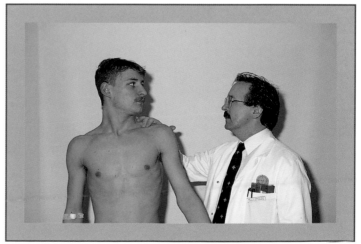

Figure 1.31 – *Adson's test. The surgeon checks whether the radial pulse fades as the patient looks to the side and upwards and holds a deep breath.*

of rotator cuff and acromioclavicular disorders. There are two phases to each injection: the early phase when the local anaesthetic is acting, and the late or therapeutic phase when the corticosteroid is acting.

Three sites can be predictably injected: the subacromial space, the glenohumeral joint and the acromioclavicular joint.

Subacromial injection: the impingement test

The patient is seated comfortably with the arm at the side, and the procedure is explained to them. The skin is cleaned and prepared with an alcohol wipe. A 5 ml syringe is used with 2 ml of 2% Xylocaine (lignocaine) and 1 ml hydrocortisone acetate (25 mg/ml). The hydrocortisone is heavier than the Xylocaine and therefore layers out in the bottom of the syringe, hence the Xylocaine is injected until the the needle has reached the correct position at which point the cortisone can be injected with no fears of it being in the wrong place or causing fat necrosis.

The surgeon washes his hands and sprays them with alcoholic skin preparing solution. The surgeon kneels to the side of the patient and palpates the anterolateral point of the acromion with the non-dominant hand.

The needle then enters from this spot aiming just under the anterolateral angle of the acromion (Fig. 1.32). The point of the needle can be felt to puncture the gritty coracoacromial ligament, and then the resistance suddenly gives and the needle falls into the subacromial potential space. At this point the 1.25" 23 G needle will be buried up to its hilt. The Xylocaine is then injected and should flow without undue pressure into the space.

The patient is then allowed 5 minutes for the block to work and the impingement tests are performed once again. The percentage relief is noted. If the impingement pain is blocked by 80–100% the diagnosis of cuff pathology is confirmed. The therapeutic phase, or late phase, takes some 4 weeks to work. The patient is re-examined at that stage to judge the effect of the steroid.

Glenohumeral injection

The injection, once again of 2 ml 2% Xylocaine and 1 ml hydrocortisone acetate (25 mg/ml), in a 5 ml syringe with a 23 G needle, is performed from the posterior approach (Fig. 1.33). This approach is identical to the posterior approach for shoulder arthroscopy. If the patient is either obese or muscular then the joint will not be reached with a 1.25" 23 G needle and an 18 G needle, or even a spinal needle, may be needed.

Once again the skin of both surgeon and patient are prepared with alcoholic preparation. The patient is seated and the surgeon kneels behind the patient and palpates the posterior angle of the acromion with the non-dominant hand. The needle is inserted, one thumb's breadth below and medial to the posterior angle of the acromion, the tip being angled towards the coracoid process. There is a slight give when the posterior capsule is punctured, and the capsule is always quite well innervated so the patient winces as the capsule is breached. Confirmation of entry is given by ease of fluid both entering the joint and the ability to draw it back into the syringe. Again the patient is left for 5 minutes after the injection and then the percentage relief is noted.

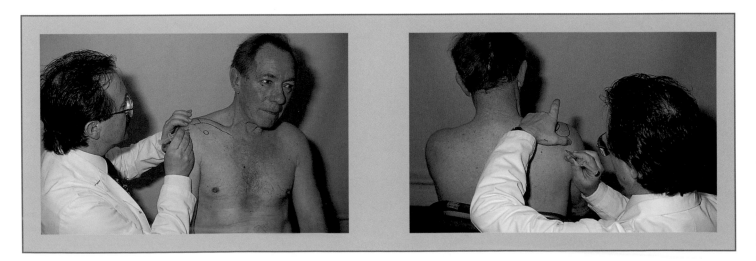

Figure 1.32 – *Injecting the subacromial space (see text).*

Figure 1.33 – *Injecting the glenohumeral joint (see text).*

Acromioclavicular joint injection

The acromioclavicular joint is a small joint which will only accept some 2 ml of fluid. The injection is therefore scaled down to 1 ml 2% Xylocaine and 1 ml of hydrocortisone acetate (25 mg/ml). The patient is seated. The skin of both surgeon and patient are prepared with alcoholic skin preparation. This time the surgeon stands. This injection is more difficult than the subacromial injection or shoulder joint injection. Look at the true anteroposterior (AP) radiograph of the acromioclavicular joint to judge the angle of obliquity of the joint and try to maintain this angle during the injection. Palpate the clavicle and the acromion. Try depressing the clavicle and finding where the joint is from the relative movement between both bones. If the joint is stiff and arthritic feel the osteophytes and go for the top of the hill. For the worst scenario where the joint is stiff, of small volume, and difficult to enter, use local anaesthetic liberally and then walk the needle from acromion to clavicle. Confirmation of entry is given by ease of flow of solution and the ability to draw it back (Fig. 1.34). Note the response of the patient to the injection itself because this is a small volume joint, and the injection may cause joint distension and temporary increase in pain. Wait the prescribed 5 minutes, and re-examine the patient to establish the percentage benefit.

Rheumatologists will have you believe that injection studies can be used for biceps and to differentiate between a lesion of supraspinatus at its insertion or 7 mm from the insertion. In my view this is not the case. The pragmatic and wise surgeon will stick to the three reliable tests described above.

Special tests

There are some special tests which should be mentioned for the acromioclavicular joint, subscapularis and biceps.

Acromioclavicular joint

The acromioclavicular joint may be stressed by cross-body adduction, taking the arm as far across the chest as possible and by placing the arm into full internal rotation — the half-Nelson position.

Subscapularis: the 'lift-off' test

Complete rupture of subscapularis is rare. The largest collection in the world literature is of 16 cases. Gerber

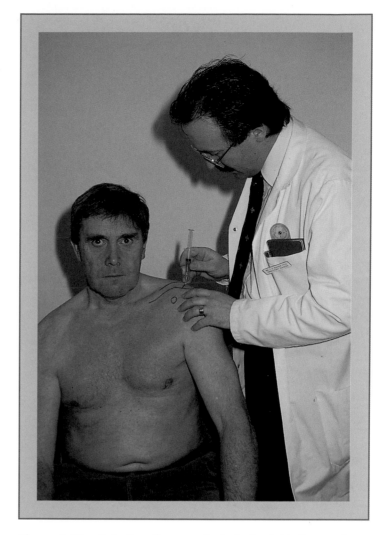

Figure 1.34 – *Injecting the acromioclavicular joint (see text).*

described his lift-off test in this condition. The arm is placed in internal rotation with the dorsum of the hand resting on the L5 vertebra. The patient is then asked to 'lift off' the hand away from the back against resistance (Fig. 1.35). If subscapularis is ruptured the patient is unable to lift off.

Biceps

Various tests have been designed to stress biceps. Yergason's test is often quoted, but Yergason only described one patient and this test has been copied from text-book to text-book. It is not reliable and should not be used. Speed's test is likewise unreliable, although the best test we have available for biceps. Biceps tendon is, however, rarely affected on its own in shoulder disease, and this should be born in mind by the prudent surgeon.

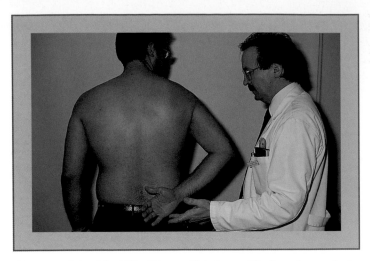

Figure 1.35 – *The 'lift-off' test. This is specific for subscapularis.*

Summary

A careful history and clinical examination will unravel the mystery of the shoulder in some 80–90% of patients. However, this still leaves some 10–20% of patients where the diagnosis remains a mystery, or the surgeon has made a differential diagnosis, but is still unsure of the definitive diagnosis. Investigation of the mystery shoulder, which is considered in the next chapter, will unravel the differential diagnosis down to a definitive diagnosis in the great majority of these patients.

CHAPTER 2

Investigating the mystery shoulder

T. Bunker

Introduction

The investigative procedures currently available to shoulder surgeons are radiography, arthrography, computerized tomography (CT) scanning, 3-D CT scanning, ultrasound, magnetic resonance imaging (MRI) and arthroscopy. Each of these methods is able to image different tissues, in differing planes, and we need to match the best investigation for each disease of the shoulder.

Plain radiographs

The story of the discovery of X-rays by Roentgen in 1895 is well known. It was the fateful juxtaposition of a cathode-ray tube and a plate of barium platinocyanide that led to this extraordinary event. The cathode-ray tube was inside a black cardboard box, but every time it was switched on the barium-platinocyanide plate fluoresced. From this Roentgen deduced that an 'invisible ray' was emitted from the cathode-ray tube — the X-ray. Wilhelm Roentgen became the first holder of the Nobel Prize for physics in 1901, and the first in a line of Nobel Laureates whose inventions have been incorporated into the science of medical imaging.

Less well known was the involvement of Codman, the grandfather of shoulder surgery, with the early application of X-rays in the diagnosis of bone diseases. Codman immediately saw the potential of X-rays in the

diagnosis of bone disease and did a great deal of research into their use at the turn of the century. The only lasting legacy of this work is 'Codman's triangle' in the diagnosis of osteosarcoma.

Plain radiographs remain the primary mode of imaging the shoulder. Three main views are used to image the glenohumeral joint. The first is the true anteroposterior (AP) view of the shoulder; this is a 45° oblique AP view (Fig. 2.1). The beam of X-rays is placed in line with the surface of the glenoid, giving a true AP

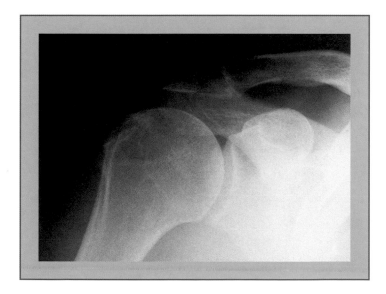

Figure 2.1 – *The normal true AP radiograph of the shoulder.*

view of the scapula. Without doubt this is the most useful radiograph of the shoulder. This radiograph shows the scapula in a standard, reproduceable fashion, along with the coracoid and acromial processes. It shows the humeral head and the tuberosities of the humerus. It shows the acromioclavicular joint and the distal clavicle.

It is mandatory to take a second radiograph perpendicular to the true AP radiograph in any patient who has sustained an injury sufficient to cause a dislocation or fracture. This is called the trauma series. Since the true AP radiograph is a square plate or sheet this second radiograph can be aligned perpendicular to either edge of the plate (Fig. 2.2). Thus we can get an axillary radiograph or a lateral scapular radiograph, each of which is perpendicular to the true AP radiograph and to each other.

To take an axillary view (Fig. 2.3) the arm needs to be abducted to 90°, a situation which is impossible in the traumatized patient. However, there are modifications of the axillary view such as the 'trauma axillary lateral', the 'Stripp view' and the 'Nottingham modified axillary view', which can be taken with the patient in a sling and with the arm at the side. The axillary view gives a good view of the relation of glenoid to humerus, and acromion to clavicle.

The lateral scapular view shows the relationship of humeral head to glenoid but is more difficult to interpret than the axillary view to inexperienced eyes (Fig. 2.4). A modification of the scapular lateral view is the 'Neer outlet view'. The Neer outlet view is a 10° caudally angled radiograph which shoots the beam straight out of the supraspinatus tunnel. This shows any bony obstruction to the outlet, such as a hooked anterior morphology to the acromion, or a spike of bone in the coraco-acromial ligament (Fig. 2.5).

The Stryker notch view is espoused by some surgeons for the assessment of anterior dislocation. This view shows the Hill–Sachs lesion.

The acromioclavicular joint is best imaged by using an AP view in the plane of the thorax, a 10° cephalic tilt AP and an axillary view. The beam and the plate should be centred on the acromioclavicular joint with the beam coned down.

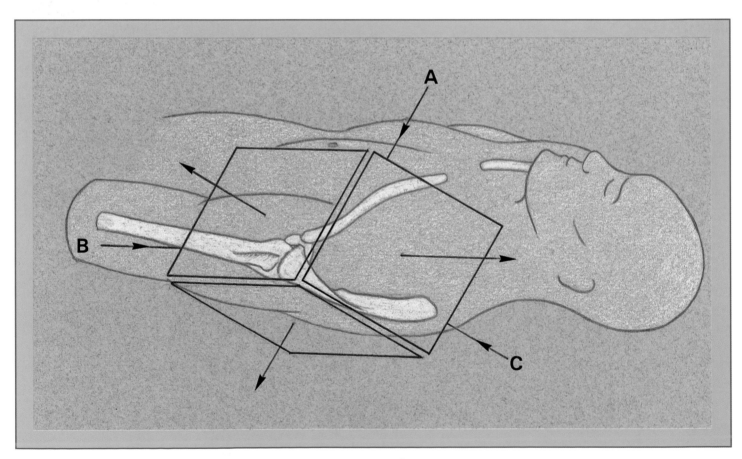

Figure 2.2 – *The trauma series. This must have two films at 90° to each other. This means a true AP (A) with either an axillary view (B), or a true lateral view (C), or both.*

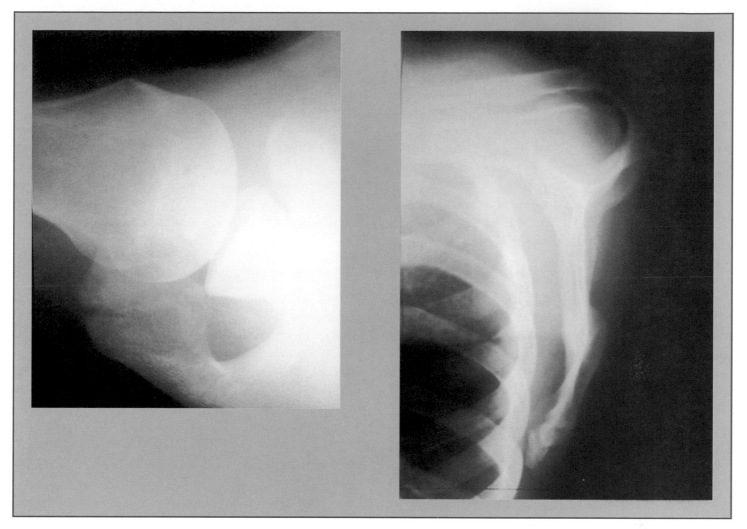

Figure 2.3 – *The axillary view of the shoulder. This clearly shows the relation of the humeral head to the glenoid and the relation of the clavicle to the acromion. (This patient has an Os Acromiale).*

Figure 2.4 – *The lateral-scapular view of the shoulder. (This patient has an old scapular fracture).*

The clavicle is best imaged with an AP view and two oblique views taken with a 30° cephalad beam and a 30° caudal beam.

The sternoclavicular joint is difficult to image with plain radiographs. The best view is the 'Serendipity' view (a 40° cephalic tilt radiograph). However, CT scans or MRI are often superior for imaging this joint.

Let us now see how plain radiographs can best help us to back up our diagnosis in the mystery shoulder.

Impingement syndrome (Mandatory; true AP shoulder. Optional axillary and Neer-outlet)

Plain radiographs may be normal in patients with impingement because this is a soft-tissue disease. In time, adaptive changes occur in the bone which will be seen on radiographs. Pressure on the acromion leads to sclerosis of the undersurface of the anterior acromion.

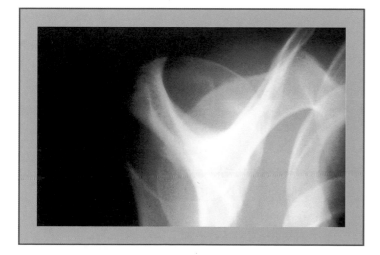

Figure 2.5 – *The Neer outlet view. A caudally angled lateral-scapular view shows the morphology of the anterior acromion.*

This is called the 'sourcil sign' (sourcil being French for eyebrow) because the acromion takes on the appearance of an eyebrow above the humerus (Fig. 2.6).

Calcific deposits and acromial apophysis may cause impingement; both can be seen on plain radiographs. The Neer-outlet view may show a hook shaped (Type III) anterior acromion, or an adaptive spike of new bone formed in the insertion of the coraco-acromial ligament.

Rotator-cuff tears (Mandatory; true AP view. Optional; axillary and Neer-outlet views)

Once again this is a soft-tissue disorder and the existence of a rotator cuff tear is a possibility even though the radiograph appears to be normal. However, the majority of patients present after adaptive changes have occurred and these will show up on plain radiographs. The sourcil sign is often present. Adaptive changes occur in the greater tuberosity with small osteophytes, an irregular margin, osteopenia and cysts (Fig. 2.7). These cysts are not in fact cysts, but merely look like cysts because they appear as sclerotic rings. They are in fact reparative osteophytic bumps seen end-on or obliquely. A decrease in the acromiohumeral interval to less than 7 mm is highly suggestive of a cuff tear. Even better is a break in 'Shenton's Line' of the shoulder. The cortical border of the medial humeral metaphysis and the lateral border of the scapula should form an unbroken elliptical arch. If the humerus is subluxed upward, due to a cuff tear, there will be a break or step in this line.

Dislocation (Mandatory; trauma series. Optional; Stryker-notch view)

In acute dislocation, and after relocation, a trauma series is required to establish direction of dislocation and then to demonstrate relocation by checking the relative position of head and glenoid in two planes. Associated fractures of the greater tuberosity or glenoid rim may be seen. The Stryker-notch view is used in patients with recurrent dislocation to establish whether there is a Hill–Sachs lesion. The value of this may be questioned. If there is a Hill–Sachs lesion will it change your surgical approach to repairing the recurrent dislocation? If the answer is no, why do it? Do you need a Hill–Sachs lesion to diagnose recurrent anterior dislocation? The answer is no, but in the difficult case it may help. However, there are better ways of investigating difficult cases in order to diagnose dislocation, examination under anaesthetic and arthroscopy being the foremost.

Frozen shoulder (Mandatory; true AP view)

The radiograph in frozen shoulder is normal by definition, so why order a radiograph at all? The answer is to differentiate the other causes of the painful shoulder with restriction of external rotation, arthritis, locked posterior dislocation, cuff tear and bone tumour of the proximal humerus.

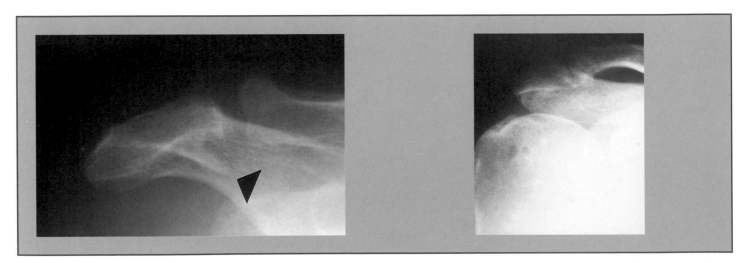

Figure 2.6 – *The 'sourcil' sign. Sourcil is French for eyebrow. If there is sclerosis of the undersurface of the acromion due to chronic rotator-cuff disease this gives the appearance of a white 'eyebrow' above the humeral head. This patient has a prominent spike of bone which has formed in the coraco-acromial ligament.*

Figure 2.7 – *A full-thickness rotator-cuff tear. Note the sourcil sign, osteophytes on the greater tuberosity, pseudocysts, decreased acromiohumeral interval and break in 'Shenton's line' of the shoulder.*

Arthritis (Mandatory; true AP shoulder. Optional; axillary)

In osteoarthritis the usual quartet of reduced joint space, osteophyte, cysts and sclerosis will be seen (Fig. 2.8). The earliest sign is the inferior osteophyte on the articular margin of the humerus. There are certain radiographic peculiarities with some forms of secondary arthritis. Avascular necrosis of the head shows the usual sequence of subchondral cresent, articular irregularity, and segmental collapse with a normal glenoid in the early stages. Acromegalic arthropathy shows as arthritis with a widened joint space in the early stages. Pigmented villonodular synovitis appears as a somewhat bizarre erosive arthritis. Synovial chondromatosis presents with multiple loose bodies.

Rheumatoid arthritis follows two distinctive patterns in the shoulder which have been termed the 'wet' form

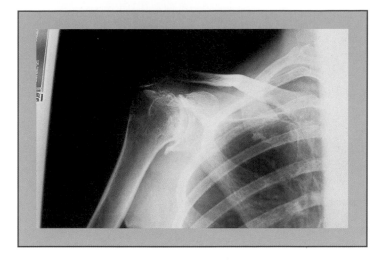

Figure 2.9 – *Wet erosive rheumatoid arthritis. This shows severe periarticular erosions and marked glenoid erosion.*

and the 'dry' form by Neer. The wet form is an aggressive type where the synovium is highly active, there is a lot of synovial fluid (hence wet), there are marked periarticular erosions and the arthritis is rapidly progressive (Fig. 2.9). In contrast the dry type acts much more like osteoarthritis, the synovium is less active, there is little joint fluid, no periarticular erosions and the disease is much slower to progress.

Fractures (Mandatory; trauma series)

Two radiographs must be taken perpendicular to each other. The true AP radiograph is always taken and this may be accompanied by a modified axillary or a lateral scapular or both.

Arthrography

The arthrogram lends a soft-tissue element to the plain radiograph. Although judged archaic by some, it is simple and cheap. Contrast material is injected under image-intensifier control into the glenohumeral joint itself. The investigation can be improved by using double-contrast with contrast material and air. On the down-side the investigation uses expensive radiologist's time, and is invasive.

The soft tissues that can be imaged are the rotator cuff, the labrum and the capsule.

Arthrography is the only investigation (with the exception of arthroscopy) which can demonstrate a partial-thickness tear of the articular surface of the rotator cuff, and the only investigation which

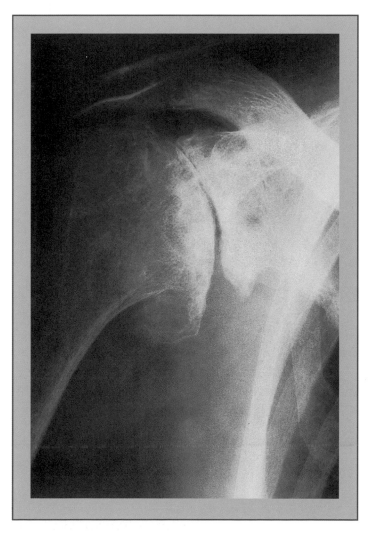

Figure 2.8 – *Radiograph of an osteoarthritic shoulder. Note the inferior osteophytes, sclerosis, narrow joint line and cysts.*

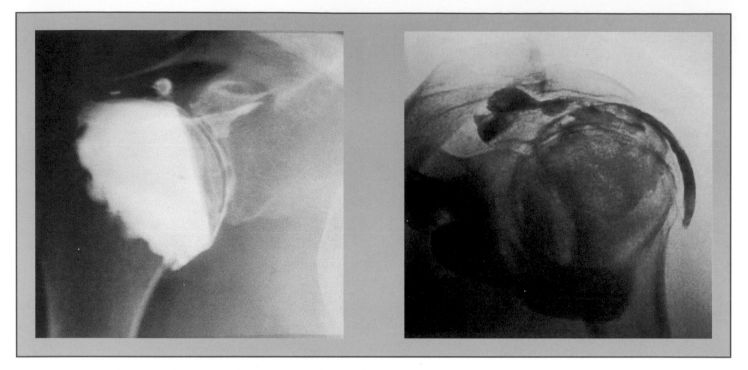

Figure 2.10 – *Arthrogram of frozen shoulder. Note the degree of contraction of the capsule. The infraglenoid and subscapular recesses have disappeared.*

Figure 2.11 – *Arthrogram of a full-thickness rotator-cuff tear. The contrast material can be seen to have escaped from the joint into the subacromial bursa.*

demonstrates the reduced joint volume of frozen shoulder (Fig. 2.10). Examination of the labrum is difficult with arthrography and has been superseded by double-contrast CT arthrography.

Full-thickness tears of the rotator cuff can be seen easily on arthrography (Fig. 2.11) because there is escape of contrast through the cuff tear into the subacromial bursa, a feature which can only occur in the presence of a tear. However, the shoulder surgeon needs to know how big the tear is, its site and shape, the quality of residual cuff and how dystrophic the muscle belly of supraspinatus is, all of which can be shown by MRI scanning, but not by arthrography. Double-contrast arthrotomography has been used to make up for these deficiencies. Certainly tear size, and the thickness of residual cuff, can be judged by double-contrast arthrotomography, but not the quality of supraspinatus.

Computerized tomography scanning

Godfrey Hounsfield was awarded the Nobel Prize in 1972 for determining how to improve upon conventional tomograms. He felt that if he could fire a pencil-thin beam of X-rays through a patient at 160 set points around the circumference of a circle, then he could position crystals opposite the beam which would measure the absorption of X-rays at all 160 points and these figures could then be fed into a computer to build up a picture of that axial slice through the body.

The benefit of CT is that it gives excellent pictures of bone, far better than MRI (Fig. 2.12). The problem is that it is not as good at imaging soft tissue as is MRI, and it is difficult to get accurate slices in anything but an axial plane.

However, if the radiologist takes slices at close enough intervals, three-dimensional pictures of the bone can be built up using specialized computer programs (3D CT) (Fig. 2.13).

CT can be used with a double-contrast arthrography technique to enhance the appearance of tissues such as the labrum.

The main uses of CT are in fracture work. CT and 3D CT are the best ways to image complex fractures such as those of the glenoid.

Care must be taken in interpreting CT arthrograms of the glenoid labrum. The reason for this is that there are normal variants of the labrum, at the 2 o'clock position on the face of the glenoid, which can be misinterpreted

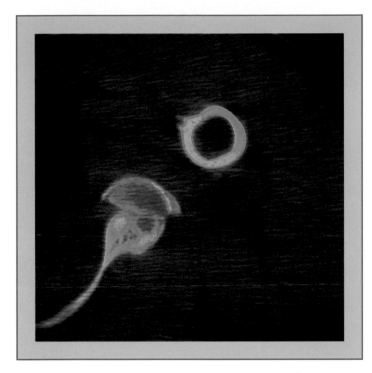

Figure 2.12 – *CT scan of a fractured glenoid. Half the glenoid has fractured off and is lying perpendicular to its proper position.*

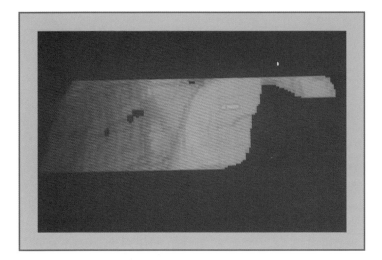

Figure 2.13 – *3D CT of fractured glenoid. There is a small step in the joint surface. (With permission from Shoulder Arthroscopy, Bunker and Wallace (eds), Dunitz).*

as Bankart tears (which occur at the 3 o'clock to 7 o'clock position). Hill–Sachs lesions show up very well on CT scans.

CT scanning is of no use in diagnosing impingement syndrome or rotator-cuff tears because these are soft-tissue lesions which need to be assessed in the oblique coronal plane. Oblique coronal reconstruction is extremely crude on CT.

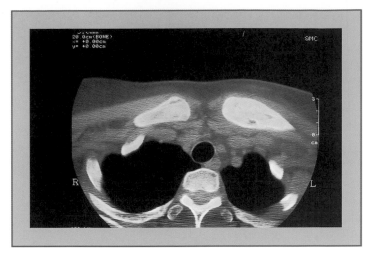

Figure 2.14 – *CT scan of the sternoclavicular joint in a patient with sternocostoclavicular hyperostosis.*

CT is very useful in imaging the sternoclavicular joint. CT shows the relative position of medial clavicle to manubrium, so it will easily detect anterior and posterior subluxation and dislocation. It is helpful in those awkward differentials of the swollen sternoclavicular joint, arthritis, infection and oddities such as sternocostoclavicular hyperostosis (Fig. 2.14).

Ultrasound

The Curies (Nobel Laureates, 1903) discovered the piezoelectric effect, upon which ultrasound is based. Two of their pupils, Chilowsky and Langevin, developed an apparatus using the piezoelectric effect to generate high energy ultrasound waves which could detect obstacles underwater in 1916. The development of the U-boat in the last years of World War I made this discovery a red hot military secret. Ultrasound was kept a military secret with the development of 'sound navigation and ranging' (SONAR) in the second World War; it was first used medically to detect gall stones in 1949.

The problem with the first ultrasound machines was that the patient had to be immersed in a water bath in order to be scanned. Professor Donald in Glasgow had the bright idea that the full bladder could mimic a water bath in order to scan the uterus — a method called direct contact scanning.

The modern ultrasound scanner uses the piezoelectric effect of a disc of lead zirconium titanate to generate and record ultrasound waves, and to detect their returning echoes. In the shoulder, frequencies of 5–10 MHz are the most effective.

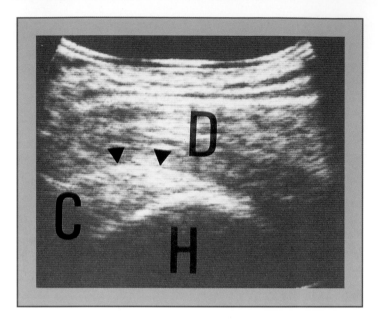

Figure 2.15 – *A focal echogenic area in supraspinatus insertion on ultrasound is one of the signs of rotator-cuff tearing (with permission from Bunker T., Shoulder Ultrasound, Seminars in Orthopaedics, 1987).*

A small-parts 7.5 MHz probe is used to scan the shoulder in an oblique coronal plane and in an oblique sagittal plane. The oblique coronal plane shows the hill and valley appearance of the greater tuberosity and articular margin. The supraspinatus tendon can be seen inserting into the bone.

Rotator-cuff tears can be diagnosed if there is non-visualization of the rotator cuff, focal thinning, focal discontinuity or focal echogenic areas (Fig. 2.15).

Ultrasound can be used to examine the cuff as the shoulder is moved (dynamic ultrasound), but its disadvantage is that it requires skilled interpretation of the images.

The other way ultrasound can be used in diagnosis around the shoulder is the use of duplex ultrasound to examine the subclavian artery and vein in suspected thoracic outlet compression. Duplex ultrasound can show velocity shifts and turbulence in the subclavian artery, as well as flow reduction or even obstruction of the axillary artery. Duplex ultrasound can also be used to examine the subclavian vein.

MRI

The principle of MRI was discovered by the physicist Felix Bloch, a finding which led to his winning the Nobel Prize for physics in 1952.

MRI has revolutionized the field of imaging in the shoulder because it can image muscle, tendon and ligaments — the very soft tissues that account for 70% of shoulder disease.

The MRI scan can be aligned in the plane of the shoulder. The routine planes for scanning are oblique coronal, in the line of the supraspinatus muscle; oblique sagittal, in the line of the glenoid, and axial.

The downside of MRI scanning is the initial outlay for the scanner, the fact that the patient has to be loaded into the bore of the magnet head first (which leads to claustrophobia) the noise of the scanner (which is quite alarming for many patients), the time taken to gain a scan (which can lead to movement artifacts), and the need for special shoulder coils to counter the shoulder not being in the centre of the bore of the magnet.

Against this the anatomy demonstrated by MRI is quite astonishing. Every tendon, every ligament, every blood vessel and nerve can be imaged, allowing the surgeon a fantastic new view of the shoulder. T1-weighted images, T2-weighted images and fat-suppression techniques are routinely used.

MRI in impingement

Unfortunately, with present techniques, MRI is not able to accurately differentiate a normal supraspinatus tendon from a tendon affected by impingement. The appearance of the tendon is graded 0 to 3 according to the MRI signal observed by the radiologist. Grade 0 is a normal tendon, a homogeneous low-signal intensity structure. Grade 1 is a tendon that exhibits a focal, linear or diffuse intermediate signal throughout the tendon. Grade 2 is a tendon with a high signal within the tendon, but not across its full width. Grade 3 is a tendon that shows a high signal right across its width. The problem is that intermediate signal intensity can occur in normal tendons and this should not be considered pathological, unless it is combined with tendon thinning, or irregularity. The so-called 'angle phenomenon' may make interpretation of changes in signal intensity within the supraspinatus tendon difficult to interpret.

Rotator-cuff tears

Full-thickness tears are seen as an area of focal discontinuity in the tendon (Fig. 2.16). These are best seen on the coronal oblique T2-weighted images. T2-weighted images show synovial fluid as a distinctive white area extending from the joint, through the tear and into the subacromial bursa. There is very good correlation between

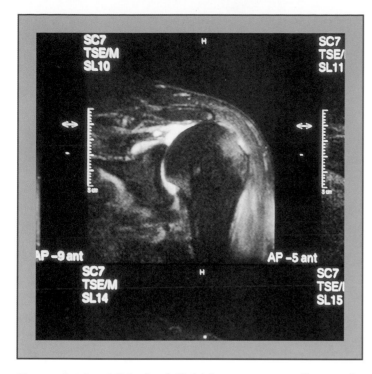

Figure 2.16 – *MRI of a full-thickness rotator-cuff tear. The tendon of supraspinatus can be seen to have a large gap from the greater tuberosity. Fluid is seen in the subacromial bursa. A Shenton's sign of the shoulder is visible.*

the size of tear measured on MRI and at surgery as well as the quality of the torn edges. The muscle belly of supraspinatus can be imaged to see whether there is disuse atrophy, which will have a direct bearing on the success of repair. The sensitivity of detection of full thickness rotator-cuff tears ranges from 69% to 100% and the specificity between 88% and 100%. Gadolinium-enhanced MRI arthrography may enhance the results of MRI but is presently not sanctioned for use in humans, except in the experimental situation, and changes a non-invasive procedure into an invasive one.

Dislocation
The labrum can be imaged quite well with MRI using T1-weighted axial views. The labrum is a fibrous structure that produces a low-signal intensity image. In patients with recurrent dislocation the labrum may be rounded off, or separated from the glenoid by a Bankart tear. Hill–Sachs lesions and secondary changes can be seen as for CT scanning.

Frozen shoulder
There are, as yet, no specific MRI changes which are pathognomonic for frozen shoulder. Thickening of the capsule of the infraglenoid recess has been found in one study.

Arthritis
MRI has no advantages over plain radiographs in arthritis with the exception of its ability to image the rotator cuff in cuff arthropathy, and in the early stages of avascular necrosis of the head of the humerus. Computerized tomography is better for analysing glenoid deficiency than MRI.

Fractures
Fractures are better imaged by CT scanning than MRI scanning.

Arthroscopy

Diagnostic arthroscopy is the gold standard of investigation for the shoulder surgeon. The present status of arthroscopy is given by Professor Ogilvie-Harris in Chapter 3.

Summary

The shoulder surgeon is in a privileged position, having at his or her disposal a whole range of diagnostic-imaging techniques. Many of these have followed a major breakthrough in physics and have led to the highest scientific award — the Nobel Prize — being bestowed upon their discoverers.

Because most problems relating to the shoulder are mechanical in nature, imaging has become the investigation of choice for the shoulder surgeon. However, there are occasions when the surgeon needs to invoke the aid of haematologists, chemical pathologists, microbiologists, neurophysiologists and even pathologists.

However, they are rarely needed in the diagnosis of impingement, cuff tear, dislocation or frozen shoulder, for these are truly mechanical. Having said this, amyloid can occasionally be deposited in the coraco-acromial ligament in renal failure, leading to impingement, and frozen shoulder is associated with diabetes (and thus elevated blood sugar levels as well as raised serum lipids) but generally these mechanical conditions need no haematological or biochemical workup. However, when we come to consider arthritis of the glenohumeral joint, the neuropathies, myopathies, tumours and infections, biochemical investigations are vital.

Arthritis

Secondary osteoarthritis is common in the shoulder. Avascular necrosis may be caused by steroid therapy, which used to be given in high doses after renal transplantation (high urea and creatinine); sickle cell disease (sickle cell anaemia); alcohol abuse (high γ-glutamyl-transferase (γGT) and abnormal liver function tests); lymphoma (abnormal white cell count); and decompression disease (blood parameters normal).

Acromegalic arthropathy (elevated growth hormone, elevated blood sugar level in 25%, elevated prolactin in 4%)

This commonly presents with arthritis in the shoulders and hips. The sella turcica is enlarged on skull radiographs. The patient has a typical acromegalic clinical appearance.

Ankylosing spondylitis

The erthrocyte sedimentation rate (ESR) is elevated in 75% of cases but the C-reactive protein level (CRP) may be a better marker of disease. Mild elevation of immunoglobulin A (IgA) is frequently seen. There is a high prevalence of human leucocyte antigen (HLA) B27. Serum complement is normal or elevated. Fifteen percent of cases have a normochromic normocytic anaemia. There may be mild elevation of alkaline phosphatase and creatine phosphokinase (CPK). Radiographs of the sacroiliac joints will show postage-stamp serrations, sclerosis or ankylosis.

Haemophiliac arthritis

Patients have an abnormal clotting screen. Factor-VIII levels are usually below 20% of normal. Those patients treated with blood products between 1980 and 1985 have a high incidence of being human immunodeficiency virus (HIV) positive and hepatitis B or C positive.

Septic arthritis (raised white cell count, ESR and CRP)

The sternoclavicular joint is a site of predeliction for many bizarre infections, particularly in intravenous drug users.

Rheumatoid arthritis

Rheumatoid factors are antibodies directed against the patient's gamma-globulins. The most common rheumatoid factor is an IgM antibody directed against IgG. Fifty to eighty percent of patients with rheumatoid arthritis are seropositive. Increased levels of IgM are associated with severe disease and extra-articular disease. However, rheumatoid factor is positive in 25–50% of patients with systemic lupus erythematosus (SLE) and leprosy; positive in 10–25% of patients with juvenile chronic arthritis, pulmonary disease and tubercle; positive in 5–10% of patients with ankylosing spondylitis, rheumatic fever, osteoarthritis, psoriatic arthritis and gout and positive in less than 5% of the normal population. Low complement levels (a low CH50) may be associated with several immune complex mediated diseases, such as severe rheumatoid arthritis, SLE, and bacterial endocarditis. The ESR and acute-phase protein levels tend to reflect disease level. Patients with rheumatoid arthritis often have a mild normochromic normocytic anaemia.

Neuropathies

The differential diagnosis of a patient presenting with a peripheral neuropathy is compression of the nerve, or a toxic-, metabolic-, deficiency-, radiation- or infection-induced neuropathy.

Toxic neuropathy

This may be caused by lead, mercury or arsenic poisoning (elevated levels can be detected in the blood), by alcohol poisoning (high serum alcohol, elevated γGT and abnormal liver function tests), and by poisoning with dichloro-diphenyl-trichloro-ethane (DDT) or organophosphorus pesticides.

Metabolic neuropathies

These may be caused by diabetes (raised blood sugar level), uraemia (raised serum urea and creatinine), and porphyria (raised serum porphyrins).

Deficiency disease

Deficiencies leading to peripheral neuropathy include vitamin B_{12} deficiency (macrocytic anaemia, low B_{12} levels).

Neuralgic amyotrophy

This may be caused by infection with human parvovirus 19, in which case acute-phase and convalescent-phase viral titres can confirm the diagnosis.

Neurophysiological testing

Neurological symptoms can be vague and difficult to diagnose. For instance, the patient may present with vague neurology in the ulnar side of the forearm and wrist. Is this ulnar nerve compression at the elbow, or a thoracic outlet compression of the lower trunk of the plexus, or is it due to C8 root compression in the neck? In this situation the neurophysiologist may be of invaluable help.

Electromyography can determine whether a muscle is partially or totally denervated. Partial denervation gives low voltage potentials, polyphasic units, fibrillation and sharp positive waves. Total denervation shows no voluntary potentials on attempted movement.

Nerve-conduction velocity is helpful in determining the site of nerve compression. The nerve can be stimulated at various levels along its course and the conduction velocity measured over each segment. This is invaluable in the peripheral nerves. However, since it requires stimulation at one end of the nerve and detection at the other this leads to difficulties in examining nerves around the shoulder. Nerve conduction is helpful in this situation by excluding distal compression. The suprascapular nerve can be examined by measuring latency between Erb's point and infraspinatus, and comparing the affected side with the unaffected side.

Determination of nerve conduction above the axilla, for instance in thoracic outlet syndrome, is best demonstrated by using the F response. This is a late muscle potential elicited from antidromically activated anterior horn cells. A stimulus is applied transcutaneously to the motor nerve in the hand, which travels antidromically to the anterior horn cell, and an impulse is then sent back down the axons to the muscle, giving a late response (Fig. 2.17).

Dystrophies and myopathies

Generalized myopathies are not usually seen in the shoulder clinic. Patients presenting with weakness should be investigated; serum CPK and aldolase should be determined and 24-hour urine samples should be tested for creatinine; myoglobin, thyroid function, sodium, potassium, calcium, phosphate, magnesium, full blood count and an ESR.

Localized muscular dystrophies do present to the shoulder surgeon, the commonest being fascioscapulo-humeral dystrophy.

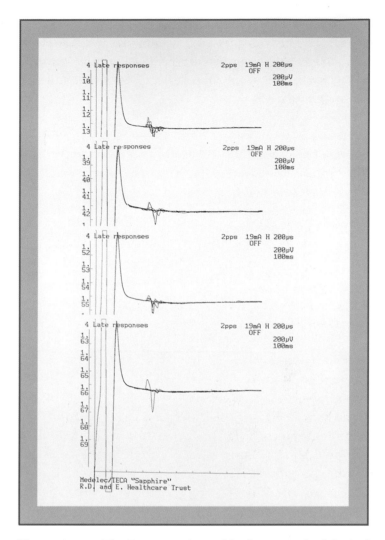

Figure 2.17 – *The F response is used in the neurophysiological test for thoracic outlet syndrome (TOS). Since the nerve compression is so proximal, it cannot be stimulated proximal to the lesion. The nerve is stimulated, therefore, distal to the compression; the stimulus travels antidromically to the anterior horn cell and an impulse is then sent back down the axon to the muscle, giving a late response — the F wave.*

Infection

Joint infections can commonly occur in the glenohumeral and sternoclavicular joints. Osteomyelitis is common in the proximal humerus and the proximal clavicle. The microbiologist can usually identify the causative organism from blood cultures, culture of synovial fluid or biopsy material.

Septic arthritis and osteomyelitis

The most common causative organisms are *Staphylococcus aureus, S. epidermidis, St. pneumoniae,*

S. pyogenes; Haemophilus influenzae; Klebsiella pneumoniae; Proteus mirabilis; Pseudomonas aeruginosa; Mycobacterium tuberculosis; Neisseria gonorrhea; Enterococcus faecalis and *E. faecium; Escherichia coli; Bacteroides fragilis* and the Salmonella species.

Tumours

Benign and malignant tumours may present around the shoulder. Diagnosis depends upon critical examination of plain radiographs, CT scans and MRI. Biopsy is essential to the confirmation of tumour type, but should be performed at the centre where definitive surgery is to be carried out. Thus most shoulder surgeons are happy to tackle all benign tumours around the shoulder, and to offer palliative surgery for secondary tumours, but will refer on potential primary-bone and soft-tissue tumours to a regional orthopaedic oncology unit.

CHAPTER 3

Profit and loss: an account of the present state of shoulder arthroscopy

D.J. Ogilvie-Harris and E. Sarrosa

Diagnostic arthroscopy

The arthroscope is a valuable tool in the shoulder surgeon's diagnostic armamentarium. Its relevance must be measured against physical examination (both in the clinic and under anaesthesia) and imaging techniques which include plain X-rays, ultrasound, arthrography, computerized tomography (CT) scanning, CT arthrography, magnetic resonance imaging (MRI) and MRI arthrography.

When shoulders were screened, using routine radiographs, to detect massive rotator-cuff tears, by looking for superior migration of the humerus and deformity of the greater tuberosity, they were found to have a 78% sensitivity, and specificity of 98% (Kaneko *et al.*, 1995).

Brenneke and Morgan (1992) concluded that ultrasonography is an effective method for the assessment of full-thickness rotator-cuff tears, but not partial-thickness tears. They found a sensitivity of 95% for the full-thickness tears and a sensitivity of 41% for the partial-thickness tears and specificities of 93% and 91% for full-thickness and partial-thickness tears, respectively. However, Van Holsbeeck *et al.* (1995) found that ultrasound can depict most partial-thickness tears with a sensitivity of 93% and specificity of 94%.

Arthrography is very useful in demonstrating the presence and site of a rotator-cuff tear, but is less successful in determining the size of the tears (Farin & Jaroma, 1995).

CT arthrography is useful in instability; it is accurate in showing capsular redundancy, loose bodies, hardware around the joint and bony glenoid rim abnormalities. However, it has low accuracy in detecting partial rotator-cuff tears. Kneisl *et al.* (1988) considers CT arthrography a reliable test for shoulder instability, but not for patients without instability. Conventional MRI was found to be only moderately reliable in evaluating labral tears and Hill–Sach's lesions and inaccurate in evaluating capsulolabral lesions (Suder *et al.*, 1995).

Reinus *et al.* (1995) compared conventional MRI with a fat-saturated technique in detecting rotator-cuff tears. He found an improved detection rate of both partial- and full-thickness tears with a fat-saturated technique, but detection of partial-thickness tears was still low at 50% sensitivity. Palmer *et al.* (1994) had excellent results for detection of both partial- and full-thickness rotator-cuff tears using fat-suppressed MR arthrography.

Chandnani *et al.* (1993) evaluated glenoid labral tears comparing MRI imaging, MRI arthrography and CT arthrography and found that MRI arthrography was the most sensitive. It detected detached labral fragments and degeneration and afforded the best visualization of the inferior part of the labrum and the inferior glenohumeral ligament.

There is unanimity that arthroscopy is the best method of evaluating pathology in the glenohumeral and the subacromial space. The accuracy of the above mentioned imaging techniques were compared on the basis of arthroscopic findings. With a good history, physical examination and with the aid of imaging techniques if necessary, a diagnosis can be made on most shoulder problems. We believe that there is little role for the arthroscope as a purely diagnostic tool. The surgeon should have a clear idea as to the pathology before committing to arthroscopy. The arthroscope nowadays is really an operative tool and should be used appropriately in this way. We find that using the arthroscope to try to elucidate unknown shoulder pathology is not a useful exercise.

Technique

Most shoulder arthroscopists place the patient in the lateral decubitus position. Distraction of the joint is obtained, with the arm suspended from a two-pulley system, using skin traction. The shoulder is placed in traction with the arm in abduction and forward flexion. There are differing opinions about the position of the arm in traction. The degree of abduction varies between 30° and 70° while the degree of forward flexion varies from 15° to 30°. Most surgeons feel that no more than 7 kg should be used. Concern over the arm position and traction weight has been generated by reports of neurovascular injury, especially to the brachial plexus. Paulos (1985) reported a 30% incidence of transient neuropraxia from shoulder arthroscopy with traction.

Pitman *et al.* (1988) used somatosensory-evoked potentials (SEP) to monitor patients undergoing shoulder arthroscopy with traction. They found abnormal SEPs in all patients, with two patients developing transient clinical neuropraxia. The musculocutaneous nerve was the most sensitive. Klein *et al.* (1987) applied strain gauges to the brachial plexus in cadavers and determined that the positions for best visualization and minimal strain were 45° of flexion with either 0° or 90° of abduction.

Gross and Fitzgibbons (1985) modified this straight lateral position by rolling the patient 30° to 40° posteriorly, placing the plane of the shoulder joint parallel to the horizontal. The traction is applied perpendicular to the long axis of the humerus with the arm in an adducted position. Skyhar (1988) advocated the beach-chair position citing improved arm mobility and traction just by gravity. The patient is positioned so that he is sitting up at least 60° and a bolster is placed between the scapulae to elevate the affected side.

Following sterile draping technique, with the arm free, a standard posterosuperior portal, just medial and inferior to the acromion, is usually chosen (Fig. 3.1). Surgical procedures are performed through

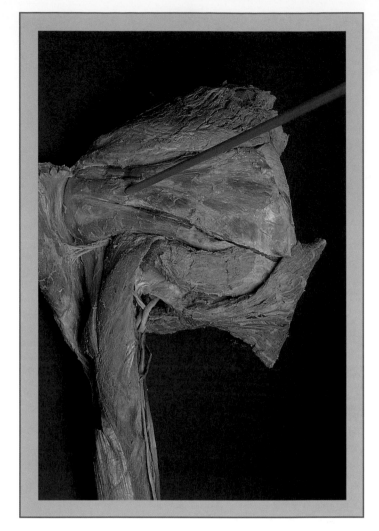

Figure 3.1 – *Anatomy of the standard posterior portal. The arthroscope passes through the deltoid, and then through the muscle of infraspinatus. Note the position of the axillary nerve (reproduced with permission from Shoulder Arthroscopy, Bunker and Wallace (eds), Dunitz).*

accessory anterior, lateral and posterior portals. The anterior portal is determined by passing the arthroscope across the joint and transilluminating the anterior structures. The portal is placed just superior to the subscapularis tendon. The lateral portal used for subacromial surgery is placed approximately 2 cm from the tip of the acromion. Nevasier (1987) described a superomedial portal which penetrates the supraspinatus muscle, allows the portals to be spread apart, and does not violate the area at risk in the rotator cuff. Wolf (1989) describes an accessory antero-inferior portal which is located inferior to the tip of the coracoid process. This has been utilized mostly in stabilization procedures.

Frozen shoulder

Frozen shoulder is a condition of pain in the shoulder accompanied by stiffness in all directions, especially in abduction and external rotation, with no obvious cause. Primary frozen shoulder is caused by a fibrous contracture of the capsule of the shoulder (see Chapter 8). It is important to rule out other significant intra-articular pathology, with a thorough history and physical examination, before establishing a diagnosis of frozen shoulder.

The initial treatment of patients with primary frozen shoulder is physiotherapy accompanied by oral analgesics and non-steroidal anti-inflammatory medication. If the patient does not respond over a 3–6 month period, an intra-articular cortisone injection, combined with local anaesthetic, can be given. Most investigators indicate that a certain percentage of patients will not recover, about 10% in most studies. If the patient remains refractory to conservative therapy for more than 6 months to 1 year then surgery may be indicated. Surgical treatment includes manipulation under general anaesthesia with or without arthroscopy and arthroscopic release.

Arthroscopy has been shown to be of diagnostic value in frozen shoulder. Arthroscopy allows the identification and treatment of alternative pathology, such as impingement lesions and secondary subacromial space inflammation, calcific deposits, and acromioclavicular arthritis.

Wiley (1991) arthroscopically evaluated 37 patients, who had primary frozen shoulder, prior to manipulation under general anaesthesia. The arthroscopic appearance was uniform with a patchy vascular reaction around the biceps and the opening into the subscapularis bursa (Fig. 3.2). In no patient was the infraglenoid recess obliterated, and no adhesions were seen. Uitvlugt *et al.* (1993) arthroscopically evaluated 20 patients selected for manipulation under general anaesthesia. The main intra-articular finding was vascular synovitis without intra-articular adhesions or degenerative changes. More than a dozen studies have now confirmed these findings (see Chapter 8).

The technique of manipulation under anaesthesia followed by arthroscopy offers a safe and reliable treatment for the resistant frozen shoulder. Inspection of the joint following manipulation reveals rupture of the inferior capsule and sometimes even the anterior

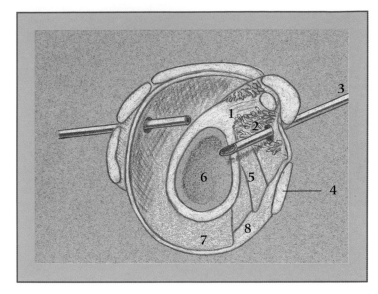

Figure 3.2 – *The shaver has been introduced anteriorly. The typical features of frozen shoulder are seen. (1) biceps ensheathed in inflammatory tissue; (2) the interval area is completely filled with inflammatory tissue obliterating the space; (3) the shaver; (4) subscapularis; (5) middle glenohumeral ligament; (6) glenoid; (7) contracted infraglenoid recess; (8) inferior glenohumeral ligament.*

capsular structures. Patients in whom conservative treatment has failed, benefit substantially from manipulation (Wiley, 1991; Uitvlugt *et al.*, 1993; Andersen *et al.*, 1996).

Recently, considerable interest has been shown in arthroscopic surgical procedures for frozen shoulder. Pollock *et al.* (1994) achieved satisfactory results in 83% of patients, using arthroscopically guided sectioning of the coracohumeral ligament in addition to manipulation under general anaesthesia. Segmuller (1995) was able to achieve excellent or good results in 87% of patients who underwent an arthroscopic release of the inferior capsule.

We compared manipulation versus surgical release in a prospective cohort study (Ogilvie-Harris *et al.* 1995). The arthroscopic division procedure was conducted in four sequential steps (Fig. 3.3): (1) resection of the inflammatory synovium in the interval area between the subscapularis and supraspinatus, (2) progressive division of the anterosuperior glenohumeral ligament and anterior capsule, (3) division of the subscapularis tendon but not the muscle, and (4) division of the inferior capsule. Patients treated with arthroscopy and manipulation did as well as patients treated with arthroscopic division for restoration of range of movement. However, the patients in the arthroscopic

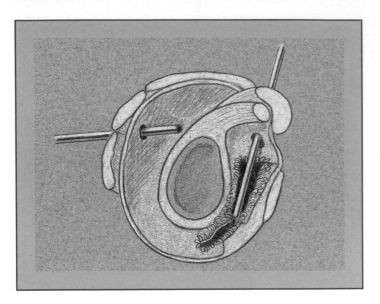

Figure 3.3 – *Arthroscopic release of frozen shoulder. The inflammatory tissue in the interval is resected. The anterior capsule is sequentially released. The infraglenoid recess is released.*

division group had significantly better pain relief and restoration of function. Patients with diabetes did worse initially, but the outcome was similar to patients without diabetes. Patients with diabetes in particular may benefit from early intervention.

Rotator-cuff pathology and impingement

Impingement syndrome refers to a spectrum of subacromial pathology, ranging from tendonitis to rotator-cuff tearing, and is the most common cause of shoulder pain (Green, 1995). Compression of the rotator cuff by the overlying acromion causes 95% of impingement (Esch, 1993). Impingement secondary to anterior or multidirectional instability accounts for the other 5% (Jobe and Kvitne, 1989).

It has been established that arthroscopy is a useful procedure for diagnosis of rotator-cuff pathology. It permits a detailed intra-articular and subacromial visualization and classification of rotator-cuff problems (Fig 3.4). During arthroscopy, the arm is placed at 60° of abduction, then passive elevation, internal rotation and adduction to reproduce the position used in the clinical test for impingement.

Most rotator-cuff disorders can be diagnosed with a careful history, physical examination and evaluation of the patient. Although the arthroscope is the most accurate diagnostic investigation for rotator-cuff pathology, isolated diagnostic arthroscopy is rarely

indicated. Its most frequent use is in overlap patients, especially throwing athletes, in whom the relative contributions of instability and impingement are unclear (Yamaguchi and Flatow, 1995). One of its important roles is in the evaluation of both the glenohumeral joint and subacromial bursa when the diagnosis is unclear. This condition is frequently found in the overhead athlete with silent atraumatic glenohumeral instability. When instability is present it should be addressed as the primary lesion; impingement symptoms due to rotator-cuff fatigue should be considered as a secondary problem (Glousman, 1993).

If symptoms persist, following conservative treatment with anti-inflammatories, steroid injections and physiotherapy, an arthroscopic acromioplasty is indicated. Arthroscopic acromioplasty is generally performed on an outpatient basis. Initially, arthroscopy of the shoulder and subacromial space is carried out. The patient is placed in the side-lying position elevated approximately 45° from horizontal. Pressure irrigation is employed. A standard posterior portal is used for initial visualization. The cuff is debrided through the arthroscope and at the same time the cuff can be evaluated to see if there is a rotator-cuff tear, and if so, the amount of retraction of the tendon. A 5.5 mm full-radius resector is used to remove soft tissue from the subacromial space. A 5 mm acromionizer is then used to remove bone from the undersurface of the acromion (Fig. 3.5). Bone is resected from as far medially as the acromioclavicular joint, to the lateral side of the acromion, and as far anteriorly as the coracoacromial ligament and hook. The coracoacromial ligament is detached from the anterior acromion with the burr to resect sufficient bone. The acromioplasty is considered complete when the deltoid muscle can be visualized clearly all the way around the acromion. In a recent study (Fig. 3.6), the posterior portal was demonstrated to be more effective in removing the anterior acromial hook as compared to the lateral portal (Ogilvie-Harris *et al.*, 1993).

The results of the subacromial decompression are dependent on the state of the rotator cuff at the time of arthroscopy. Most investigators report 80–90% satisfactory results for stage-I and -II impingement (Van Holsbeeck *et al.*, 1992; Sachs *et al.*, 1994; Olsewski and Depew, 1994; Roye *et al.*, 1995). We would consider this to be the procedure of choice for patients, with impingement syndrome, who have failed to respond to conservative treatment.

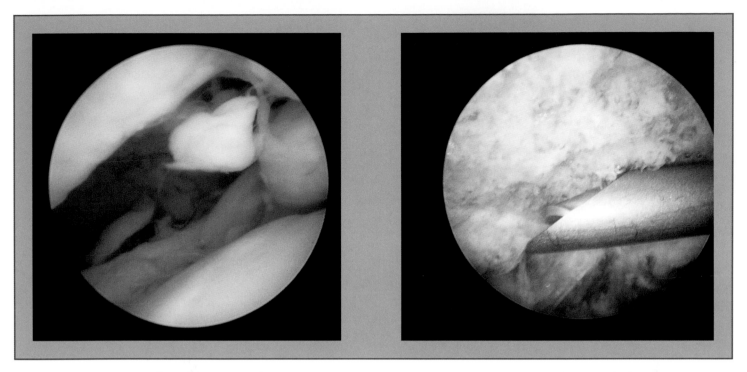

Figure 3.4 – *A rotator-cuff tear as seen at arthroscopy.*

Figure 3.5 – *Arthroscopic subacromial decompression. An arthroscopic view of the acromionizer burr removing the undersurface of the acromion.*

The results in patients with complete tears of the rotator cuff (stage III) have been less satisfactory. The results range from 50 to 68% satisfactory (Ellman, 1987; Ogilvie-Harris & Demaziere, 1993; Zvijac *et al.*, 1994). We compared arthroscopic subacromial decompression and rotator-cuff debridement with open-repair and acromioplasty for rotator-cuff tears 1–4 cm in size (Ogilvie-Harris & Demaziere, 1993). Pain relief was approximately equal in both. However, open-repair gave significantly superior results in strength and function. We recommend the use of arthroscopic subacromial decompression and debridement for low-demand patients who require mainly pain relief and range of movement. Open-repair is necessary if strength and functional recovery are the prime objectives.

Recently, Imhoff and Lederman (1995) compared laser-assisted arthroscopic subacromial decompression (Holmium:YAG-laser) with the conventional arthroscopic procedure. They found better results, especially for early pain relief, activity and movement, and better values for abduction power in the laser group.

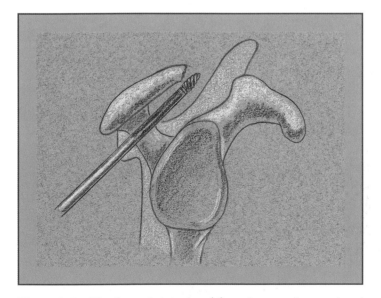

Figure 3.6 – *The shaver is introduced from the posterior portal and the acromion is used as a jig for removal of the anterior hook.*

Acromioclavicular joint disease

Acromioclavicular joint pain is a relatively common cause of shoulder disability. It can occur as an isolated lesion, or can coexist with other shoulder pathology, such as impingement syndrome. Traditionally, open resection of the distal clavicle is the procedure of choice for patients refractory to conservative management. With recent advancements in arthroscopic techniques, resection of the acromioclavicular joint can be done with minimal morbidity. Gartsman *et al.* (1991) compared open and arthroscopic resection of the acromioclavicular joint using cadaveric models and found no difference in terms of the amount of bone resection. Flatow *et al.* (1992) compared open and arthroscopic resection for osteolysis of the distal clavicle and found earlier relief of pain, and return to activities and sports, in the arthroscopic group. Conventional open techniques require detachment and reattachment of the deltoid which causes postoperative weakness and subsequently prolongs rehabilitation.

There are two basic approaches to the acromioclavicular joint, the direct superior and the bursal approach. Bigliani *et al.* (1993) uses the superior approach for isolated acromioclavicular joint pathology and in patients with narrow or medially inclined overriding clavicles. In their series of 42 patients, who underwent arthroscopic resection of the acromioclavicular joint through the direct superior approach, 91% had resolution of their symptoms and returned to full activity. The bursal approach is beneficial for patients with both subacromial and acromioclavicular joint pathology. Snyder *et al.* (1995) reported a 94% success rate in 50 patients who underwent arthroscopic acromioclavicular joint resection using a special clavicle burr.

Biceps tendon

Biceps tendon pathology can be managed well with the arthroscope. Degeneration of this structure usually parallels the severity of rotator-cuff degeneration. According to Neer (1972), 95% of biceps-tendon pathology is caused by impingement. However, in many cases, especially in the younger patients, isolated bicipital tendonitis is found at arthroscopy. In some of these patients there may be an impingement syndrome, but in some cases the tendon has degenerated as the primary pathology. Arthroscopic evaluation for diagnosis is important for determining the extent of the lesion (Fig. 3.7), and in many cases obviates the need for open surgical exploration .

At arthroscopy, a frayed tendon can be debrided and this should achieve good results in about 80% of cases. Good results drop to 60% if mild glenohumeral degeneration is present (Ogilvie-Harris, 1987).

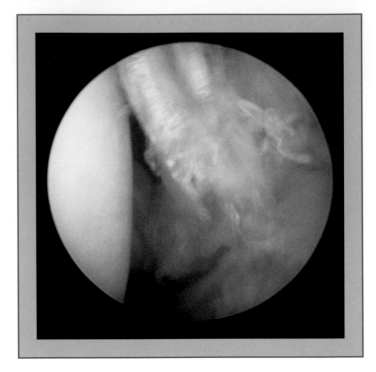

Figure 3.7 – *Arthroscopic view of a partial tear of the long head of biceps.*

Glenoid labrum tears and instability

Arthroscopy is not a substitute for a thorough clinical evaluation and physical examination of the shoulder in patients with instability. It provides confirmation of the clinical impression, especially in subtle cases of instability (Caspari & Geissler, 1993).

Karzel and Snyder (1994) classified glenoid labrum pathology into three types (Table 3.1).

The classic findings in a dislocating shoulder are the Bankart lesion, Hill–Sachs impaction fracture, loose bodies, and tears of the anterior inferior glenohumeral ligament. Hintermann and Gachter (1995) arthroscopically evaluated 212 patients who had at least one documented shoulder dislocation. They

Table 3.1 Types of labral tear.

(1)	Labral tear associated with instability
(2)	Isolated tear within a meniscoid labrum
(3)	Biceps anchor tears (SLAP lesion).

found that 87% had anterior glenoid labral tears, 79% had ventral capsule insufficiency, 68% had Hill–Sachs compression fractures, 55% had glenohumeral ligament insufficiency, 14% had complete rotator cuff tendon tears, 12% had posterior glenoid labral tears, 7% had superior labrum anterior and inferior lesions (Fig. 3.8). Wolf *et al.* (1995) found a lesser known entity — the humeral avulsion of glenohumeral ligaments (HAGL) — to be present in 6 out of 64 patients (9.3%) with anterior instability. They recommended that HAGL should be ruled out in patients with documented anterior instability, but without a demonstrable primary Bankart lesion.

In stable shoulders, tears of the glenoid labrum can be resected and this is successful in relieving symptoms. These patients often complain of clicking in the shoulder when tested by gentle internal and external rotation with the arm at 90° of abduction, and applying longitudinal compression to the shoulder (Ogilvie-Harris & D'Angelo, 1990). Similarly, Martin and Garth (1995) had good results with arthroscopic debridement of glenoid labral tears when there was gross instability or Bankart lesion.

In unstable shoulders, resection without stabilization led to poor results in all patients (Ogilvie-Harris & Wiley, 1986). Cordasco (1993) reported less than satisfactory

results with arthroscopic treatment of glenoid labral tears in 52 patients without clinical instability or history of dislocations. They concluded that occult instability is frequently present in patients with glenoid labral tears. They believe that arthroscopic labral debridement may have an indication for short-term goals in competitive athletes, or those who are willing to accept some compromise in function.

There have been recent advances in the field of arthroscopic stabilization in shoulder instability. Most of these procedures are based on the concept of repairing the antero-inferior capsulolabral complex back to the glenoid rim (Bankart lesion) (Fig. 3.9). The methods available at the present time include capsulorrhaphy using staples, transglenoid sutures, bioabsorbable tack and suture anchor (Table 3.2).

In 1982, Johnson was the first to perform an arthroscopic shoulder capsulorrhaphy, by using metal staples. Although this has its inherent advantages as an arthroscopic procedure, it has many disadvantages. These include technical difficulties, with a slow learning curve, an average failure rate of 12%, and the use of a metal staple which may itself be a major source of complications (Detrisac & Johnson, 1993).

Caspari and Savoie (1996) have utilized the trans-glenoid suture technique for arthroscopic Bankart repair (Fig. 3.10). Their series gave a 94–96% satisfactory success rate. However, they found an age-related association with failure of this procedure. They do not recommend this technique for individuals aged 16 or under. Youssef *et al.* (1995) reported a 27% failure rate with the transglenoid arthroscopic Bankart procedure.

Warren *et al.* (1996) has developed a cannulated bioabsorbable tack to stabilize the Bankart lesion

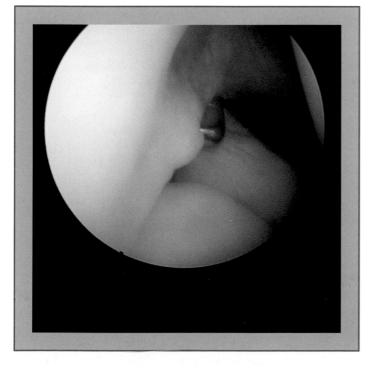

Figure 3.8 – *Arthroscopic view of a SLAP tear.*

Table 3.2 Techniques of arthroscopic repair.		
Staple capsulorrhaphy	Johnson	1982
Transglenoid suture	Morgan	1987
Transglenoid suture	Caspari	1989
Mulberry knot suture	Maki	1991
Suretac device	Warren	1995
Slalom screw technique	Resch	1992
Intra-articular suture anchor	Wolf	1991
Laser assisted capsulorrhaphy	Hardy	1996

(Fig. 3.11). This eliminates some of the dangers of metallic fixation devices and has eliminated the necessity for suturing over the infraspinatus muscle posteriorly. Warner *et al.* (1995) was able to do a 'second look' arthroscopy on 15 patients who had failures from this procedure with pain or recurrent

instability. They concluded that the high failure rate for this procedure appears to result from improper patient selection and errors in surgical technique. Two concerns relating to the use of bioabsorbable implants are non-infectious inflammatory responses to the implant, and premature loosening due to absorption (Berg 1996).

Wolf (1993) used the Mitek GII suture anchor to restore the anatomic integrity of the inferior glenohumeral ligament labral complex. Although the follow-up was short, in 50 patients he had only one recurrence. Hoffman and Reif (1995) were able to follow up 30 patients stabilized with Mitek anchors and had three poor results. They concluded that patients with more than 10 dislocations are not suited for this procedure even if a Bankart lesion is present.

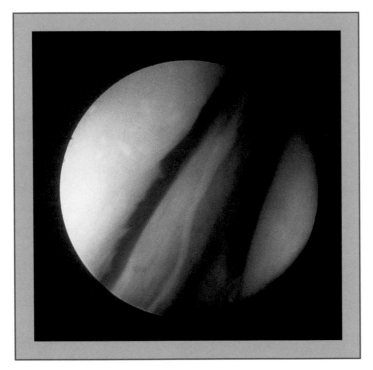

Figure 3.9 – *The Bankart lesion (with permission from Shoulder Arthroscopy, Bunker and Wallace (eds), Dunitz).*

Most of these investigators emphasize appropriate patient selection as an important factor for success. Ideally, patients should have a traumatic anterior instability with a discrete Bankart lesion and with strong ligamentous tissue.

Treatment of shoulder instability with the arthroscope is still evolving. These new arthroscopic techniques are technically demanding, with slow learning curves, and should be performed only by physicians with superior arthroscopic skills. Apparently, the success of the original authors was not consistently duplicated by independent investigators. Generally, the rate of redislocations after arthroscopic treatment is higher than with open surgical repair. At present, open

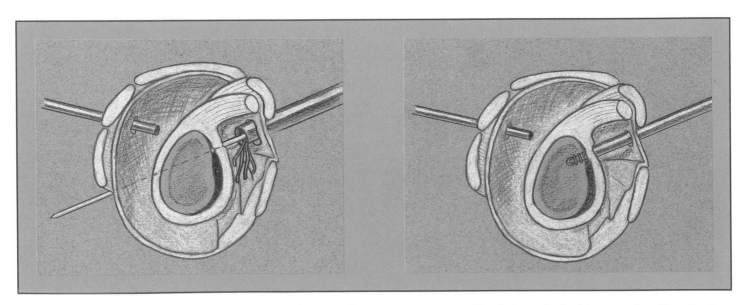

Figure 3.10 – *The Caspari transglenoid suture technique. The bed has been prepared and the sutures placed in the capsule.*

Figure 3.11 – *The Suretac device being used to fix a Bankart lesion.*

surgery is still the gold standard for treating shoulder instability.

Hardy *et al.* (1996) used laser-assisted capsular shrinkage (LACS), in addition to arthroscopic labral reattachment, in 18 patients with recurrent anterior dislocation. Short-term results revealed no recurrence with 7 of 18 patients returning to their previous sports activity at the same level. Recurrences from arthroscopic stabilization for anterior instability are probably due to capsular redundancy and laxity of the glenohumeral ligaments. They believe capsular shrinkage together with labrum reattachment will provide long-term results comparable to open methods. Markel *et al.* (1996) studied the effects of non-ablative lasers in the joint capsule of animal models and found significant capsular shrinkage, without affecting the relaxation properties of the tissue. They pointed out the potential of the laser in multidirectional and unidirectional shoulder instability.

Snyder *et al.* (1990) described the superior labrum anteroposterior (SLAP) lesion. This is a lesion involving the superior aspect of the glenoid labrum, beginning posterior to the biceps tendon and extending anterior to the biceps tendon, stopping at or above the midglenoid notch. With the widespread use of shoulder arthroscopy this lesion is becoming increasingly recognized. SLAP lesions are usually associated with other pathology, such as instability and rotator-cuff tears. Although relatively uncommon, they are said to be a source of significant shoulder disability. Four types of SLAP lesion have been described (Fig. 3.12). In type I, there is extensive fraying of the superior labrum without biceps instability. In type II, in addition to the fraying of the superior labrum there is avulsion of the labrum/biceps anchor of the superior glenoid. Type III involves a bucket-handle tear of the superior labrum with an intact biceps anchor. Type IV has a similar bucket-handle tear, but it extends to a variable extent into the substance of the biceps tendon. Arthroscopic treatment depends on the type of SLAP lesion. In type I, the frayed labrum is debrided back to intact labrum. Type-II lesions are treated with arthroscopic repair of the biceps attachment to the labrum using similar techniques to those used in anterior instability (Fig. 3.13). In Type-III lesions, the bucket handle is excised. Type-IV lesions are treated similarly, but excision extends to the torn portion of the biceps tendon. If the biceps-tendon tear involves more than 50% of the tendon, tenodesis of the tendon can be performed.

Yoneda *et al.* (1991) reported 80% success with arthroscopic stapling for 10 patients with SLAP lesions. Field and Savoie (1993) reported 100% success in 20 patients with SLAP lesions (Snyder Types II and IV) using multiple sutures into the torn labrum-biceps tendon complex. Snyder *et al.* (1996) used permanent anchor screw with non-absorbable sutures to fix the biceps anchor into the glenoid rim. They re-inspected eight patients arthroscopically at an average of nine months and found seven firmly re-attached to bone.

Although follow up studies are available, considerable confusion still exists as to the pathological significance of the SLAP lesions. In our own hands we would rarely repair such a lesion. We have had good results with simple excision of the loose or unstable portions. It may be that surgical stabilization is too radical a treatment. Further follow up studies need to be carried out to determine if the documented pathology really translates into functional problems, and whether repair of the unstable labrum is of benefit compared to excision or just rehabilitation.

Loose bodies

The most common cause of loose-body formation in the shoulder is glenohumeral instability (Fig. 3.14). Other causes are osteoarthritis, osteochondritis dissecans, and foreign bodies. There is unanimity in the literature that the arthroscope is the ideal method for managing loose bodies of the shoulder joint, and the results are excellent. Most loose bodies can be removed with the arthroscope but arthrotomy can be an option when the loose body is too large to be removed through a standard portal. The most common area for finding loose bodies is in the axillary pouch of the shoulder joint. Other possible sites include the subscapularis bursa, posterior recess, and deep to the middle glenohumeral ligament. McGinty (1982) made two good points about the arthroscopic management of intra-articular loose bodies. Firstly, as soon as a loose body or fragment is identified the surgeon should immediately stop all movement, turn off the irrigation and then stop and think for 30 seconds. Secondly, if a loose body cannot be found with the arthroscope it is not likely that an arthrotomy will be successful; the procedure should be abandoned and the patient observed or a further attempt made on another day.

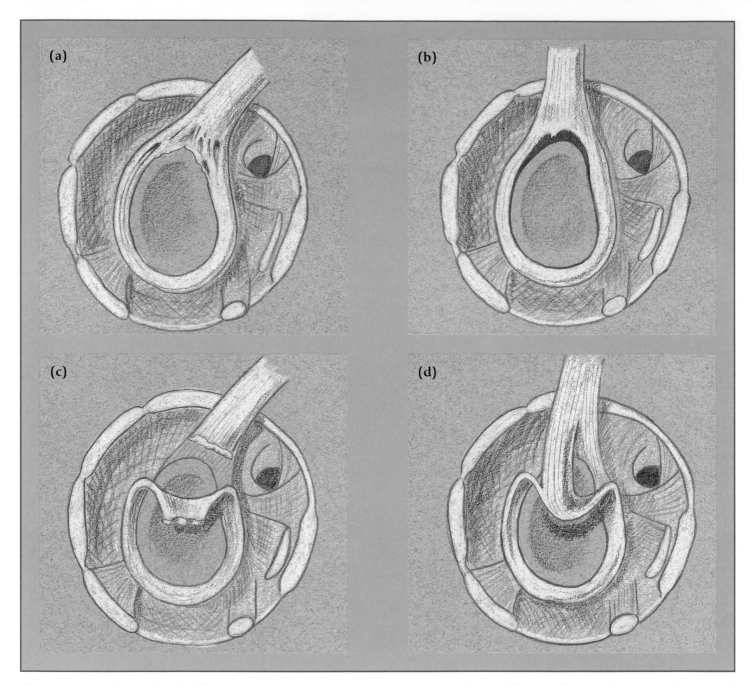

Figure 3.12 – *The Snyder classification of SLAP tears: I fraying of the superior labrum (a); II avulsion of the superior labrum and biceps (b); III bucket handle avulsion of the biceps (c) and IV the bucket handle extends into the biceps (d).*

Infection

The septic shoulder can be successfully treated using arthroscopic techniques, thus avoiding morbidity from open drainage. Infection in the shoulder usually occurs by direct inoculation from knives, gunshot wounds or following arthroscopy. In the elderly, and the very young, it may present spontaneously.

The diagnosis is made when there is pain accompanied by fever, swelling and an increased erythrocyte sedimentation rate (ESR). The arthroscope is used to perform a thorough lavage and debridement of fibrinous or foreign material followed by placement of drains. D'Angelo and Ogilvie-Harris (1988) and Cofield (1983) used suction-irrigation catheters followed by broad-spectrum antibiotics. Parisien and Shaffer (1992)

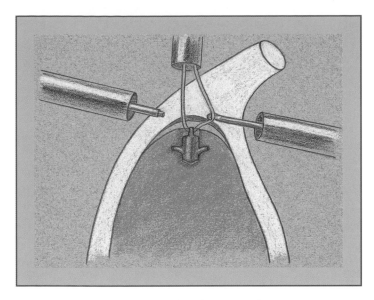

Figure 3.13 – *A suture anchor being used to repair a SLAP lesion.*

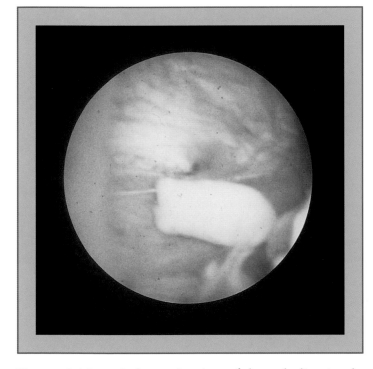

Figure 3.14 – *Arthroscopic view of loose bodies in the infraglenoid recess.*

used only suction drains without irrigation. The use of irrigation is not necessary if the tubes are removed within 48 hours. Success has been reported in all cases with prompt diagnosis and treatment. Ogilvie-Harris and D'Angelo (1990) reported on two cases with poor results which were explained by a delay in referral which resulted in joint damage.

Symptoms resolve within 2 or 3 days and antibiotics are continued intravenously for 1 week and then orally for at least 6 weeks. It is not necessary to perform a synovectomy unless the involved tissue is necrotic. Continuous passive motion may aid in maintaining range of motion and increasing patient comfort.

Synovectomy

Arthroscopic synovectomy can be helpful in the diagnosis and treatment of inflammatory arthritis as well as a variety of primary synovial disorders affecting the shoulder (Matthews & Labudde, 1993). Patients with rheumatoid arthritis, pigmented villonodular synovitis and synovial chondromatosis of the shoulder are ideal candidates for arthroscopic synovectomy. Following adequate conservative therapy, persistent pain and weakness in the shoulder is an indication to perform a synovectomy. Patients best suited for synovectomy demonstrate minimal bony destruction and an intact cuff. The benefits of synovectomy appear to diminish in relation to the severity of articular involvement (Matthews & Scerpella, 1996). Partial and complete synovectomy can be performed by rotating the power shaver, arthroscope and drainage cannula through three portals as described by Nevasier (1987). Debridement of the pannus invading bone can be accomplished and both the subacromial space and glenohumeral joint can be debrided (Johnson, 1987). The procedure can be technically difficult because of bleeding but this is reduced by using a pressure irrigation system or adding adrenaline to the irrigation fluid. Arthroscopic synovectomy results in minimal tissue disruption and morbidity compared to open synovectomy.

The results of this procedure are generally satisfactory. We reported significant improvement in 12 out of 15 rheumatoid patients (Ogilvie-Harris, 1990). Covall and Fowble (1993) stated that in cases of synovial chondromatosis, the results in terms of efficacy and recurrence rates of the arthroscopic and the open method appear comparable. Takenaka *et al.* (1992) reported on eight patients with haemodialysis-related shoulder arthropathy who underwent arthroscopic synovectomy. The therapy was effective for pain relief, and improvement of shoulder function for 6 months, but in 1 year the shoulder pain reappeared in most patients. Johnson stated that the rehabilitation process can be initiated immediately and that its duration is shorter when compared to the equivalent open procedure.

Complications

There are definite risks associated with arthroscopic surgery of the shoulder. The overall complication rate reported by the Arthroscopy Association of North America in 1988 was 0.76%. This must not be taken out of context as certain procedures such as staple capsulorrhaphy have a complication rate of 3.3–5.3% (Small, 1986, 1988). Wall and Warren (1995) reported complications of shoulder instability surgery, including recurrent instability, limitation of motion, inability to return to the previous level of sport, problems related to hardware, pain, development of osteoarthritis, and neurovascular injuries.

We studied patients who had an arthroscopic acromioplasty using pressure irrigation and found significant extravasation of fluid into the deltoid muscle (Ogilvie-Harris & Boynton, 1990). Pressure in the deltoid went up during the procedure but returned to baseline with 4 minutes of the end of the procedure. No patients showed evidence of muscle damage during electromyography (EMG) studies conducted 4–6 weeks postoperatively.

Lee *et al.* (1992) reported a rare subcutaneous emphysema, pneumomediastinum and tension pneumothorax in three patients who underwent arthroscopic subacromial decompression. They thought that these complications were associated with the extravasation of air that may be drawn in when the arthroscopic infusion pump and power-shaver with suction are turned on. We reported a 3% complication rate in 439 procedures (Ogilvie-Harris & D'Angelo, 1990). This series included fluid extravasation, articular cartilage damage, infection and musculocutaneous-nerve palsy, none of which resulted in serious sequelae.

Summary

Diagnostic arthroscopy is currently the best method for assessing glenohumeral and subacromial pathology. However, we feel very strongly that it should only be undertaken when a specific pre-operative diagnosis has been formulated. There is no substitute for a careful history and diligent examination.

With the advent of modern imaging techniques, most shoulder disorders can be diagnosed with accuracy. Shoulder arthroscopy initially confirms or rejects that diagnosis, and can usually be followed by therapeutic arthroscopy, or open surgery if needed. Successful shoulder arthroscopy necessitates familiarity in the set-up, positioning of the patient and the different portals, and an awareness of the anatomy at risk.

The diagnosis of frozen shoulder is established clinically, but arthroscopic evaluation of the intra-articular structures is valuable. The arthroscopic sequential release of the tight structures resulted in better pain relief and restoration of function than that achieved using manipulation. Patients with diabetes may benefit from early intervention.

Arthroscopic decompression of the subacromial space is the treatment of choice for impingement syndrome, if unresponsive to conservative means. Low-demand patients with significant full-thickness rotator-cuff tear can undergo subacromial decompression and debridement if they require only pain relief and range of movement. Young patients would need an open repair if strength and functional recovery are the prime objectives.

Instability should be ruled out for throwing athletes presenting with symptoms similar to impingement syndrome. The biceps tendonitis can be successfully debrided and decompressed arthroscopically. Concomitant impingement syndrome should be ruled out as this is very common.

Acromioclavicular joint pain refractory to conservative means can be effectively treated with arthroscopic acromioclavicular resection. It has distinct advantages over the traditional open resection.

Glenoid labral lesions can be debrided in stable shoulders. Further evaluation of the SLAP lesions is necessary to determine their role in causing shoulder pain, and the most effective treatment. In unstable shoulders, resection without stabilization leads to poor results. There have been recent advances in arthroscopic stabilization of the traumatic anterior instability with typical Bankart lesions. The different techniques are generally, technically demanding. Proper patient selection is related to the success of the procedure. Generally, the rate of redislocation after arthroscopic treatment is higher that with open methods. Arthroscopic techniques should not be carried out in contact athletes. Promise is shown in the management of multidirectional instability with lasers.

Loose bodies are best managed by arthroscopic removal. Septic shoulder can be managed by arthroscopic lavage and debridement combined with antibiotics. Arthroscopic synovectomy can be performed on patients with rheumatoid arthritis and other synovial disorders, to relieve persistent pain and weakness that is unmanageable using conservative means.

CHAPTER 4

Impingement: needle, scope or scalpel?

T. Bunker

Introduction

Rotator-cuff disease is the commonest cause of shoulder pain. Impingement and rotator-cuff tears may cause pain, sleepless nights, loss of work, loss of income and, all too often, a crippling and permanent loss of function to the patient.

The surgeon is in a privileged position because only he can see, and feel, the living pathology of the rotator cuff. There appears to be a continuum of rotator-cuff disease (Table 4.1). The surgeon is able to counter this continuum with a selection of therapeutic techniques ranging from injection to fusion. On the one hand, the surgical management of impingement syndrome, by the simple operation of anterior acromioplasty, can lead to the most grateful of patients, and the most satisfied of surgeons. On the other hand, the surgical management of massive rotator-cuff tears can be the most demanding

test of surgical aptitude and, if the surgeon is not careful in selection and counselling of his patients, may lead to the most dissatisfied of patients and the most frustrated of surgeons.

Diseases of the rotator cuff also pose an intellectual challenge to the surgeon. Many research papers have been written on the rotator cuff over the last decade, which have raised as many questions as they have answered. Controversy looms large in virtually every area studied. The aetiology of impingement and rotator-cuff tears is controversial; abnormal morphology, diminished blood supply to the cuff, age related changes in the tendons, and repetitive trauma each have their champions. Imaging techniques have evolved rapidly over the last decade, with ultrasound taking over from arthrography which itself is being superseded by magnetic resonance imaging (MRI).

Surgical treatment is even more controversial. Should impingement be managed by arthroscopic or open decompression? How should massive tears be managed: by debridement or by attempts at repair? If repair is attempted, should direct repair be used, or should tendon transfers be used? What approach should be used? How should the patient be managed postoperatively; in a sling or abduction splint? How should cuff arthropathy be treated: by hemiarthroplasty, bipolar arthroplasty or even by fusion?

This chapter will discuss impingement, and the following chapter will consider rotator-cuff tears. Neither chapter claims to have all the answers, as this field is changing rapidly, but each chapter will analyse these controversies in a logical manner, such that the reader will be able to act as an enlightened advocate for each patient referred to him.

Table 4.1 The continuum of rotator cuff disease.		
Overused normal tendon		
Tendonitis		
Partial-thickness tear	Deep surface	A
	Bursal surface	B
	Interstitial	
Full-thickness tear	Small	1 cm
	Moderate	1–3 cm
	Large	3–5 cm
	Massive	> 5 cm
Cuff-tear arthropathy		

Aetiology of impingement

Adams (1852) first proposed an extrinsic cause of rotator-cuff disease, the cuff rubbing on the acromion until it tore. He stated: 'The explanation of the circumstances why the superior and external part of the capsular ligament has been found perforated by a large circular opening, through which the head of the humerus can pass, appears to be ... that the head of the humerus is at once elevated by deltoid, and kept habitually pressed up against the acromion'.

Meyer (1931) popularized this theory of attrition-lesions of the cuff. This led Smith Peterson (1943), McLaughlin (1944) and Armstrong (1949) to attempt to treat these lesions by complete acromionectomy. However, complete acromionectomy led to weakening or detachment of the deltoid. It was disappointment with the results of this operation that stimulated Neer to study the role of the undersurface of the acromion in impingement syndrome.

Neer (1983) stressed that the function of the shoulder is to place the hand in space where the eyes can see what the hand is doing, and then to maintain a stable platform whilst the hand carries out its function. The important functional movement of the shoulder must therefore be forward elevation.

Neer (1972) stated that his observations at surgery consistently showed that the area of degenerative tendonitis and tendon rupture was centered in the supraspinatus tendon. Moreover, this area lay anterior to the acromion (Fig. 4.1), and on forward elevation abutted against the coraco-acromial ligament and anterior acromion, and on occasion the acromioclavicular joint.

Neer (1972) examined 100 cadaver scapulae. Eleven had abnormalities of the undersurface of the acromion. All these changes only affected the anterior acromion. Eight had a characteristic ridge of proliferative spurs on the undersurface of the anterior acromion, caused by repeated impingement leading to traction on the coraco-acromial ligament. In three cases there was eburnation of the undersurface of the anterior acromion, which he felt was a later stage of the same process.

A pattern thus emerged: tears were anterior, movement was forwards, abutment was anterior and the bone changes only occurred on the anterior acromion.

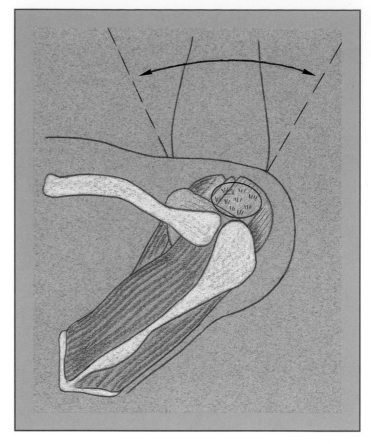

Figure 4.1 – *The impingement lesion. The shoulder is designed as a stable base which supports the hand in positions where it can be seen by the eyes. In this position impingement occurs between the tendon of supraspinatus and three structures, the anterior acromion, the coraco-acromial ligament and the acromioclavicular joint. (After Neer, reproduced with permission from Clinical Orthopaedics and Related Research.)*

Based on these clinical observations, Neer restricted his acromioplasty to the anterior and antero-inferior acromion alone and found that the results were far superior to those of total acromionectomy. At a single stroke, shoulder surgery leapt from the dark ages into the scientific age.

Over the next decade Neer refined his theory of impingement. Based upon observations of 400 patients with rotator-cuff disease he came to believe that 95% of cuff tears were caused by impingement.

Neer (1983) went on to state that there were three stages of impingement (Table 4.2). **Stage I.** A reversible oedema and inflammation of the supraspinatus tendon. Characteristically, this was caused by excessive overhead use in sports or work. This was found in young patients,

Table 4.2 Classification of impingement.

Stage I	Age	< 25 years
	Pathology	Oedema and haemorrhage
	Course	Reversible
	Treatment	Conservative
Stage II	Age	25–40 years
	Pathology	Fibrosis and tendonitis
	Course	Recurrent pain on activity
	Treatment	Acromioplasty
Stage III	Age	> 40 years
	Pathology	Bone spurs and cuff tears
	Course	Progressive disability
	Treatment	Acromioplasty and cuff repair

from 25 to 40 years of age. Treatment should be conservative, with a good prognosis for return to normal.

Stage II. With repeated impingement the changes in the bursa and cuff become permanent, with fibrosis and tendonitis. The patient has pain on exercise, which does not recover with rest, and may require subacromial decompression. The patient is usually around the age of 40.

Stage III. Further impingement will cause bony alteration, with spurring of the anterior acromion, and partial or full-thickness tears of the supraspinatus.

Having come to the conclusion that impingement is caused by rubbing of the cuff upon the acromion and coraco-acromial ligament, we now need to take a step backwards and ask the question 'why'?

Impingement can either be functional or anatomical. Functional impingement means that there is some loss of control of normal shoulder movement. The humeral head loses its ability to self-centre on the glenoid, causing impingement of the supraspinatus against the roof of the subacromial canal. Thus the patient with shoulder instability may present with an impingement-type pain.

The commonest presentation of functional impingement is in the young athlete. The athlete performs repetitive tasks close to the maximum tolerance of the shoulder (Jobe, 1982). Because athletes demand 110% of their body, the level of tolerance of the tissues is exceeded and injury occurs. Often, this injury is a repetitive microtrauma that causes tearing of fibres, either in the muscle or at the tendon–bone junction. Healing will occur but, in the body which is continually being abused by sport, may be 'pathological'. The tendon–bone junction is an area of transition from highly elastic and mobile tendon to stiff bone. This rapid change in stiffness leads to a stress riser. The body has an elegant way of reducing the stress-riser effect, which depends on the junction having four layers, each layer being slightly stiffer than the preceding layer. The layers are: (1) tendon, (2) unmineralized fibrocartilage, (3) mineralized fibrocartilage, and (4) bone (Fig. 4.2). If fibres are injured at this junction they will heal, but they may heal abnormally, leading to an enthesopathy. The stages of healing are: (1) oedema, haemorrhage and inflammation, (2) granulation-tissue formation, (3) tissue calcification, and (4) ossification. Healing may stop at any stage, which can leave abnormal areas within the tendon–bone junction, in particular areas of failed healing (microtears) and overhealing (bone spurs). Both the microtears and the bone spurs may extend right across the four layers of the normal tendon insertion, and play havoc with nature's elegant stress-protection mechanism; and this will lead to a vicious circle of decreased tolerance against further athletic insult.

Functional impingement is thus the cause of Stage-I and Stage-II impingement. These changes occur most often in athletes, but they can occur in anyone who stumbles, falls or injures their shoulder. Thus, by the age of 40, many people will have enthesopathic changes around the shoulder, both in the cuff insertion and in the coraco-acromial ligament.

Functional impingement can occur with other diseases that interfere with the normal proprioceptive loop (Table 4.3). Nerve injury at any level from the neck to individual nerves, such as suprascapular nerve entrapment, will cause deranged movement and impingement. Similarly, instability and scapulothoracic weakness can lead to functional impingement.

Any space-occupying lesion within the subacromial tunnel will cause anatomical impingement. Such stenosing lesions may originate from the acromion, the coraco-acromial ligament, the acromioclavicular joint or the coracoid. Lesions taking up space within the tendon itself can also cause anatomical impingement such as calcific deposits, or the swollen edges of cuff tears. Each

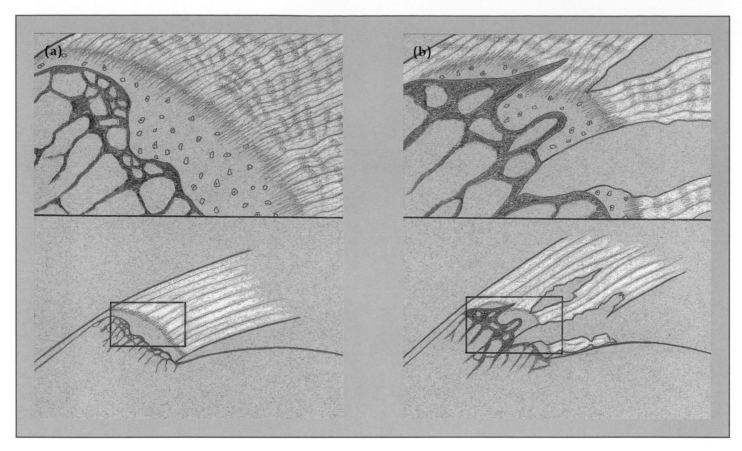

Figure 4.2 – *The tendon–bone junction. (a) The healthy tendon bone junction shows a gradual transition through bone, mineralized fibrocartilage, unmineralized fibrocartilage and then tendon. (b) The overused tendon heals with bone spikes and tears which transgress the junctional layer, leading to stress riser areas.*

Table 4.3 Aetiology of impingement.

● Functional	Overuse	Sports		Acromioclavicular joint	Osteophytes
		Overhead work			Instability
		Wheelchair user			Malunited fracture
		One-armed man		Cuff	Partial tear
	Instability				Full-thickness tear
	Cervical spondylosis				Calcific tendonitis
	Suprascapular-nerve entrapment			Tuberosity	Osteophyte
					Malunited fracture
	Thoracoscapular-weakness			Bursa	Rheumatoid nodule
				Capsule	Tight posterior capsule
● Anatomical	Acromial	Abnormal morphology			Tight interval (frozen shoulder)
		Acromial apophysis			
		Malunited fracture			Instability (loose capsule)
	Coraco-acromial	Hypertrophy		Glenoid	Posterior impingement
		Amyloid		Iatrogenic	Misplaced humeral prosthesis
	Coracoid	Malunited fracture			
		Post surgery			Prominent plate or screws
		Anterior offset prosthesis			

of these points of origin, which can lead to stenosis of the supraspinatus tunnel, are considered in detail below.

The acromion

Understanding the variations in shape of the acromion is essential for the surgeon involved with rotator-cuff disease.

The acromion is only well developed in man, and to a lesser extent in the chimpanzee. Most primates have a small acromion, which allows brachiation through the trees. The fact that the human acromion is large may account for damage to the rotator cuff arising from overhead activities in man.

Bigliani *et al.* (1986) studied the cross-sectional shape of the acromion in the sagittal plane and found that there were three different shapes. Type I has a flat undersurface, Type II has a curved undersurface, and Type III has a downward pointing spur on the anterior surface of the acromion, the so-called hooked type (Fig. 4.3). This hooked shape was associated with rotator-cuff tearing in 70% of cases presenting with cuff injury (Morrison & Bigliani, 1987) and this observation has been confirmed in more recent studies (Tiovonen *et al.* 1995). The relevance of this study is that if a hooked shape causes damage to the rotator cuff, then removal of the hook (thereby changing the shape from Type III to Type I) should arrest progression of this damage. This is the basis of the operation of anterior acromioplasty.

However, Edelson and Taitz (1992) examined 280 scapulae and found a far lower proportion of hooked acromions than did Bigliani, and made the point that it is difficult to distinguish a curved from a hooked acromion. They also examined the acromions from the point of their axial cross-sectional shape and found three types. These were a square shape, a cobra shape and an intermediate type. The significance of this lies in the cobra type, which extends forwards beyond the plane of the anterior border of the clavicle, as seen on an axillary radiograph. These cobra shaped, or long acromions showed degenerative changes in 26% of cases, whereas the shorter acromions only had degenerative changes in 11% of cases. If the cobra shape is present then the protruding bone must be removed as a first stage of the acromioplasty, the underlying hook is removed as a second stage of the operation (Rockwood & Lyons, 1993).

Edelson and Taitz found two types of degenerative change on the acromion. The first resembled a traction spur and the second an eburnated facet, like a

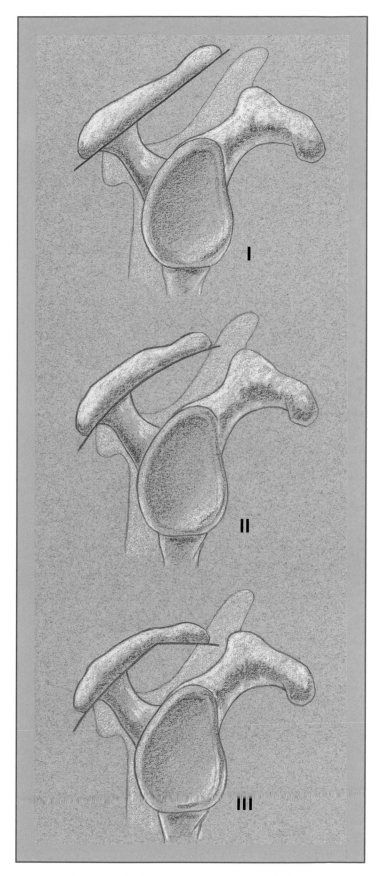

Figure 4.3 – *Morphology of the acromion. Bigliani describes three shapes of acromion: flat, curved and hooked.*

pseudoarticulation for the humeral head. The traction spur actually forms within the coraco-acromial ligament and is a form of enthesopathy, resulting from the transmission of tensile forces.

These studies have been conducted on dry bones and therefore do not show the soft-tissue changes which are also occurring, and which lead to further narrowing of the tunnel. Ogata and Uhtoff (1990) studied these soft-tissue changes and confirmed that the majority of the fibres of the coraco-acromial ligament insert into the undersurface of the acromion over a crescent-shaped area, an area which we may term the footprint of insertion of the ligament. The rest of the undersurface of the acromion is covered in fibrofatty tissue. Ogata and Uhtoff found four grades of change in the soft tissue.

Grade-1 change was loss of areolar tissue. Grade 2 showed localized thickening of the coraco-acromial ligament and thickening of the fibrocartilage pad. This thickening can be seen well on MRI scanning (Fig. 4.4). Bone spurs can occur at this stage. Grade-3 changes were irregularity of the undersurface of the acromion and breakup of the fibres of the coraco-acromial ligament, as though it had been ground up. Grade-4 changes were eburnation of the bone and loss of the coraco-acromial ligament insertion.

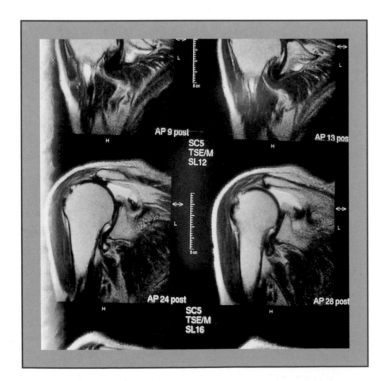

Figure 4.4 – *A MRI scan of the acromion showing thickening of the insertion of the coraco-acromial ligament into the undersurface of the acromion, in a patient with a full thickness tear.*

Banas *et al.* (1995) examined the acromion in the coronal plane. In an MRI study they found an increase in rotator-cuff changes associated with an increase in acromial slope in the coronal plane.

Os acromiale

The incidence of os acromiale is 7% (Grant 1951) (Fig. 4.5). Neer (1983) has suggested that os acromiale may be associated with rotator-cuff tears because the unfused section impinges upon the cuff as it moves down, hinging on the pseudarthosis.

Edelson *et al.* (1993) found an os acromiale in 8% of 270 scapulae. Two-thirds of the specimens had a distinctive pattern of osteophytic lipping, suggesting impingement against the rotator cuff.

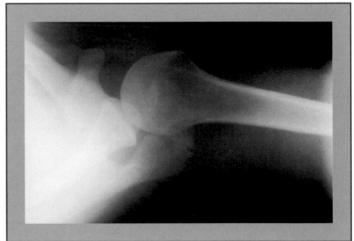

Figure 4.5 – *An axillary radiograph to show the acromial apophysis.*

The coraco-acromial ligament

The coraco-acromial ligament is a true ligament which passes from the coracoid to the acromion (Fig. 4.6). Holt and Allibone (1995) describe three shapes of ligament. The commonest was the quadrangular ligament (47%), followed closely by the 'Y' shaped ligament (41%), and then the broad-band type (12%). The first two types are wider at the coracoid than at the acromial end. The 'Y' shaped ligament consists of two bands with a diaphenous membrane linking them. One variant of the 'Y' shaped ligament is the multibanded type. The ligament inserts onto the undersurface of the acromion.

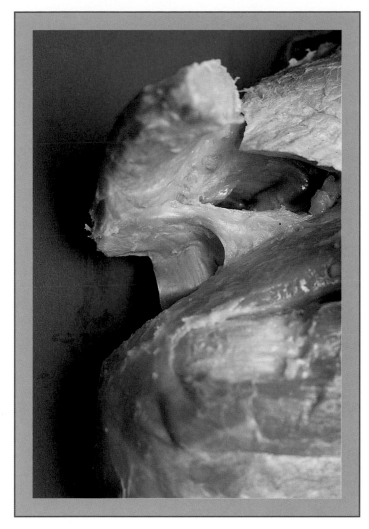

Figure 4.6 – *The insertion of the coracoacromial ligament into the inferior surface of the acromion (reproduced with permission from Bunker and Wallace, 1991).*

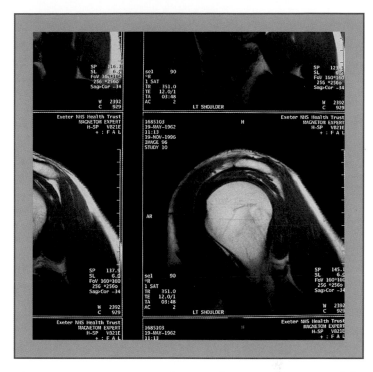

Figure 4.7 – *A MRI scan showing the anterior margin of the acromion. The coraco-acromial ligament inserts into the undersurface of the acromion and the deltoid inserts into the superior surface of the acromion. Between the two lies the acromial artery.*

The lower free edge of the coraco-acromial ligament blends with the clavipectoral fascia, indeed the ligament is really a thickening of the clavipectoral fascia.

The acromial branch of the thoraco-acromial trunk passes obliquely over the superior surface of the coraco-acromial ligament and then passes along the anterior surface of the acromion. It thus lies in a triangular space whose floor is the coraco-acromial ligament, whose roof is the deltoid and whose posterior wall is the anterior border of the acromion. The relationships of this artery are vital to understand because this is the vessel which, once damaged by an arthroscopic burr, causes 'red out' during arthroscopic acromioplasty (Fig. 4.7).

Golser *et al.* (1995) has shown histologically that the coraco-acromial ligament is a highly innervated structure,

an interesting observation which may relate to its function and may relate to the pain of impingement syndrome, and even perhaps to the relief of this pain following acromioplasty. Ide *et al.* (1994) have demonstrated Pacinian corpuscles, Ruffini end organs, unclassified receptors and free nerve endings clustered around the coraco-acromial ligament and the greater tuberosity. They suggest that the Ruffini end organs transmit information on joint position sense to the central nervous system, whilst the Pacinian corpuscles and Golgi–Mazzoni corpuscles recognize compression within the subacromial space. Information from these receptors allows the brain to control the balance of muscle strength, to elevate the arm, and to centre the humeral head. They have found substance P, as well as calcitonin gene related protein (CGRP), and protein gene product 9.5, all of which are nociceptive polypeptides, in this area. Such neuropeptides, released into the subacromial space, cause vasodilitation and primary hyperalgesia, the final elements of impingement pain.

Due to its anatomical position the coraco-acromial ligament plays a pivotal role in impingement syndrome. Uhtoff and Sarkar (1991) have shown that the changes which take place in the ligament are most likely secondary to increased strain within the ligament, produced by changes taking place in the tissues within the subacromial space.

Renal patients on chronic dialysis can develop amyloid within the coraco-acromial ligament, leading to impingement.

The acromioclavicular joint

The acromioclavicular joint could be considered to be of faulty design because the articular surfaces are made of fibrocartilage, rather than hyaline cartilage, which leads to an accelerated rate of degeneration. DePalma (1973) found degenerative changes of the joint surface, and the intra-articular disc, to be the norm over the age of 40. The acromioclavicular joint is a diarthrodial joint, the two halves separated by the fibrocartilagenous disc, which is often perforated.

The clavicle is joined to the acromion by the acromioclavicular ligament. Superiorly the ligament is much thicker and is contiguous with the deltotrapezius fascia and periosteum on the superior surfaces of the clavicle and the acromion. This fact is utilized in the 'Matsen deltoid-on' approach to the rotator cuff. The inferior ligament is much thinner and is well perfused by tiny branches from the acromial artery.

The accessory ligaments of the acromioclavicular joint pass between the corocoid process and the clavicle. The conoid ligament is pyramidal, and the trapezoid ligament is the more lateral. Often a small bursa lies between the two.

Petersson and Genz (1983) looked at the association between rotator-cuff tears and inferior osteophytes, both radiologically and histologically (Fig. 4.8). They found that normal shoulders had acromioclavicular joint osteophytes in 14% of cases radiographically, and 10% of cases histologically compared with shoulders with proven rotator-cuff tears which had osteophytes in 51% of cases radiologically, and 54% of cases histologically. This study strongly suggests an association between cuff tears and inferior osteophytes, with the osteophytes causing impingement upon the cuff.

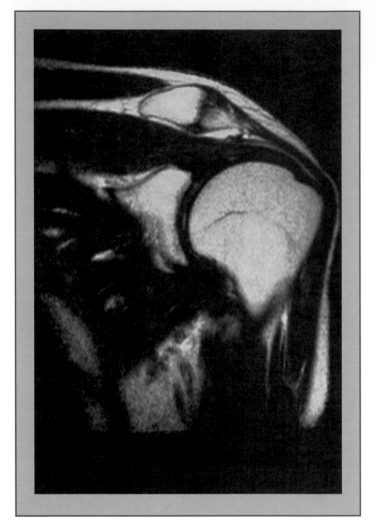

Figure 4.8 – *A MRI scan showing the critical position of the acromioclavicular joint in relation to the supraspinatus tendon.*

Subcoracoid impingement

Gerber *et al.* (1985) described the syndrome of subcoracoid impingement. Pain is caused by impingement of the coracoid upon the anterior rotator cuff and is reproduced by internal rotation of the arm which has been flexed to 90°. This is called the coracoid impingement sign (Dines *et al.*, 1986). Coracoid impingement is rare and is often diagnosed only after failure of acromioplasty or in patients with iatrogenic injury to the coracoid.

Posterior impingement

Walch *et al.* (1992) described a new form of impingement where the articular surface of the cuff impinges against the posterosuperior glenoid rim (Fig. 4.9) when the arm goes into a position of extreme abduction and external rotation, such as during the cocking phase of throwing. This form of impingement occurs in young sporting patients and may commonly lead to partial-thickness tears of the deep surface of the cuff. Posterior glenoid osteophytes may be seen both on plain radiographs and on MRI scanning.

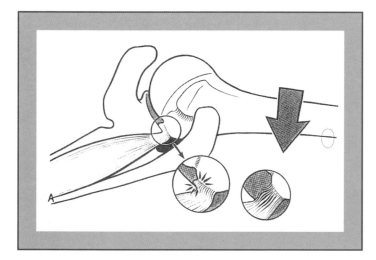

Figure 4.9 – *The method of posterior impingement of the supraspinatus tendon on the postero-superior glenoid rim (reproduced with permission from the Journal of Shoulder and Elbow Surgery).*

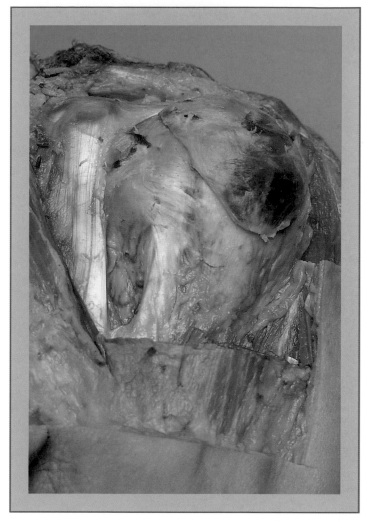

Figure 4.10 – *The subacromial bursa sits on the front of the humerus like a Frenchman's beret. Note the anterior position of this bursa.*

The subacromial bursa

The subacromial bursa is really misnamed because the majority of it lies under the deltoid and the coraco-acromial ligament. The bursa sits on the front of the humeral head like a Frenchman's beret (Bunker and Wallace, 1991) (Fig. 4.10). Understanding the position of the bursa, is vital for surgeons undertaking arthroscopic procedures within the subacromial space. If the arthroscope is within the bursa, the view of the coraco-acromial ligament and undersurface of the acromion is excellent, but if the arthroscope is not in the bursa the surgeon can not see what he is doing. How would you react to being operated on by a blind surgeon? Johnson (1983), in his paper on the uses and abuses of arthroscopy, stated 'I am shocked to learn that it is not uncommon for surgeons who are unable to see in the subacromial space, to remove the arthroscope and continue the procedure by feel to complete the acromioplasty'. The bursa often has small septae within it.

The clinical presentation of a patient with impingement

The principle presenting complaint of a patient with impingement is pain. This is true shoulder pain, felt around the shoulder and radiating down into the muscles of the upper arm.

The patient is usually over 40 years of age. If the patient is under 40 they may have impingement, but it will be secondary to instability or sporting overuse, and the prime cause (the instability or the sports technique or training) must be treated. This is Wallace's aphorism.

The pain comes on insidiously, although the patient may associate it with some form of repetitive overhead movement, such as racquet sports, swimming, throwing or working overhead (Table 4.4).

The pain is made worse by reaching, typically putting on a coat, reaching a high shelf, reading a newspaper, using the gearstick on a car. The pain is worse at night. The pain is exacerbated by the internal rotation required to wash the back or do up the bra.

The patient starts by being optimistic that the pain will go away, and of course often it does, and those patients are never seen by the surgeon. As the condition drags on, or gets worse, the patient presents to the general practitioner who usually prescribes analgesia or anti-inflammatory medication. If the general practitioner is enlightened they will inject steroid into the subacromial bursa. It is important to ask whether this gave immediate or short-term relief. If it did not, consider that the injection may not have been placed into the bursa; some practitioners will inject trigger spots, and I have even had one patient who allowed his practitioner to inject the asymptomatic shoulder without complaining that it was the wrong one! The general practitioner may elect to send the patient to physiotherapy. If so, question the patient as to what methods were used, whether they helped, and if so how much they helped. Patients may often go to alternative therapists, such as osteopaths or chiropractitioners, or have acupuncture. Eventually, when every other option has been tried they present to the shoulder surgeon, usually some months since the onset of symptoms. Clearly, this is time well spent because the shoulder surgeon does not want to operate on patients who are going to recover spontaneously, and unlike the patient with a rotator-cuff tear, the patient with impingement is not going to come to any lasting harm by this trial of conservative management.

On examination the patient with impingement does not usually have a great degree of wasting of the supraspinatus and infraspinatus. There may be some prominence of the acromioclavicular joint. The patient will usually have tenderness over the greater tuberosity, but not at any other site.

The key finding is a painful arc of movement. The American Shoulder and Elbow Surgeons (ASES) research committee suggest that impingement is recorded in three movements. Firstly, the painful arc may occur in elevation with slight internal rotation. Secondly, the arm is elevated passively to 90° and then internally rotated. Thirdly, the arm is actively abducted, the classic painful arc. External rotation is unlimited but internal rotation is reduced with end-point pain. Minor soft subacromial crepitus may be felt.

If this is primary impingement then the shoulder will be stable. Strength of abduction, and to a lesser degree external rotation, may be slightly reduced and may cause mild pain on resistance.

Plain radiographs in impingement are often normal. Sometimes an anterior traction spur on the acromion, or a small area of sclerosis may be seen. This area of sclerosis is called the 'sourcil sign' (sourcil being French for eyebrow) (Fig. 4.11). Plain films may show an os acromiale, which is best seen in the axillary view. Calcific deposits (Fig. 4.12) show well on plain films. The Neer outlet view is used by some as a measure of the bony stenosis of the supraspinatus tunnel.

Table 4.4 Clinical presentation of impingement.

- Insidious onset of pain
- Associated with overhead movement
- Increased on reaching
- Worse at night
- Increased on internal rotation
- Minimal wasting of infraspinatus
- Prominent acromioclavicular joint
- Tender greater tuberosity
- Painful arc of movement
- Normal power
- Sourcil sign, Type III acromion
- Impingement test positive

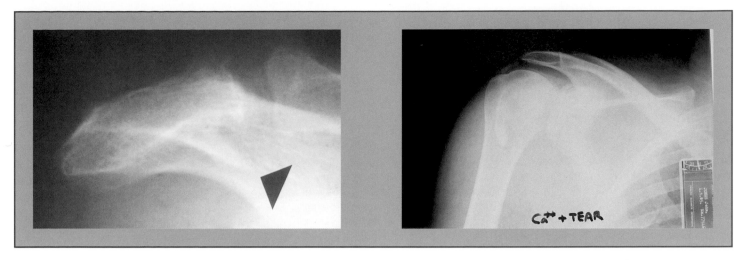

Figure 4.11 – *Sclerosis of the undersurface of the acromion. This is termed the 'sourcil' sign.*

Figure 4.12 – *Calcification of the rotator cuff.*

Confirmation of impingement can be obtained using the impingement test.In the impingement test a small dose (2 ml) of 2% Xylocaine is placed in the subacromial bursa, just under the free edge of the coraco-acromial ligament. After 5 minutes the three tests for impingement are carried out again, and marked relief of the patient's pain signifies that the diagnosis of impingement is correct.

Investigations

Shoulder arthroscopy

Shoulder arthroscopy and bursoscopy is the gold-standard investigation. However, the arthroscopy must always be performed in a well ordered and careful manner, so as to visualize every part of the shoulder, as in the standard textbooks (Bunker & Wallace, 1991). Particular attention must be used to search the supraspinatus insertion, as small tears can be hidden from view until the arthroscope is advanced right up to the insertion (Fig. 4.13).

Shoulder bursoscopy requires a different portal (lateral, or posterolateral) to gain access to the bursa. Once in the bursa the top surface of the cuff can be seen and the impingement lesion (Fig. 4.14), and its partner the attrition lesion of the acromion, can also be seen.

It is vital that the sequence of tests for instability are carried out under anaesthetic, to see if the impingement is secondary to instability.

MRI

MRI is rapidly becoming the imaging technique of choice in the shoulder. It is less invasive than arthrography, more accurate than ultrasound, gives a clear view of the soft-tissue anatomy around the shoulder and does not subject the patient to ionizing radiation. However, there are problems with MRI of the shoulder. The first are purely technical considerations.

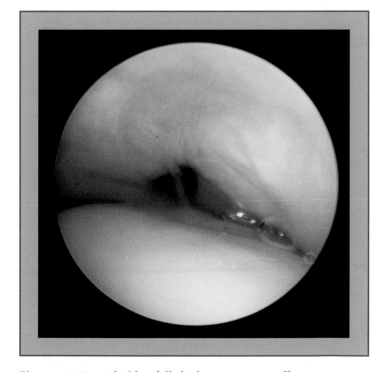

Figure 4.13 – *A hidden full-thickness rotator-cuff tear.*

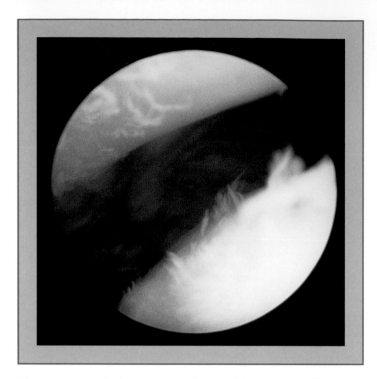

Figure 4.14 – *An impingement lesion of the rotator cuff.*

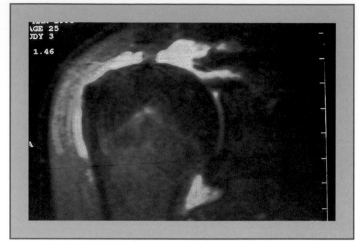

Figure 4.15 – *An MRI scan of a full-thickness rotator-cuff tear. There is tendon discontinuity and interposed fluid. (T2 sequence.)*

When the patient lies within the scanner the shoulder is not central within the bore of the magnet. This necessitates an off-centre field of view, and there is decreased magnetic field homogeneity in the periphery of the magnet. In order to get high-resolution images, special shoulder coils need to be used. The planes of visualization must be oblique rather than orthogonal. For instance to visualize the supraspinatus an oblique coronal view is used, which is centred down the line of supraspinatus; the sagittal view is also oblique, centred down the face of the glenoid. For MRI of the shoulder the patient has to go into the scanner head first, making the examination extremely claustrophobic and very noisy. Whereas for MRI of the knee patients go in feet first, which is much less stressful. Keeping the patient calm and still during the scanning sequence to prevent movement artifacts can be difficult.

Interpretation of the MRI can also be difficult. Complete tears are reasonably easy to interpret (Fig. 4.15) as there is tendon discontinuity, with interposed fluid. The changes of partial-thickness tears or tendonitis are far more difficult to interpret because of such esoteric effects as the 'angle phenomenon'. In a recent study (Miniaci *et al.*, 1995) 20 asymptomatic volunteers had their shoulders scanned and reported on blind by a radiologist; every one was reported as having an abnormal rotator cuff and 30% were reported as having a partial tear. Even with fat-saturation techniques detection of partial thickness tears is unreliable (Reinus *et al.*, 1995.)

Future developments such as fat-suppressed images may reduce artefacts from respiration and hybrid rapid aquisition relaxation enhancement (RARE) images may allow rapid-image aquisition and thus decrease motion artefacts.

Treatment options for the patient with impingement

The surgeon understands that impingement varies from mild and reversible (Neer Stage I) to irreversible (Neer Stage II) and must tailor the treatment according to the severity of the disease.

Conservative management

There are two conservative treatment regimes that work — steroid injection and physiotherapy.

Steroid injection

Whenever the rotator cuff is damaged, either by impingement or tear, an inflamatory response is set up within the subacromial bursa. The rationale of steroid injection is to reduce this inflamatory reaction, and thus to decrease the swelling and volume of the contents of the subacromial canal. The effectiveness of steroid injection is coming under increasing pressure by those exponents of evidence-based medicine. Withrington *et al.* (1985) showed no benefit of steroid over placebo in a prospective controlled study.

Against this Blair *et al.* (1996) performed a prospective controlled study of steroid versus placebo injection and concluded that subacromial corticosteroid is effective, in the short term, in relieving pain and improving movement in patients with impingement.

The steroid must be injected into the subacromial bursa. It has already been shown how the bursa is on the front of the humeral head, under the coraco-acromial ligament, and this is where the injection is deposited. The exact preparation used is up to the surgeon, all of them work and none of them work better than the other. Simple hydrocortisone acetate (25 mg in 1 ml) is cheap and works. It is preferable to mix the steroid with 2 ml of 2% Xylocaine so that an impingement test can be performed with the one needle (23 G).

After skin preparation with spirit the injection is performed using the anterolateral approach (Fig. 4.16).

The needle is aimed at the leading edge of the coraco-acromial ligament, which can be felt as a gritty obstruction which the needle then pops through. The syringe is aspirated, firstly to make sure no blood is drawn back, but also to see if any joint fluid can be withdrawn from the subacromial bursa — a sure sign of a cuff tear.

The steroid and local anaesthetic solution is then injected. Usually the needle (23 G) will be inserted up to the hub, if it is correctly positioned. The patient is warned that the injection may be mildly uncomfortable that night and that it does not work immediately.

The mixture is left for a full 5 minutes and then the impingement test is performed again. The result is recorded, and the patient seen 4–6 weeks later.

Physiotherapy

The rationale for physiotherapy treatment is that the rotator cuff is dysfunctional, allowing superior translation of the head during elevation and therefore impingement. Treatment is therefore aimed at strengthening the rotator cuff, improving scapular rotation and improving proprioception and control of movement.

Strengthening the rotator cuff is the mainstay of physiotherapy treatment. Exercises may be isometric, isotonic or isokinetic. In practice isotonic exercises using TheraBand graduated elastic exercise bands, are the most commonly used method.

TheraBand is used as an isotonic resistance to external rotation, internal rotation and abduction. A useful tip regarding rotational exercises is to ask the patient to hold a book under the armpit, squeezed between the arm and the chest wall, whilst using the TheraBand. This has two effects, firstly it ensures that the patient does not cheat and abduct the arm during the exercise, and secondly since the adductors are used to hold the book in place (pectoralis major and latissimus) this means that the deltoid can not be used (as it is antagonistic to the adductors) and thereby the exercises do not strengthen the deltoid.

It is important that the scapular muscles work properly and that the scapula rotates normally, as one-third of the elevation originates from the scapula.

Finally, the patient should be instructed in proprioceptive neuromuscular facilitation (PNF). PNF involves using specific spiral and diagonal patterns of movement; these patterns of movement result in the

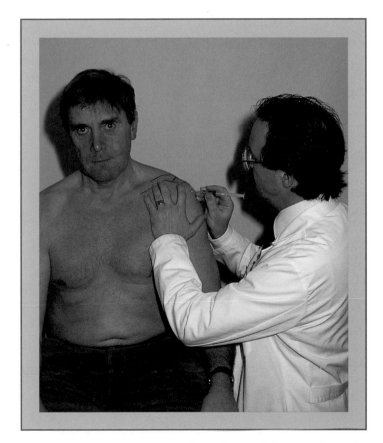

Figure 4.16 – *Injection of the subacromial space from the antero-lateral approach.*

whole arm being exercised. By applying resistance, and invoking stretch reflexes, the skilled therapist can lead to an improvement in shoulder fuction and reduction in impingement symptoms. Brox *et al.* (1993) performed a prospective randomized trial comparing arthroscopic acromioplasty against a supervised exercise regime including PNF and found that both were equally effective, and both were superior to placebo treatment.

Surgical treatment of impingement

The surgical treatment of impingement involves acromioplasty, which can be performed arthroscopically or by open surgery. Arthroscopic acromioplasty is described in Chapter 3.

Open acromioplasty

Indication

Open acromioplasty is indicated in the patient with impingement of over 1 year's duration and that has been unresponsive to conservative treatment. The patient must have shown a good response to the impingement test.

Pre-operative preparation

It is vital that the patient is counselled about the objectives of surgery, and postoperative rehabilitation, prior to undergoing surgery. The objective of the operation is to relieve pain and restore the function of the shoulder to normal. However, this does not occur immediately and the patient must be told that the objective of surgery is to enlarge the tunnel through which the supraspinatus passes so that the muscle can heal itself, a process that takes between 6 and 8 weeks, depending on how bad the damage to the muscle has been.

The patient is told that the surgical scar will be over the top of the shoulder and will be quite fine, but that there is always a numb patch on the skin lateral to the scar because fine filaments of the supraclavicular nerve are always divided with this approach.

The patient is told that there will be a course of rehabilitation physiotherapy after the surgery, how quickly and completely they recover is up to them, and depends on how well they comply with the rehabilitation programme. The patient is given a printed acromioplasty protocol with advice about the surgery and recovery.

Anaesthesia

It is essential that the patient is intubated and ventilated with a circuit that allows the anaesthetist to be at the foot-end of the patient. Venous access must be established in the opposite arm or in the foot. The course of the incision is infiltrated by the surgeon with bupivacaine 0.25%, and with adrenaline 1:200 000 before the patient is transferred from the anaesthetic room to the operating room.

Positioning

Every element of this operation is important. Correct positioning is critical. The patient is positioned supine on the operating table. A head ring is positioned under the occiput and a sand bag under the medial border of the scapula. The patient must have the eyes taped and protected prior to skin preparation and should wear a nurse's theatre cap, so that the adhesive drapes do not stick to their hair.

Preparation

The skin is prepared from the earlobes, down the neck, the chest to below the nipples and to the midline, the shoulder, back of the shoulder and the arm as far as the wrist. The skin is then dried and an adhesive drape is placed around the shoulder to seal the area. The hand is then double gloved in a sterile manner and the arm covered in a sterile stocking. Draping is then completed to the satisfaction of the surgeon.

Using a sterile skin-marking pen, the outlines of the acromion, the acromioclavicular joint, the clavicle, and the coracoid are marked; the course of the coraco-acromial ligament is also marked (Fig. 4.17). The skin incision is then marked and, finally, the surgeon draws a face on the drapes over the patient's head to alert the surgical team against leaning on this area while working. A plastic adhesive seal is then placed on the skin and the anaesthetist's permission sought to start the operation. At this stage the table can be angled into the deckchair position.

The incision

The incision extends for 8 cm. The incision is placed in Langer's lines and runs along the course of the acromioclavicular joint to the coracoid process. This line is slightly medial to Neer's original description, but allows better exposure and the ability to extend to repair even a large rotator-cuff tear if needed. The skin is

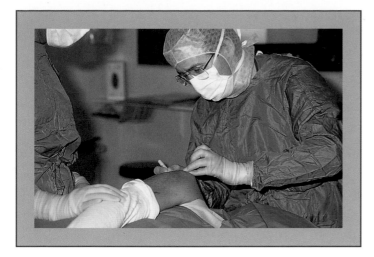

Figure 4.17 – *An operative photograph of the position for acromioplasty.*

undermined to expose the acromion, acromioclavicular joint and anterior deltoid. The incision can be held open with a sharp self-retaining retractor (Irwin's retractor), but even better is to use stay-stitches through the skin to hold the flaps back, as stay-stitches do not get in the way like a self-retaining retractor.

The deltoid split

Every master shoulder surgeon will describe his own particular way to negotiate the deltoid. The aim is to split the deltoid and to expose the anterior acromion from its lateral border to the acromioclavicular joint (Fig. 4.18) and then to repair it such that none of its strength is lost. Some surgeons detach the deltoid from the anterior acromion (Neer, 1983; Rockwood, 1993; Craig, 1995), but the author's preference is the 'Matsen deltoid-on approach'. The Matsen deltoid-on approach makes use of the fact that the trapezius and deltoid make up one continuous sheet of muscle connected by the periosteum over the acromion and clavicle and the superior acromioclavicular ligament. The approach depends upon making a split in this layer and then raising a medial and lateral flap. This is similar to the direct lateral approach to the hip which makes use of gluteus medius and vastus lateralis being in continuity with the periosteum, over the trochanter of the hip, such that an anterior flap can be raised of the two muscles in continuity.

Matsen actually describes this split as being sited across the acromion centred on its anterolateral corner. The problem with centring the split so far lateral is that

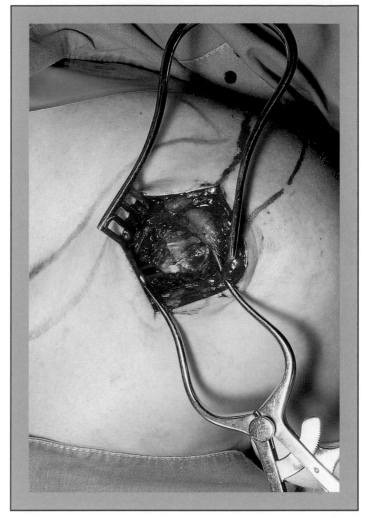

Figure 4.18 – *An operative photograph of the exposure of the coraco-acromial ligament.*

the periosteum over the acromion is at its thinnest here and therefore closure can be difficult, particularly in the small female. For this reason we centre the split along the line of the acromioclavicular joint. This has four advantages. Firstly, the split is actually through the superior acromioclavicular ligament, the thickest part of the sheet of tissue, which connects the trapezius to the deltoid, and therefore is the best tissue to hold sutures for repair. Secondly, it allows exposure of the acromioclavicular joint, so enabling inspection of the joint surfaces and enabling a decision to be made regarding whether the joint should be resected. Thirdly, it allows resection of the joint if indicated. Fourthly, it allows an extensile exposure into the supraspinatous fossa if a sizeable rotator-cuff tear is found. The modified Matsen deltoid-on split is then extended down, splitting the deltoid in the direction of its fibres for a length of

4 cm. The axillary nerve may lie as high as 5 cm from the acromion and is therefore at risk of being injured.

The deltoid split is held open with a small self-retaining retractor (West's retractor) and three structures can be seen. The first is the coraco-acromial ligament, and the second is the clavipectoral fascia which blends with it. Because they blend with each other it is sometimes difficult to be precise regarding where one starts and the other ends. The third structure is the acromial artery, which lies in protective fat on top of the ligament, and closely adjacent to the bony edge of the acromion.

The artery is diathermied, and the coraco-acromial ligament is further visualized by using a swab to push the deltoid off it. The 'deltoid-on' flap is then developed using electrocautery to peel it off the bone of the acromion making sure to keep the flap as thick as possible, until the anterior acromion is exposed as far as its anterolateral corner.

The free edge of the coraco-acromial ligament (where it blends with the clavipectoral fascia) is then incised, so that the ligament edge can be seen from acromion to coracoid. The bursa is adherent to the inferior surface of the ligament and is incised at the same time. If synovial fluid emerges then a cuff tear is always present. The coraco-acromial ligament is then surgically removed from the undersurface of the acromion, exposing the inferior surface of the acromion from the lateral border to the acromioclavicular joint. The ligament is not excised from its coracoid attachment, for reasons which will become apparent later.

The two-stage acromioplasty

The objective of the operation is now in view — i.e. the abnormally shaped anterior acromion and its bony spur. The surgeon has to remove the anteriorly protruding spur, or 'cobra-shaped extension', and the inferior spur or Bigliani Type-III 'hook'.

Most surgical texts suggest using a sharp osteotome for the acromioplasty, but in reality a fine reciprocating saw is far more controllable, more accurate and easier to use.

The first cut is in the coronal (vertical) plane, in line with the anterior border of the clavicle, from the acromioclavicular joint to the lateral acromion. A bevelled axial (horizontal) cut is then made, removing a wedge of the antero-inferior acromion including the hook, aiming to exit the inferior acromion 1.5 cm posterior to the first coronal cut (Fig. 4.19).

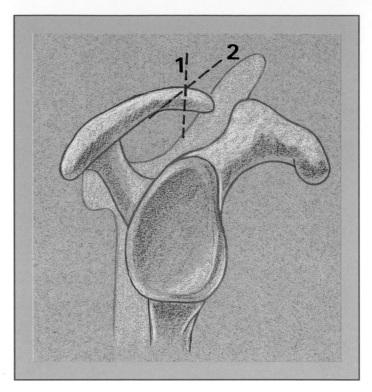

Figure 4.19 – *The first saw-cut is vertical. The second saw-cut removes a wedge of the antero-inferior surface of the acromion.*

The acromioclavicular joint

The inferior osteophytes should always be removed from the acromioclavicular joint as part of the acromioplasty. However, there is a great deal of contention as to whether the acromioclavicular joint should be formally excised. On the one hand Rockwood and Lyon (1993) urge great caution in excising the acromioclavicular joint. In his personal series of 37 acromioplasties and 34 cuff repairs, performed over an 8-year period, he only excised the acromioclavicular joint in four cases. His rationale for such caution came from two studies (Thorling, 1985; Daluga, 1989) that stated the results of acromioplasty were inferior if the acromioclavicular joint was excised, and recovery took longer.

On the other hand Neviaser *et al.* (1982) recommends that the acromioclavicular joint is resected in every case. Stuart *et al.* (1990) concluded that resection of the distal clavicle did not impair the final result.

So what are the indications for resection of the acromioclavicular joint? The first indication is a cuff tear, the repair of which requires the surgeon gaining access to the supraspinatus. The second indication is significant arthritic change, with irregularity of the joint surface and fibrillation of the cartilage. The danger in excising the acromioclavicular joint is that in doing so it will unmask a severe instability of the joint. This is why we left the coraco-acromial ligament attached to the coracoid and stored it; if the surgeon finds that, after the acromioclavicular joint is excised, there is marked instability of the clavicular stump, then a Weaver–Dunn repair can be performed to stabilize it.

How should the excision be performed? Neer suggests excising the distal 2.5 cm of the clavicle. For access to a major cuff tear it is easier if the excision is carried out 20% from the acromial side and 80% on the clavicular side. The cuts should be in the oblique coronal plane (Fig. 4.20).

Examination of the rotator cuff

The cuff must now be examined by moving the freely draped arm, taking particular care to examine the distal insertion of the supraspinatus. If there is any doubt, then a Fukuda test can be performed. The Fukuda test involves injecting sterile methylene blue into the joint and looking for any egress from the joint, or staining of the cuff from a bursal side tear.

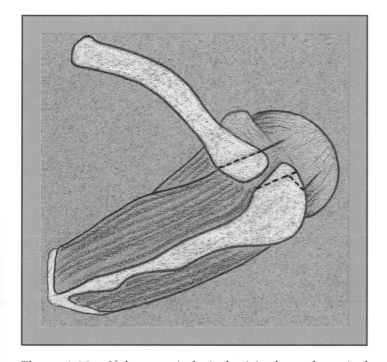

Figure 4.20 – *If the acromioclavicular joint has to be excised then the cuts should be parallel with the supraspinatus tendon. A total of 2 cm should be excised taking the majority from the clavicular side and a sliver from the acromial side.*

Closure

The cuff is now washed out prior to closure. Remember the aphorism 'the answer to pollution is dilution with solution'. If the clavicle is unstable a Weaver–Dunn reconstruction, using No 2 absorbable suture taken through drill holes in the clavicle and 'Bunnelled' down the coraco-acromial ligament, is performed. The medial and lateral flaps of the deltoid-on approach are now carefully repaired with No 1 absorbable suture. Bupivacaine, 0.5% (10 ml), is now injected under the reconstructed flap and the subcutaneous tissue, and skin closed in layers using a subcuticular suture to the skin. A Seton polysling is then applied.

Rehabilitation

The patient must be motivated to recover as rapidly as possible and must take responsibility for this. The patient is given a written protocol emphasizing that how quickly and fully they recover is, to a large degree, up to them. The patient is encouraged to take mild pain-relieving tablets regularly, for the first postoperative week, in order to allow them to do the rehabilitation exercises more easily.

Phase one: protective phase (1–6 weeks)

The goals of this first phase are to re-establish a good range of movement, and to prevent muscle wasting, whilst protecting the surgical repair to the deltoid. The sling should be worn at night over the first 3 weeks to protect the deltoid repair from unusual arm positioning during sleep. However, by day the patient is told that the sling is there purely for their comfort, and they should be weaned off it as soon as possible. The only exception to this is if the acromioclavicular joint has been excised and stabilized with a Weaver–Dunn-type repair; in this case the sling should be worn by day for 3 weeks in order to protect the stabilization procedure.

Elbow extension exercises

These should be performed from day one. Twenty repetitions should be performed, three times per day.

Pendulum exercises

These should also be started from day one. The patient should be told that pendulums must be done slowly and gently. This exercise must not hurt. Five pendulums (grandfather clock) should be alternated with five circumductions ('stirring the porridge') and the exercise should continue for 5 minutes, three to five times per day.

Rotation exercises
With the elbow to the side and flexed to a right angle, the hand is taken from touching the abdomen to pointing straight ahead. This is performed with 10 repetitions, three times per day.

After 1 week the pain of surgery should be reduced enough to add closed-chain elevation exercises and TheraBand cuff-strengthening exercises.

Closed-chain elevation exercises
The concept of closed-chain exercises actually applies to the lower limb. Closed-chain exercises mean that the leg is in contact with the floor. When we apply the principle of closed chain to the arm it does not mean that the hand is fixed to the ground, but that the hand is supported, either by the therapist, the patient's other hand, or the environment (bench, wall, pulley handle), thus forming a closed chain. In distinction an open-chain exercise means that the arm is unsupported.

Supine-assisted elevation
With the patient lying supine on a bed the operated arm is held by the unoperated side and elevated as far as discomfort will allow. Once again none of these exercises should hurt, pain signifies that the stitches are under undue tension.

Pulley exercises
Using a skipping rope over a hook on the back of a door, the patient once again uses the unoperated arm to pull on the pulley thereby passively elevating the operated arm. This exercise moves from passive to assisted active, as discomfort allows, over the first 3 weeks.

TheraBand exercises
With a book clamped in the armpit (this relaxes the deltoid and ensures that no tension is placed upon the deltoid repair), a weak yellow TheraBand is used for resisted active internal and external rotation exercises.

Phase two: strengthening phase (7–12 weeks)
The repair of the deltoid and re-attachment to the acromion should be fully established and strong by 6 weeks. Open-chain exercises can now be commenced in abduction and forward flexion. The goals of this phase are to regain and improve strength around the shoulder, and to improve neuromuscular control.

Closed-chain exercises should continue as above. To these should be added TheraBand isotonic exercises to strengthen the deltoid in elevation and abduction. TheraBand isotonic programme to biceps and triceps.

Scapular strengthening exercises and mobilizations should be carried out. Upper extremity endurance exercises can be started.

Dumbell training can start, or build up strength of TheraBand until the power of resistance changes the exercise from isotonic to isometric.

Initiate PNF pattern exercises.

Phase three: return to sport (3 months)
The goals of this phase are return to work, full activities of daily living and sport. Entry to this phase requires a full range of motion, no pain or tenderness, and the blessing of both physiotherapist and surgeon.

High speed/high energy strengthening exercises are initiated. Endurance exercises and sport specific exercises are added to phase two exercises under the supervision of a physiotherapist.

Complications

Complications are uncommon, but do occasionally occur after acromioplasty. They include wound infection, failure of the deltoid repair, and continuing pain following the procedure.

Deltoid avulsion should not occur. It is a reflection of poor surgical technique and repair (Fig. 4.21). The surgeon must be satisfied that the repair is adequate at the end of the procedure. If there is any question that it is not then drill holes must be made in the acromion and further sutures used from bone to deltoid to back up the repair. The other reason for deltoid avulsion is that too much acromion has been excised (a subtotal acromionectomy), or that it has been thinned so much as to precipitate fracture of the remaining acromion.

Once the deltoid has avulsed from the acromion this is a surgical disaster, of major proportions, from which it is difficult to salvage a functioning shoulder! Such a patient should be sent on to a specialist shoulder surgeon, there is no benefit from an occasional shoulder surgeon attempting to extricate himself from this complication. Re-repair may be undertaken, protecting

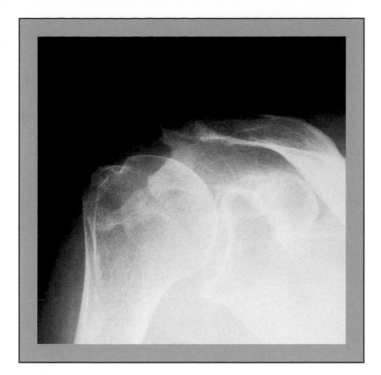

Figure 4.21 – *This patient has had too much clavicle excised; the deltoid is detached and unable to function and the patient is consequently crippled.*

the repair in an aeroplane splint. If a large area of acromion has been removed in error then a complex graft of pelvic brim and fascia lata can be used to replace the acromion and repair the deltoid. However, it should be recognized that this is a disaster from which recovery is difficult, and the patient may even end up with a shoulder fusion in the face of an irreparable deltoid. Prevention is better than cure!

Failure to relieve pain

Operative failure may be a consequence of incorrect diagnosis, incomplete subacromial decompression, missed cuff tear, or failure of rehabilitation.

Incorrect diagnosis

This is the commonest reason for failure. The surgeon should consider three areas: (1) pain eminating from the acromioclavicular joint, (2) impingement from developing frozen shoulder, and (3) impingement from instability.

Pain eminating from the acromioclavicular joint can be confirmed by injecting the acromioclavicular joint and observing the proportion of pain relief achieved. If this test confirms that the acromioclavicular joint is the culprit, then re-operation may be necessary to perform an excision arthroplasty with or without stabilization.

A frozen shoulder may mimic impingement pain in the early phase. By the time the patient has gone through an acromioplasty, and failed to gain relief, the pathognomonic sign of reduced passive external rotation has usually become apparent, and manipulation under anaesthetic cures the problem.

The young patient may have impingement secondary to instability; run through the tests for instability, and investigations for instability. This patient may not be cured until the shoulder has been stabilized.

Ogilvie-Harris and Demazaire (1993) studied 65 patients with a failed acromioplasty. In 27 patients there had been a diagnostic error, and in 28 an operative error. All the patients underwent shoulder arthroscopy. Of the 27 errors of diagnosis, 7 were found to have referred pain, 11 had intra-articular pathology (early arthritis in 2 patients, a labral tear in 2 patients and instability in 7 patients). Nine patients had extra-articular pathology (3 with frozen shoulders and 6 with cuff pathology).

Failure to detect a cuff tear

The inexperienced surgeon may fail to find a lurking cuff tear, either through not looking hard enough, or through mistaking a thickened bursa for an intact cuff. The patient will continue to have pain, weakness, wasting and subacromial crepitus. This is where an arthrogram or MRI can be very useful.

Operative errors

In Ogilvie-Harris' series there were judged to be 28 operative errors. Of these five had acromioclavicular joint pain and needed an excision arthroplasty. Eleven patients had subacromial scarring, a condition now termed 'captured cuff syndrome', and finally 12 had had insufficient surgery.

Twelve of the 65 patients were judged to have had both a correct diagnosis and correct surgery and were referred to the pain clinic.

Summary

Impingement is the first stage in a continuum of disease to the rotator cuff muscles. We are beginning to understand that the aetiology is more complex than we had previously thought. There are many different aetiologies which may lead to impingement. These causes can be subdivided into functional and anatomical causes, although often functional abnormality will lead on to secondary anatomical features which cause stenosis of the subacromial space.

The diagnosis of impingement is clinical and must be confirmed by the 'impingement test'; the transient freedom from pain induced by injection of local anaesthetic into the subacromial space.

The treatment of impingement is by subacromial decompression, which can be performed either arthroscopically or by open surgery.

CHAPTER 5

The management of rotator-cuff tears: tricks of the trade

T. Bunker

Introduction

The repair of rotator-cuff tears is one of the most challenging and rapidly developing areas within orthopaedic surgery. For the surgeon, repair of cuff defects is physically demanding, involves rapid decision making, is highly time consuming, has a long learning curve, and depends on the backup of a highly skilled and developed team of nurses and physiotherapists. To the patient, rotator-cuff repair is a painful operation which is demanding on motivation and persistence, and that involves considerable time off work.

There is some dispute over the incidence, aetiology, surgical approaches, method of repair and rehabilitation of rotator-cuff tears. This chapter will critically evaluate these disputed areas and show you the 'tricks of the trade' that will allow you to cope with difficult cuff problems which you may encounter.

Incidence

The incidence of symptomatic rotator-cuff tears is difficult to estimate. Looking at my own diagnostic index, 310 out of the last 1500 patients referred to my shoulder clinic had a rotator-cuff tear.

Recent research has shown that partial tears are more common than was originally thought. Andrews *et al.* (1985) showed that 36 patients out of 106 undergoing shoulder arthroscopy had a partial tear of the cuff; all these patients were athletic and their average age was 22 years.

Many of the studies of incidence have been performed on cadavers; clearly the pathologist cannot

determine in these cases whether the tear was symptomatic during life. Most autopsy studies place the incidence of full-thickness tears at 20%. The exceptions are Fukuda at 7% and Neer *et al.* (1992) at 5%. It is well known that cuff tears can be asymptomatic. Pettersson (1942) performed an arthrogram on the asymptomatic shoulders of 71 patients and found that 13 had partial or full-thickness tears. This makes cadaver counting somewhat irrelevant. Partial thickness tears are twice as common as full thickness tears.

The cost to society of rotator-cuff tears in a working population has been studied by Savoie *et al.* (1995). The average cost of a successful repair was $50302 per patient, and the average length of time away from work was 11 months. There was a marked difference in costs if the patient was sent immediately to a shoulder surgeon where the average cost was $25870 compared to the cost of being managed initially by a general practitioner where the average cost was $100280; the length of time off work was also significantly different, 7 months in the direct route and 18 months if diagnosis and treatment were delayed by a 'gatekeeper'.

There is no doubt that the incidence of rotator-cuff tearing is related to age. We live at a time where the elderly are forming a growing proportion of the population. Increasing wealth will allow more leisure time and greater involvement in sport, which will lead to premature tendon-fibre failure and yet more rotator-cuff tears. This ageing, sporting population will have increasing expectations for their health and will expect us, their surgeons, to react by improving our skills such that we can ensure a rapid return to normality for any shoulder which sustains a tear of the rotator-cuff.

Functional anatomy of the rotator cuff

Before we can discuss the tricks of the trade used by the specialist shoulder-surgeon to achieve a successful repair, and a working shoulder, it behoves us to review the functional anatomy of the rotator-cuff itself.

The rotator-cuff is a composite of the capsule, the ligaments, and the tendons around the shoulder (Clark & Harryman, 1992). Microscopically the cuff is composed of five layers in the region of supraspinatus and infraspinatus.

Classically the rotator-cuff is thought of as the four tendons of insertion of the subscapularis, supraspinatus, infraspinatus and teres minor; however, in reality it is much more complex, being reinforced by the coracohumeral ligament and the glenohumeral ligaments, and being weakened by the rotator interval.

The long head of biceps, although not formally part of the rotator-cuff, is ensheathed by interwoven fibres from the subscapularis and supraspinatus as it enters its sulcus, and shares many of the functions of the cuff.

Supraspinatus

The supraspinatus tendon is the most vulnerable part of the rotator-cuff. The 'critical zone' (Codman, 1934) of the supraspinatus is the starting point for both impingement lesions and cuff tears.

Supraspinatus is a bipennate muscle, which originates from the whole of the supraspinous fossa of the scapula, which measures 8 by 4 cm. The tendon develops within the centre of the muscle, but then migrates towards the leading edge of the muscle where it forms a thick tendon at the level of the glenoid, as can be seen on magnetic resonance imaging (MRI) cross sections of the muscle (Fig. 5.1). This fact is important in the surgery of massive tears because this leading-edge tendon holds sutures well whereas the muscle fibres of the posterior aspect of the muscle hold sutures poorly. The leading edge of the tendon is further strengthened by the coracohumeral ligament, which ensheathes the leading edge of supraspinatus, some fibres passing over the bursal side and some passing onto the deep surface (Clark & Harryman, 1992). In massive tears the coracohumeral ligament contracts (Neer *et al.*, 1992) and pulls the leading edge of the tendon forwards and down towards the subscapularis tendon. The coracohumeral ligament must therefore be released in order to mobilize the tendon.

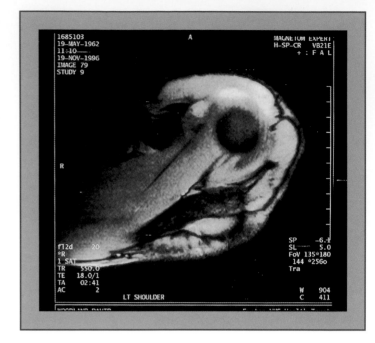

Figure 5.1 – *An axial MRI scan of the supraspinatus. Note that it is a bipennate muscle and observed how the tendon starts centrally and migrates forwards to the anterior margin of the muscle.*

As the muscle is traced beyond the joint-line a flat tendon forms from the posterior muscle fibres as well as the thick leading-edge tendon. These fibres of supraspinatus then interweave with fibres from infraspinatus making a strong, bonded, tough and flat tendinous sheet — the rotator-cuff. The merging laminations of supraspinatus and infraspinatus form the five histological layers of the cuff tendon (Fig. 5.2). The most superficial layer (layer 1) is made up of fibres from the coracohumeral ligament. Layer 2 is made of tendon fibres running parallel to the line of pull of supraspinatus and infraspinatus. Layer 3 is made of interdigitating fibres from supraspinatus and infraspinatus crossing each other at an angle of 45°. Layer 4 is made of the fibres coming from the deep surface of the coracohumeral ligament. Layer 5 is the true joint capsule made of the collagen fibres of the capsule, which originate from the glenoid rim of the scapula (Clark & Harryman, 1992).

Layer 5, that is the capsule itself, is more complex than previously thought (Gohlke *et al.*, 1994) (Fig. 5.3). The superior capsule underlying supraspinatus has both circular and radially reinforcing collagen fibres, as shown by polarized light microscopy. The radial reinforcement comes from the coracohumeral ligament fibres (layer 4).

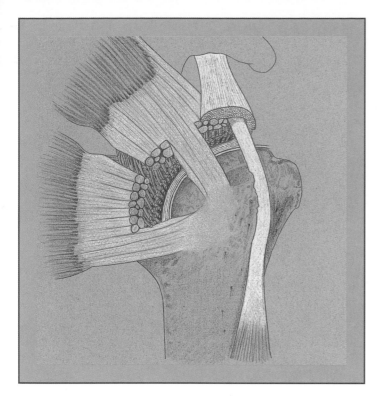

Figure 5.2 – *The rotator cuff is a composite consisting of five layers: (1) fibres from the coraco-humeral ligament; (2) tendon fibres running parallel to the muscle fibres; (3) tendon fibres running obliquely; (4) fibres running from the coraco-humeral and superior gleno-humeral ligaments and (5) the synovium.*

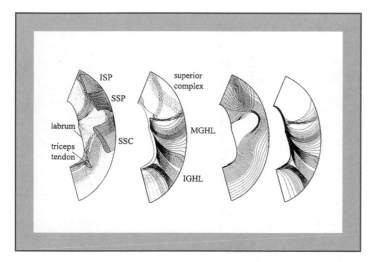

Figure 5.3 – *Examination of the capsule shows radially reinforcing layers (reproduced with permission from Gohlke F., Journal of Shoulder and Elbow Surgery, 1994)*

Nakajima *et al.* (1994) showed that the superficial (bursal) side of the rotator-cuff has greater deformation and tensile strength than the joint surface side, which concurs with the histological findings. This also agrees

with the pathological findings that cuff tears usually start on the joint surface of the supraspinatus tendon.

Blood supply to supraspinatus

The final centimetre of the tendon of supraspinatus, the 'critical zone' of Codman is the usual starting point of rotator-cuff tears and so a lot of attention has been placed on the blood supply to this area of the cuff.

Cadaveric perfusion studies (Rothman & Parke, 1965; Rathburn & MacNab, 1970) demonstrated a hypovascular area at this site of the supraspinatus tendon. More recent studies have criticized these earlier papers and contradicted their findings. Brooks *et al.* (1992) examined the blood supply of the distal tendon in a quantitative histological study. They found that although there was a reduction in the percentage of the tendon occupied by vessels in the distal 15 mm of the tendon, a similar appearance was found in the infraspinatus tendon which is much less commonly affected by tears. They concluded that factors other than vascularity are important in the aetiology of cuff tears. Clark and Harryman (1992) confirmed that the vessel diameter decreases as it is traced more distally, and that vessels run mainly in the outer layers of the cuff, parallel to the collagen fibre bundles. Gohlke (1994) found a similar pattern with the vessels running in the coracohumeral layer. In an *in vivo* study, Swiantkowski *et al.* (1989), using laser doppler flowmetry, found that the critical area of the cuff was in fact well perfused, as were the edges of cuff tears; this can be confirmed when you next trim the edges of a mature cuff tear. Clearly, there is more to tendon failure than just the blood supply.

Nerve supply to supraspinatus

Supraspinatus is innervated by the suprascapular nerve. The suprascapular nerve leaves the upper trunk of the brachial plexus at Erb's point and passes, through the suprascapular notch, under the suprascapular ligament.

The course of the nerve then becomes very important to the shoulder surgeon who must not damage it even during radical mobilization of the cuff (Fig. 5.4). The nerve runs an oblique course across the floor of the suprascapular fossa where it is relatively fixed. It supplies two motor branches to supraspinatus, the more proximal being larger. The average distance from the joint-line to the nerve is 3 cm. The nerve then passes around the angle of the spine of the scapula where again it is fixed within the spinoglenoid notch

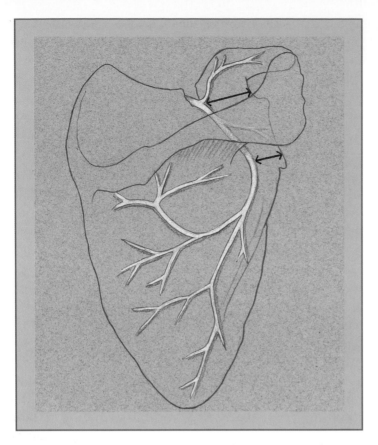

Figure 5.4 – *The suprascapular nerve follows a course from the notch to the infraspinatus fossa.*

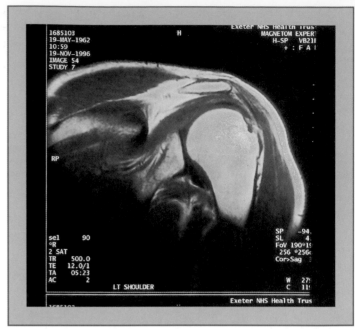

Figure 5.5 – *A MRI scan showing the suprascapular nerve and artery winding around the spine of the scapula.*

(Fig. 5.5). The nerve then supplies three or four motor branches to the infraspinatus. The nerve is an average of 2 cm from the joint-line at this point, and is therefore at risk from the normal posterior portal for shoulder arthroscopy.

Function of supraspinatus

Supraspinatus, acting in concert with the rest of the rotator-cuff, acts to stabilize and centre the humeral head (see Chapter 6). However, in this chapter we are more interested in the function of supraspinatus in powering movement of the shoulder joint, in other words the contribution of supraspinatus to the production of torque forces in the shoulder.

Supraspinatus was once believed to act in the initiation of abduction and elevation. Van Linge and Mulder (1963) demonstrated in an elegant experiment, where they paralysed the deltoid with an axillary nerve block, that supraspinatus not only initiated elevation but could also power-up a normal arc of elevation. However, the subjects fatigued more quickly than normal.

Howell *et al.* (1986) repeated this work but using a dynamometer and suprascapular blocks as well as axillary blocks. They demonstrated that paralysing either deltoid or supraspinatus led to a reduction in torque of 50%.

Blocking the suprascapular nerve clearly paralyses infraspinatus as well, but this muscle has been shown to be electromyographically silent until 120° of elevation has been achieved, beyond which it contributes about 12° of torque.

If both the axillary nerve and the suprascapular nerve are blocked, then no torque can be generated and the shoulder becomes immobile and can not be stabilized in space against gravity (Colachis & Strohm, 1971).

These findings are of vital importance in the understanding of shoulder function. Comparing the relative size of deltoid to supraspinatus, it is surprising that each generates equal torque during elevation. This can be understood more easily if we consider the normalized cross-sectional area of each third of the deltoid (area of muscle/area of supraspinatus). Howell *et al.* have shown that the normalized cross-sectional areas are: supraspinatus 1; anterior deltoid 0.91; middle deltoid 0.85; and posterior deltoid 1.07. They then worked out the relative force exerted at 90° elevation, based upon the product of the normalized cross-sectional area and the integrated electromyographic signal. Electromyography showed that during elevation the middle deltoid was active, but that the anterior deltoid was only functioning at 57% of maximal stimulation; the posterior deltoid was silent. Using this model they calculated that although deltoid is three times as big as supraspinatus, the relative force of deltoid to supraspinatus was 1.38–1.0. This would fit very well with the dynamometer studies.

However, when a tear occurs in the supraspinatus the shoulder loses not only the torque effect but also the stabilizing effect on the head, allowing anterosuperior subluxation; this effectively cripples the shoulder.

Sometimes shoulder function remains relatively normal despite a tear in the supraspinatus, this is termed a functional-cuff tear. How can this happen? Burkhart (1994) described what he termed the rotator cable (Fig. 5.6). This is a thickening within the rotator-cuff, which runs in a crescent shape from the bicipital tunnel under the supraspinatus and infraspinatus to insert into the humerus, at the posterior border of the infraspinatus. This band is 12 mm wide and 1.8 mm thick and runs for some 41 mm in length. This band can clearly be seen arthroscopically. Although Burkhart did not examine this histologically he states that it probably represents layer 4 in Clark and Harryman's (1992) study, that is the deep

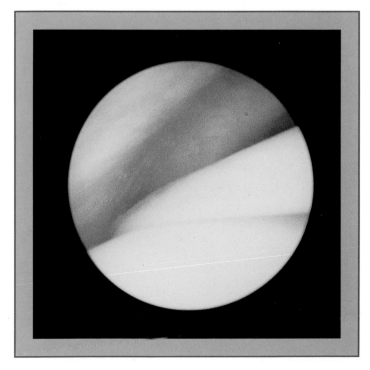

Figure 5.6 – *An arthroscopic view of the radial thickening of the superior capsule (the rotator cable).*

extension of the coracohumeral ligament. If the collagen alignment is examined in Gohlke's (1994) study the rotator cable probably represents the other circumferential band, which they show, rather than the coracohumeral band, which is also clearly shown in their paper. Burkhart states that this thick cable can take the pull of the rotator-cuff muscles even if there is a tear and allow near normal function — the so-called 'functional tear'.

The area distal to this cable has been termed the rotator crescent by Burkhart (1994), which he likens to a stress shielded area. The problem with this hypothesis is why should all cuff tears start in the rotator crescent if it is stress shielded? Surely tears must start in an area of high load. However, this is an interesting idea, and the student of shoulder surgery should at least consider the hypothesis as it is the basis of the school which believes in debridement, rather than repair, of massive cuff defects.

The coracohumeral ligament

The coracohumeral ligament is intimately associated with the anterior border of the supraspinatus wrapping both over and under the leading edge. This ligament is not without controversy, however.

Neer *et al.* (1992) found the coracohumeral ligament to be a clear, well developed structure. Its origin was consistently on the lateral aspect of the coracoid process averaging 18 mm in length. The insertion was more variable but usually blended into the rotator interval tissues.

Prior to Neer's study the coracohumeral ligament had been stated to be a prolongation of the tendon of pectoralis minor. However, in Neer's study, four cadavers, were found to have an extension of the pectoralis minor tendon, which quite clearly was entirely separate from the coracohumeral ligament and inserted into the tendon of supraspinatus. Neer discussed the contracture of the coracohumeral ligament in large retracted-cuff tears and the fact that the coracohumeral ligament needs to be divided in order to mobilize such a tear. Cooper *et al.* (1993) examined the coracohumeral ligament histologically and found no discrete collagen bundles suggestive of a true ligament. They suggested that the coracohumeral ligament was a tent-like extension of the capsule of the shoulder. It is the folded ridge of this tent which appears as a ligament when it is tensioned by external rotation of the shoulder. Edelson *et al.* (1991) concur with Cooper that the coraco-humeral ligament is not a true ligament like the coraco-acromial ligament. Histologically it is typical of a joint capsule, with a layered pattern of sheets and bundles of collagen interspersed with loose connective tissue and vascular channels. They also felt it was the strongest portion of the capsule (Fig. 5.7) and was analagous to the 'Y'-shaped iliofemoral ligament of Bigelow in the hip, which although not a true ligament is often quoted to be the strongest ligament in the body. Perhaps, as you can tell, this is a matter of semantics. Whatever the coracohumeral ligament is, it is an important structure that blends intimately with the leading edge of the supraspinatus in its distal course and with the superior glenohumeral ligament forming the mouth of the bicipital tunnel.

Infraspinatus

Infraspinatus is a strong bipennate muscle that originates from the infraspinatus fossa of the scapula. The muscle inserts into the greater tuberosity behind supraspinatus. The tendons of the two muscles converge producing a common continuous insertion. The infraspinatus tendon

has a five-layered histological appearance similar to that of supraspinatus (Fig. 5.8). The blood supply and nerve supply from the suprascapular nerve and artery have already been discussed above. The muscle is far less prone to tearing than the supraspinatus, and usually only tears as an extension of a tear which has started in the supraspinatus. The principle action of the infraspinatus is external rotation of the shoulder joint.

Teres minor

Teres minor originates from the infraspinatus fossa below the infraspinatus muscle itself. The split between the two muscles can be difficult to find at surgery, but is important because this is a watershed-plane between the territories of the suprascapular nerve and the axillary

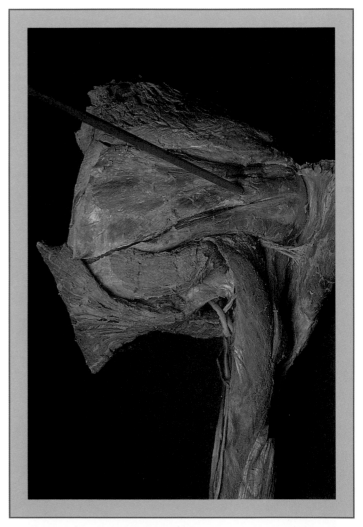

Figure 5.8 – *An anatomical specimen showing the course of the infraspinatus. The deltoid has been raised from the spine of the scapula to show the infraspinatus and Teres minor (reproduced with permission from Shoulder Arthroscopy, Bunker and Wallace (eds), Dunitz, 1991).*

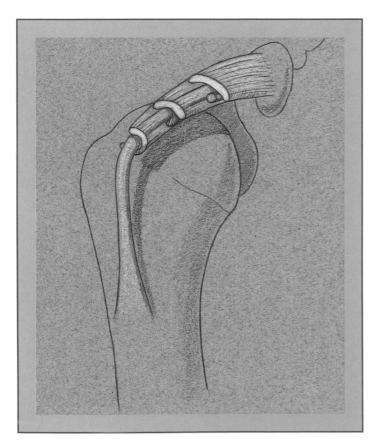

Figure 5.7 – *The coracohumeral ligament and the superior glenohumeral ligament merge distally and form the pulley at the entrance to the bicipital tunnel.*

nerve; it is a safe plane to dissect in order to approach the posterior capsule. Teres minor is supplied by the superficial division of the axillary nerve. There is a rich vascular anastomosis around teres minor, for the circumflex scapular branch of the subscapular artery anastomoses with the supraspinatus artery under the muscle, and fine branches of the posterior circumflex accompany the nerve on to its superficial surface. Teres minor also acts as an external rotator of the shoulder.

Subscapularis

Subscapularis is the largest and the strongest muscle of the rotator-cuff. This muscle accounts for 53% of the total strength of the cuff (Keating *et al.*, 1993). Hinton *et al.* (1994) noted that there was a contradiction between the classic description of the tendinous insertion of subscapularis into the lesser tuberosity and reality. The reality is that the upper 60% of subscapularis inserts into the humerus as a tendon but the lower 40% is pure muscle and inserts as such into the humerus. The anterior circumflex humeral artery, and its two veins, run at the level of the junction of the tendinous and muscular portions of the subscapularis. Thus this artery does not mark the inferior surface of subscapularis as stated in most textbooks, it marks the lower-third of the muscle. The tendon forms some 4–6 cm from the insertion into the humerus as a series of tendinous strips from the multipennate fibres and becomes truly tendinous 2 cm from its insertion. The tendon is thickest at the superior edge of the muscle. From an arthroscopic perspective this superior edge can clearly be seen as an intra-articular structure, which is the secondary landmark of shoulder arthroscopy, and is crossed obliquely by the middle glenohumeral ligament. The axillary nerve leaves the posterior cord of the brachial plexus and passes, along with the posterior circumflex artery and vein, below the lower border of the subscapularis into and through the quadrilateral space. The subscapularis muscle is supplied by the two subscapular nerves which are branches of the posterior cord. Turkel *et al.* (1981) showed how the subscapularis forms an important restraint to anterior subluxation as the arm is by the side (see Chapter 6). As the arm is elevated the subscapularis becomes less important as a passive anterior restraint. The subscapularis muscle is a powerful internal rotator of the shoulder but is dwarfed by pectoralis major, teres major and latissimus dorsi.

The rotator interval

We have described the areas of reinforcement of the rotator-cuff in some detail, but there are also areas of the cuff that are weak; weakest of all is the rotator interval. This has only recently assumed a great importance in discussions of shoulder laxity (Nobuhura, 1987) and shoulder contracture (Bunker & Anthony, 1995). The rotator interval is the area of the capsule which spans the gap between the leading edge of the supraspinatus and the superior edge of the subscapularis. Long head of biceps arcs across the humeral head under this gap. The arthroscopic view of the interval reveals a recess (Fig. 5.9) which disappears down under the coracoid process. The entrance to the recess is called the foramen of Wietbrecht. The space within this recess is like the inside of a ridge tent, and indeed the roof and ridge of the recess is the folded capsule of the rotator interval, which is the coracohumeral ligament. The rotator interval is difficult to see from outside because it lies under the coraco-acromial ligament. Only when the coraco-acromial ligament has been completely excised can the interval be seen, and often even then there is a pad of fat containing the anterior superior humeral vessel which prevents a good view. The function of the rotator interval is to allow free movement of the subscapularis and

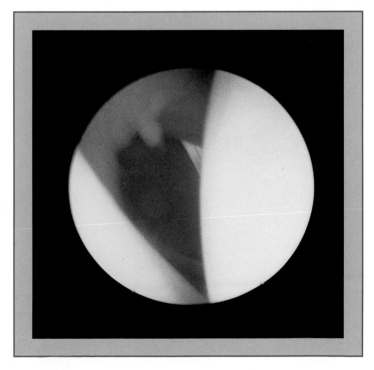

Figure 5.9 – *An arthroscopic view of the rotator interval showing the entrance to the subcoracoid recess (the foramen of Weitbrecht).*

supraspinatus around the coracoid process. Harryman *et al.* (1992) selectively incised and then imbricated the rotator-interval capsule in order to study its function in relation to movement and stability of the shoulder (Fig. 5.10). They found that release of the rotator interval improved the range of flexion and external rotation. Conversely, imbrication of the capsule helped to control posterior and inferior instability.

Long head of biceps

The tendon of long head of the biceps is actually contiguous with the glenoid labrum (Fig. 5.11). Thus it arises not only from the supraglenoid tubercle but as a direct continuation of the labrum itself. The tendon is entirely intra-articular and may have thin whispy synovial attachments to the overlying synovium. Occasionally, a continuous thin sheet of synovium

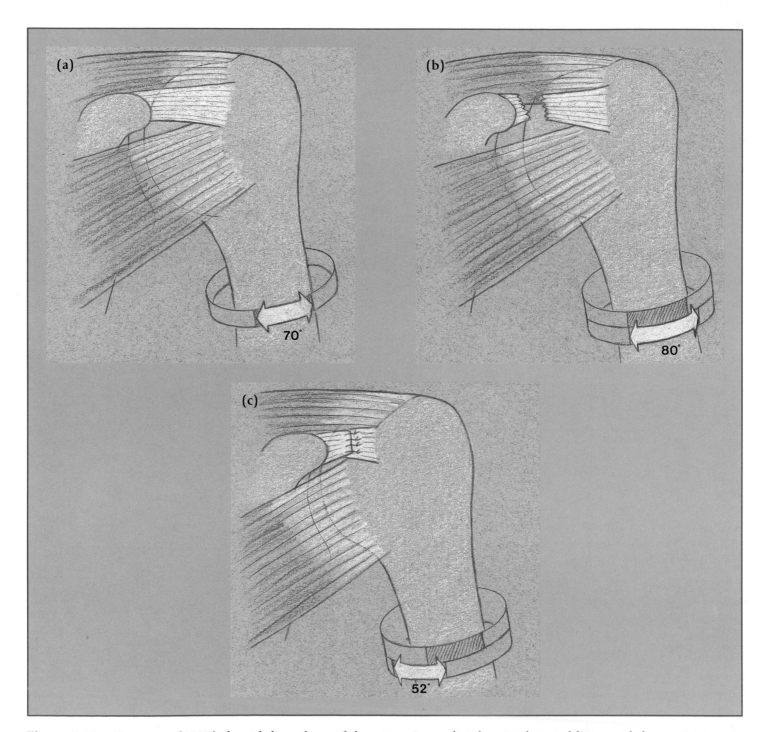

Figure 5.10 – *Harryman (1992) showed that release of the rotator interval and coraco-humeral ligament led to an increase in external rotation of 10° (b), whilst imbricating it by 1 cm led to a reduction of external rotation by 18° (c).*

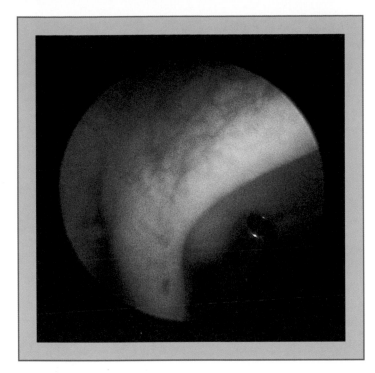

Figure 5.11 – *Arthroscopic view of the long head of biceps to show how it is contiguous with the posterior labrum.*

passes between the tendon and the synovium. We have termed this a mesentery (Bunker & Wallace 1991). Johnson terms these strands the 'vinculae' of the long head of the biceps. Unlike the vinculae to the finger flexors they do not contain any blood vessels. The long head of the biceps disappears from the shoulder by passing into its bicipital sulcus where it is encircled by layers of the rotator-cuff, the coracohumeral ligament and the superior glenohumeral ligament.

Causes of rotator-cuff tears

The aetiology of rotator-cuff tears has been debated for the best part of this century. Two schools have emerged, the extrinsic school (impingement) and the intrinsic school (tendon-fibre failure). We have discussed the extrinsic theory and shown that Neer believes that 95% of rotator-cuff tears are caused by impingement. The fact that the cuff tear and the hooked acromion occured together was taken as proof that the hook caused the cuff tear. However, recent research states that, in fact, the cuff tear may cause the hook, a finding which may turn the world of shoulder surgery upside down! Ozaki *et al.* (1988) examined 200 cadaver shoulders histologically. Examining these shoulders they found that partial tears of the cuff were most commonly seen on the deep surface of the cuff, and

without any acromial changes. However, if there were acromial changes, there were always deep-surface cuff changes. They therefore postulate that the lesion of the anterior one-third of the undersurface of the acromion is a secondary change that follows a tear of the cuff on the deep surface. In other words microtrauma causes damage to the tendon–bone junction on the joint surface of the cuff; cuff weakness leads to functional impingement and this puts increasing stress upon the coraco-acromial ligament, leading to secondary bone spurs on the undersurface of the acromion. These bone spurs then cause secondary damage to the bursal side of the cuff, and things go from bad to worse. This is certainly a unifying theory which joins the previously warring factions of the extrinsic school (impingement) and the intrinsic school (tendon-fibre failure). Codman (1934) suggested that most cuff tears started not on the superficial (bursal) side but on the deep side of the cuff, and termed this the rim rent tear. Codman actually stated 'It would be hard to explain this section...by erosion from contact with the acromion'. Codman made the study of tears of the supraspinatus his life's work, publishing his first report in 1906. Every case was thoroughly documented and he found that all his patients led a labouring life (even, or perhaps especially, the women). Because all his patients had a history of injury he stated that trauma was a major cause of rotator-cuff tears. However, this injury was small in many, for instance his first patient described in 1906 was throwing a wet blanket over a clothesline. Since the episode of trauma was quite small it was felt that there must be some predisposing weakness of the rotator-cuff. The blood supply of the cuff thus came under scrutiny. The critical area of the supraspinatus tendon corresponds to the area of anastomosis between tendinous and osseous vessels (Moseley & Goldie, 1963). This area was found to be hypovascular in the studies of Rothman and Parke (1965) and Rathburn and Macnab (1970). Lohr and Uhtoff (1989) showed that on the bursal side of the supraspinatus there was a good blood supply but the supply was much poorer on the joint surface, the area where tears originate. Most surgeons agree that tendon degeneration occurs with age. Ozaki (1988) in a cadaver study showed that there was a clear association between rotator-cuff tearing and increasing age (Fig. 5.12). The debate as to whether cuff tears are initiated by intrinsic or extrinsic causes will continue. Essentially both schools agree that the tear occurs with a traumatic insult to a cuff insertion, which is already weakened, either by a congenital weakness of the collagen of the insertion, or

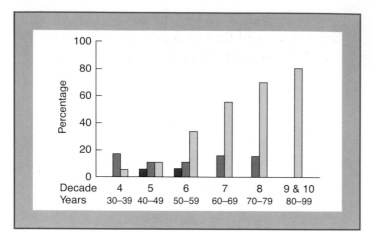

Figure 5.12 – *This graph shows how rotator-cuff tears become more numerous with increasing age (reproduced with permission from the Journal of Bone and Joint Surgery).* ■ *Stage 1,* ■ *Stage 2,* ▨ *Stage 3.*

due to natural changes in the collagen with ageing, or due to damage to the cuff from impingement. Most likely it is a combination of all three, which starts with repetitive microtrauma leading to mild muscle dysfunction, and thus on to impingement, with the secondary soft tissue and bony changes in the coraco-acromial arch. The rotator-cuff is thus weakened and a moderate injury to the tendon, whilst it is powered-up under tensile load, causes the tendon to tear away from its insertion.

Classification of rotator-cuff tears

Rotator-cuff tears come in all shapes and sizes. Shape and size has a bearing not only on the method of repair, but also upon the prognosis following repair. Because of this we have to classify the tears in some acceptable way. Most classifications depend upon operative findings, what is needed is an accurate and reproduceable method of classifying tears preoperatively, and the logical way to do this is with MRI scanning.

Partial-thickness tears

Ellman *et al.*(1993) classified partial-thickness tears (Fig. 5.13) according to the depth of the lesion and its anatomical site. Thus they are graded A or B, depending upon whether the tear is on the articular or bursal side. They are then graded further from 1 to 3 depending upon if the tear is less than quarter thickness (Grade 1), less than half thickness (Grade 2) or more than half thickness (Grade 3).

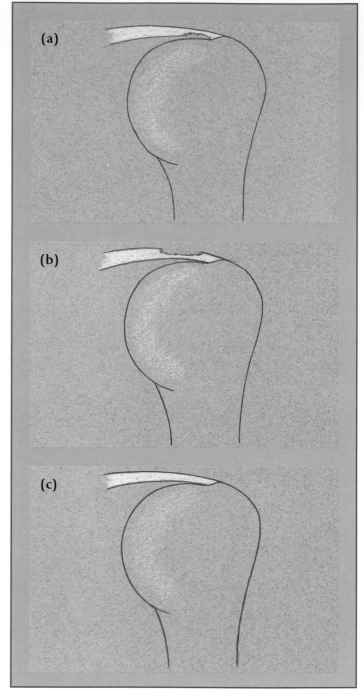

Figure 5.13 – *Ellman et al. (1993) classified partial-thickness tears according to their situation. Articular surface tears (a); bursal side tears (b) and the normal tendon (c).*

Full-thickness tears

There are many systems of classification of full-thickness tears according to their situation (which tendon), shape, and size. Virtually all tears start in the supraspinatus tendon, approximately 1 cm behind its leading edge. The tear then expands to take in infraspinatus, and more rarely teres minor and subscapularis. Most surgeons classify rotator-cuff tears according to their size. Post *et al.* (1983) classified tears as small (less than 1 cm), moderate (1–3 cm), large (3–5 cm) or massive (larger than 5 cm) (Table 5.1). This is a very useful classification because the watershed for good versus poor results following rotator-cuff repair is 4 cm. Thus we would

expect good results following repair of small and moderate tears and limited results following repair of large and massive tears. The shape of the tear (Fig. 5.14)

Table 5.1 Post *et al's* (1983) classification of rotator-cuff tears according to size (cm).

Small	< 1
Moderate	1–3
Large	3–5
Massive	> 5

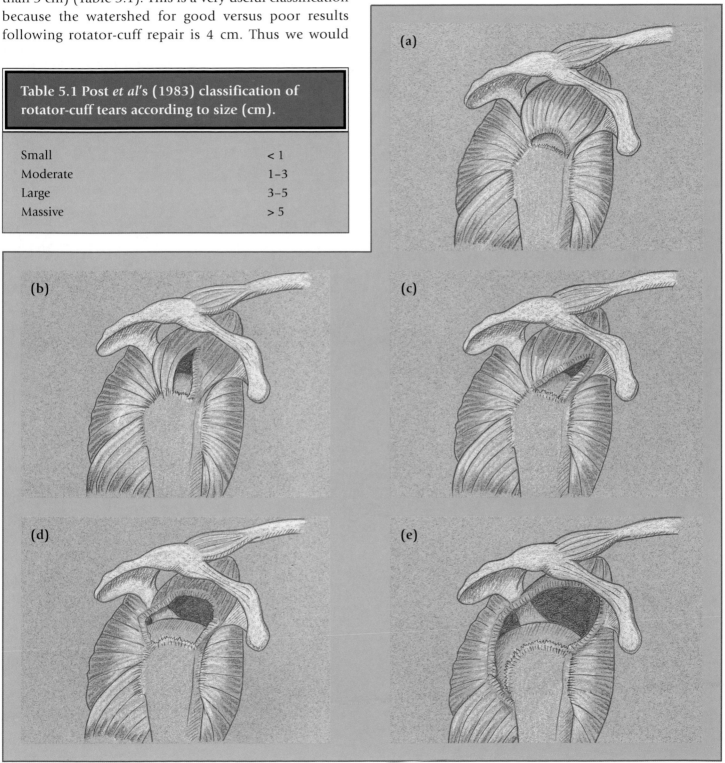

Figure 5.14 – *Rotator-cuff tears vary from a small crescent-shaped tear (a), to L-shaped (b) and reverse L-shaped (c), to trapezoidal (d) and on to massive (e).*

is just as important as its extent because, for the method of suture depends on it. Ellman (1993) describes a progression of shape from crescent, through 'L' shaped and reverse 'L' shaped, to trapezoidal and finally massive. Massive tears are sometimes called 'bald head tears' because the cuff remnant surrounding the bare humeral head is said to represent the tonsure of the monk. This ecclesiastical adjective is particularly apposite for the term 'rotator-cuff' is said to have come from the French term for the white headpiece of a nun, the 'coiffe' (Stableforth, 1995). Norwood *et al.* (1986) classified tears into single-tendon and multiple-tendon tears. Snyder (1994) has an even more complex classification where each muscle is abbreviated (SS,IS,TM,Sub) and then graded by extent; although useful for research this system is too unwieldy for general use. The final end-point of cuff tearing is cuff-tear arthropathy. In cuff-tear arthropathy the humeral head erodes the superior glenoid and the acromion and there is degenerative change leading on to a severe painful arthritis. Fortunately, cuff-tear arthropathy is rare and occurs in only 4% of patients with cuff tear.

The clinical presentation of rotator-cuff tears

Codman's (1934) description of the clinical presentation of a patient with a rotator-cuff tear still can not be bettered; 'A labourer, aged over forty, with a previously normal shoulder, injures the shoulder, has an immediate but brief pain, with severe pain the following night, loss of power in elevating the arm, but no restriction when stooping, a faulty scapulohumeral rhythm, a tender point, sulcus and eminence at the insertion of supraspinatus, which causes a jog, a wince, and soft crepitus, as the tuberosity disappears under the acromion, as the arm is passively elevated, and usually reappears on descent of the arm, with a normal radiograph.' Codman's conditions are summarized in Table 5.2. He stated that if these 18 conditions were met the patient should be immediately operated on, sound advice in 1934 which has not changed to date. Codman came to these findings on the basis of 30 years of annotated analysis of patients with rotator-cuff tears. For instance, in stating that the patient was usually a labourer he noted the occupation of 100 consecutive, proven, rotator-cuff patients and contrasted them with 300 patients with partial tears, calcific deposits and

Table 5.2 Codman listed 18 conditions associated with rotator-cuff tears.

(1)	Occupation	Manual labourer
(2)	Age	> 40 years
(3)	History	Previously normal shoulder
(4)	Onset	Injury to shoulder
(5)	Symptoms	Immediate pain
(6)		Window of relief
(7)		Severe pain that night
(8)	Signs	Loss of power in elevation
(9)		No restriction when stooping
(10)		Faulty scapulohumeral rhythm
(11)		Tender point on greater tuberosity
(12)		Sulcus at tear site
(13)		Eminence at tuberosity
(14)	Symptoms	Causes a jog
(15)		And a wince
(16)		And soft crepitus on elevation;
(17)		These reappear on descent of arm
(18)	Investigation	Normal radiograph

frozen shoulder. It is interesting to cull a few more gems from the original paper of this most observant surgeon. Codman states that as far as a previous history of shoulder problems is concerned he would rather have the history given by the man's wife because labouring men often forget, or even lie about past injury, saying the shoulder was previously normal. The patient is typically 50–60 years old. Remember the aphorism, 'grey hair equals cuff tear.' He goes on to state that the injury is often a result of sudden elevation of the weight-bearing arm, a typical example of which is the throwing a wet blanket over a washing line, as was the case with his original patient in 1906. Usually the patient has a sudden pain at the time of injury, with a snap, just like an Achilles tendon rupture. The patient will often then have a window before the severe pain comes on. In the evening the severe pain starts and the patient presents for medical help the day after the injury. This is confusing to general practitioners who think that if the patient did not report for help for 24 hours there can't be much wrong! Active elevation is always limited, but passive elevation is full. The rhythm of movement is always protective, and most noticeable as the patient brings the arm down. The patient locks the humerus to the glenoid, with considerable effort, until he reaches the horizontal, when suddenly he lets the arm go and it falls the remaining distance. This is done in order to prevent the severe impingement-type pain which he knows would otherwise occur. External rotation with the arm at the side is virtually normal, but internal rotation may be limited by end-point pain. The tear itself can sometimes be felt by the surgeon; a hole the size of a finger tip can be palpated, and below it a bump where the stump and tuberosity are more prominent than usual, can be felt. As the tear moves under the acromion there is a jog and the patient winces, and crepitus can be felt by the surgeon as the torn area passes under the acromion. After a few weeks the spinati atrophy. Not only is Codman's description unsurpassed, but the order in which he places his 18 symptoms and signs can be plotted in the same order on the American Shoulder and Elbow Surgeons assessment (ASES) form devised 60 years later. Lyons and Tomlinson (1992) showed that, using these clinical symptoms and signs alone, there was a sensitivity of 91% and a specificity of 75% in sizing the cuff tear in 42 patients who later had their rotator-cuff tears confirmed at surgery. However, this result was actually the clinical diagnosis of one professor of shoulder surgery in one of the top shoulder units in the UK. The study does not therefore guarantee that everyone will be so successful, but it does show a level of diagnostic expertise that we should all strive for. Norwood (1986) found that the characteristics of the pain, the site of tenderness, and the power of resisted abduction were poor predictors of whether the cuff was torn or not.

Investigations for suspected cuff tear

The majority of rotator-cuff tears can be diagnosed, and also sized with some accuracy, by an experienced shoulder surgeon questioning the patient and conducting an examination. However, at both ends of the scale investigation can be helpful in diagnosis and planning treatment. At the one end we have the patient in whom we have a differential diagnosis of impingement, partial-thickness tear, or small full-thickness tear, where investigations can help. At the other end of the scale we have the large tear where the question is 'Is this tear repairable, and if so what kind of

function can we expect?'. In this situation MRI can be very helpful not only in sizing the tear, but also in enabling us to look at the fatty degeneration in the muscle belly of the supraspinatus.

Plain radiographs

Four features seen on plain films can be helpful in deciding whether there is a cuff tear and how big it is.

(1) Changes on the greater tuberosity
These start with enthesopathic changes, small cysts and sclerotic rings (Fig. 5.15). Bone mineral can be resorbed leading to osteoporotic change in the tuberosity. The tuberosity then becomes irregular and finally reparative osteophytes form.

(2) Changes in the acromion
As impingement occurs bone changes become evident on the lower surface of the acromion. These changes were noted by Neer (1992), on radiographs as sclerosis (sourcil sign) and bone spurs on the anterior acromion (Fig. 5.16). These bone spurs can be seen best in the Neer outlet view.

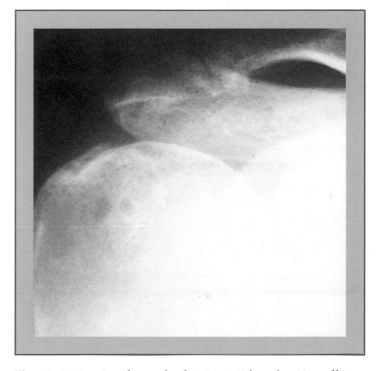

Figure 5.15 – *A radiograph of patient with a chronic-cuff tear. Note the irregularity of the greater tuberosity with sclerotic-edged cysts and osteophytes.*

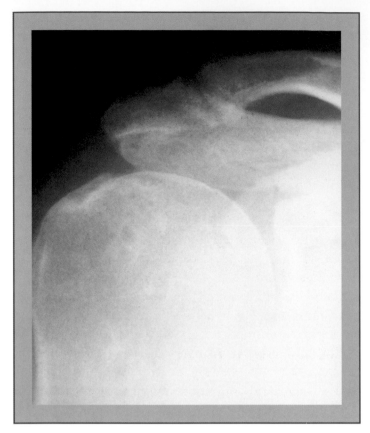

Figure 5.16 – *A radiograph of a patient with a cuff tear showing sclerosis of undersurface of the acromion — the so-called 'sourcil sign'.*

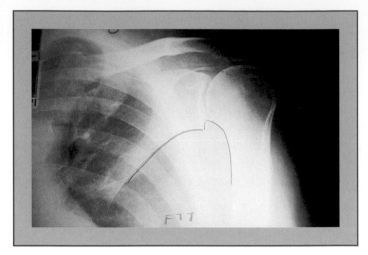

Figure 5.17 – *A radiograph of a patient with a rotator-cuff tear showing the elevation of the humeral head with a break in Shenton's line of the shoulder.*

and MRI scanning. An arthrogram will show whether a cuff tear is present (Fig. 5.18). The difficulty is in using arthrography to size a cuff tear accurately. In order to do this, double-contrast arthrotomography has to be used and interpreted by a skilled radiologist experienced in this technique. MRI, being non-invasive and far less demanding of skilled radiologist time, has now taken over this function. Arthrography may still have a place in

(3) The acromiohumeral interval

As the cuff tears, it gets weaker and the humeral head subluxes upwards. As it does so the acromiohumeral interval decreases. The cut-off level between a normal cuff and a dysfunctional cuff is said to be a humeral distance of 7 mm. Beware that the film must be centred on the subacomial space, or else this measurement will give a false result.

(4) As the cuff tear matures the humeral head rides up

This can be seen as a break in the normal arch of the medial border of the scapula to the calcar and medial border of the humerus. This is analogous to Shenton's line at the hip, and I term it Shenton's line of the shoulder (Fig. 5.17). If the line is broken this is a good predictor of cuff tear; the amount of shift relates to the size of tear.

Arthrography

The arthrogram was the gold standard for diagnosis of a rotator-cuff tear prior to the introduction of arthroscopy

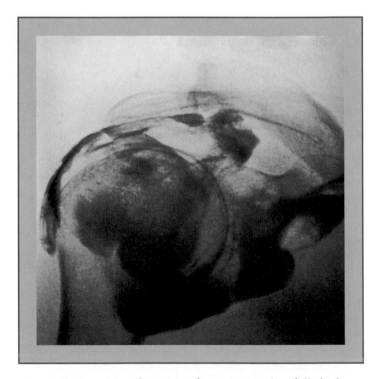

Figure 5.18 – *An arthrogram of a patient with a full-thickness rotator-cuff tear.*

the diagnosis of deep-surface partial-thickness tears, which are poorly seen on MRI, because it is less invasive than arthroscopy.

Ultrasound

Ultrasound went through a popular phase in the 1980s but has been superseded by MRI. A 7.5 MHz small-parts transducer is used, working across the greater tuberosity with the arm in slight extension. There are three features which demonstrate a full-thickness tear: (1) absence of the cuff layer, (2) a gap in the cuff layer (Fig. 5.19), and (3) focal displacement of the deltoid. Ultrasound scans are reliable and have a sensitivity of 81% and a specificity of 100%. It costs 0.19 of the cost of MRI and is less alarming to the patient. However, it is not as good at showing partial or small tears as it is at showing large tears.

Magnetic resonance imaging

MRI is the investigation of choice in the diagnosis of rotator-cuff tears. However, MRI is very poor if used to diagnose impingement and partial-thickness tears. In a recent study, thirty asymptomatic patients had an MRI of the shoulder. All were reported as abnormal by the radiologist (who was unaware of their clinical lack of history) and some were reported as having partial-thickness tears.

Impingement or tendonitis is manifested by focal areas of increased signal on proton-density images which persist on T2-weighted images. If the changes are not seen on the T2-weighted images then they may be due to an artifact called the 'magic angle effect'.

For full-thickness tears MRI is very sensitive (Fig. 5.20), although not fool-proof. The sensitivity for MRI in full-thickness cuff tears is 91% and specificity 88% compared with arthrography giving a sensitivity of 71% and a specificity of 71%.

Magnetic resonance imaging will not only show discontinuity of the supraspinatus tendon, but will also display fluid in the subacromial bursa (which means there must be a tear). It will also show the quality of residual supraspinatus muscle and whether there is fatty degeneration of the muscle. The distance between the proximal and distal stump of the torn cuff can be estimated from the scan. Intra-articular gadolinium may enhance the performance of MRI in detecting rotator-cuff tears but suffers from being an invasive, and technically more demanding, time consuming study. Patients who clinically have a massive tear, and who are biologically older than 65, should have an MRI to confirm the extent of the tear because if the tear is confirmed as massive and retracted the results of surgery will be poor; in these cases it may be in the patient's interest not to operate.

Arthroscopy

Arthroscopy is the present 'Gold standard' for the diagnosis of both partial-thickness tears and full-thickness tears

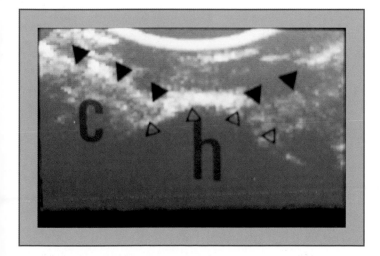

Figure 5.19 – *Ultrasound of a patient with a rotator-cuff tear showing break in line of cuff (with permission from Bunker, Seminars in Orthopaedics, 1987).*

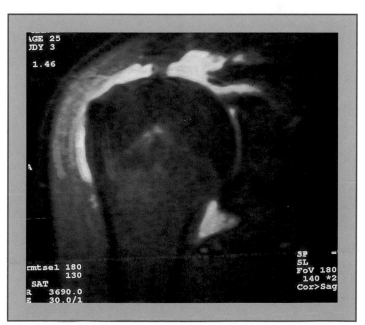

Figure 5.20 – *A MRI scan of a patient with a full-thickness rotator-cuff tear showing tendon discontinuity.*

(Fig. 5.21). Partial-thickness tears can be visualized from the joint surface, and impingement lesions from the bursal side. Full-thickness tears can be seen from both sides. Large tears can be confusing to the uninitiated as the margin may be out of view (Fig 5.22), and the defect may be mistaken for a large rotator interval. Likewise unless the arthroscope is taken up above the long head of the biceps and pushed up to the cuff insertion, a small rim rent can be missed. Bursal endoscopy is very easy in patients with rotator-cuff tears because the bursal wall is thickened and the bursa is prefilled from the joint, making it easy to enter with the arthroscope.

Indications for surgery

The surgeon must understand that treatment should be tailored to the patient. Clearly a massive cuff tear in a young patient should be repaired, but the same cuff tear in the non-dominant arm of an 84-year-old in atrial fibrillation and on warfarin would not be considered for surgery by the wise surgeon! The surgeon must also understand that treatment must be tailored to the society in which the patient lives. Rehabilitation is so important to rotator-cuff surgery that it is folly to spend hours on a difficult repair if the patient will clearly not assist in the rehabilitation programme, or if the environment in which they live prohibits them from complying. The ideal indication for surgical repair of a rotator-cuff tendon is the young, active, thin, fit patient, with a short but classic history of rotator-cuff tear. The size of the tear should be less than the watershed between good and poor results (presently 4 cm). The shape of the tear should be a split which is far easier to repair than a trapezoid tear. There should be minimal retraction and no secondary bone changes. The patient should be intelligent, employed, and determined to get back to work as soon as possible. The patient should have a supportive family to back him up, and access to a good surgeon and physiotherapist. Unfortunately, such a patient is rarely seen, which is why we need to know all the tricks of the trade for dealing with larger, trapezoid, retracted tears with secondary changes.

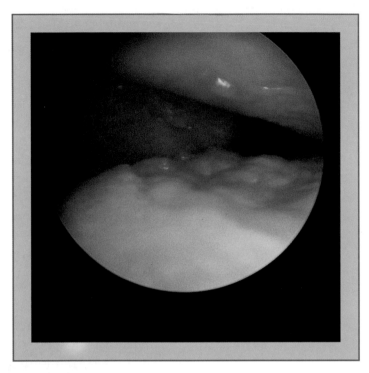

Figure 5.21 – *Arthroscopic view of a small rotator-cuff tear.*

Rotator-cuff repair

Small tears (less than 1 cm)
Approach

Small tears can be approached either arthroscopically, through a mini-open approach or open. Arthroscopic and mini-open techniques are discussed by Professor Ogilvie-Harris in chapter three. In the open technique the Matsen deltoid-on approach is used as for acromioplasty.

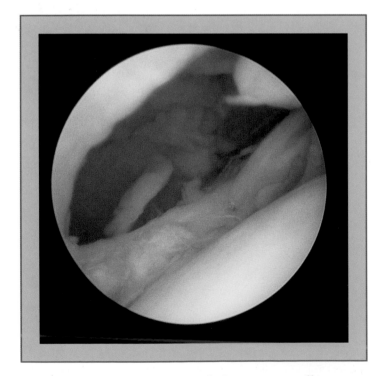

Figure 5.22 – *Arthroscopic view of a large rotator-cuff tear.*

Repair

Repair of such small tears can usually be performed by direct side-to-side repair after edge debridement to viable bleeding tendon margin. Blood is the key to the biology of healing. For this reason it is good practice to make a shallow trough in the bone under the repair to expose the bleeding cancellous bone. The repaired tendon is pulled down on to this area with interosseous sutures or suture anchors. The postoperative regime is as for acromioplasty.

Moderate tears (1–3 cm)

Approach

The Matsen deltoid-on acromioplasty incision is used, as described in the last chapter. An anterior acromioplasty must be performed to protect the repair postoperatively and to prevent further impingement. It is rarely necessary to excise the acromioclavicular joint for access. The acromioclavicular joint should only be excised if it is markedly arthritic. Any osteophytes protruding from the undersurface of the acromioclavicular joint should be excised.

The repair

The repair depends upon the shape of the tear (split, crescent, L shaped or trapezoid). In all cuff repairs there is a sequence that must be adhered to (Table 5.3). The tear is first classified and inspected. The tear may need to be extended to see if there are laminations or joint-side extensions. The novice must be careful not to mistake the bursa for the cuff edge. The edges are then mobilized. Stay-sutures are inserted in the edge of the tear and put under tension to show which structures need to be released. The release will clearly not be extensive for these relatively small tears. The bursa will often need to be mobilized because it thickens, scars and becomes adherent to everything it touches — deltoid,

acromion and coracoid. The coracohumeral ligament may need to be released from the base of the coracoid. This always causes bleeding from the anterosuperior humeral artery, a small artery that travels across the rotator interval on the undersurface of the coracoid. The bone now needs to be prepared to accept the repair. This is essential because the tendon has to be repaired into bleeding cancellous bone. Remember that we are simply replacing the tendon; nature will reattach the tendon to the bone. In order to allow this, a bleeding bed must be created and stitches placed in order to hold the tendon until nature has taken its course. A trough is created, using fine osteotomes (7 mm, Stille), at the anatomical point where the cuff should insert. The medial border of the trough is chamfered so as not to leave a sharp edge to cut into the repaired tendon (Fig. 5.23). There has recently been a study arguing that the supraspinatus tendon can repair as well directly to bone, as into a bone trough. However, this study was on goats and was in surgically divided and immediately repaired tendons, a far cry from the real situation of a 2-year-old retracted

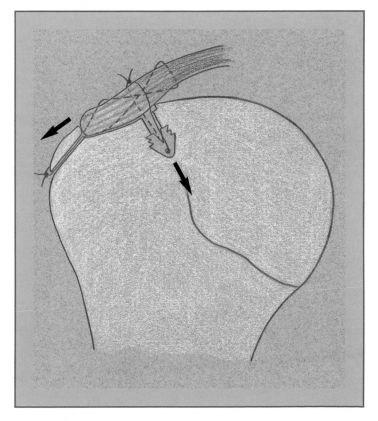

Figure 5.23 – *The edge of the rotator-cuff tear is sutured into a shallow trough in the humeral head sulcus using interosseous suture in line of tendon and suture anchor to hold the tendon down into the trough.*

Table 5.3 The sequence of rotator-cuff repair.
Inspection
Mobilization
Releases
Bone preparation
Repair

mature-cuff tear in man. A split can be sutured side to side. A crescent will be brought fully into the bone trough. An L shaped or reversed L shaped tear will have the base of the L repaired into the trough and the vertical limb side to side. Interosseous tunnels must now be created for the sutures which can be No 1, or No 2 in size. Most authors recommend non-absorbable sutures, but in reality such thick sutures made of absorbable tissue remain present for up to a year, and if the tendon has not repaired by then it never will! The technique of repair should be borrowed from the realm of hand surgery. A modified Kessler or Mason–Allen suture should be placed in the tendon. Drill holes are then made to pass the intra-osseous sutures through the tuberosity. The sutures are taken through the bone tunnels and tied. Gerber (1995) compared nine different methods of repair. Simple and mattress sutures failed at quite low loads (184 N and 269 N). A modified Mason–Allen suture took the tensile strength up to 359 N (Table 5.4). One of the problems encountered at surgery is that the bone of the tuberosity is soft, as it has not been stressed since being disconnected from the tendon, and the sutures can cut out. There are two ways around this problem. Firstly, the bone tunnels can be taken further distally, which gives more bone volume and also brings the suture exit to a point in the bone that has been stressed and therefore is much stronger. In Gerber's experiment the bone was the weakest point, the transosseous tunnel failing at 139 N to 146 N. The alternative is to use a prosthetic patch on the bone through which the suture is passed and over which it is tied (Sward *et al.*, 1992). In Gerber's experiment, using a cortical-like bone augmentation device raised the strength to failure of the bone tunnels up to 329 N. Suture anchors have been used instead of transosseous tunnels, but these are no stronger than bone tunnels, with a pull out strength of 142 N. Burkhart (1995)

suggests putting the suture anchors in at a low angle of incidence, like a tent peg, in order to give increased purchase. It is essential that, after the sutures have been tied, there is no gapping between tendon end and cancellous bone, even with the arm at the side. The bursa is then oversewn across the top of the repair. This has two effects: Firstly it covers the knots and tidies up the repair, and secondly it brings in a rich blood supply.

Closure

A meticulous closure of the deltotrapezius fascia is performed. If there is any weakness of the deltoid origin then it must be repaired through 2 mm drill holes in the acromion.

Large rotator-cuff tears (3–5 cm)

The surgery of large rotator-cuff tears is not for the novice. This type of surgery is challenging and requires a few tricks of the trade.

Indication

There is no point in attempting to repair a large tear in a patient who is biologically over the age of 65. The tissue is too poor, and the motivation and effort needed to rehabilitate are too much for someone over this biological age. Marked atrophy of the cuff muscles, severe weakness of external rotation, and dystrophic muscle with retraction on MRI are all poor prognostic factors. Upward elevation of the humeral head, both clinically and radiologically, are poor prognostic factors. The patient must be made aware of the fact that the final result may be poor and that the rehabilitation is extremely prolonged; if the tear is larger than 4 cm then the result may be poor and the patient is told so. The patient may ask what is meant by 'poor'. The answer is that they should get relief of pain, but that the function of the shoulder may not be improved. If they accept the need for repair on this basis, then any improvement in function is a bonus. The patient must be warned about the length of rehabilitation. A useful phrase for the surgeon to use preoperatively is that for the first 3 months you will wonder why you had the operation. It should then be explained that after this time improvement becomes evident and continues for up to 1 year. A pessimistic prognosis, such as this, is better given to the patient than an over optimistic prediction of outcome. In this way the patient's expectations will not be too high and if a better result is achieved it will present as a bonus to the patient.

Table 5.4 Strength of repair (N).		
Suture	Simple	184
	Mattress	269
	Modified Mason–Allen	359
Bone tunnel		146
Anchor		142

Surgical approach

Many surgeons will approach the massive tear with the standard acromioplasty incision through the bed of the acromioclavicular joint, with the patient lying supine on the operating table in the deckchair position. However, for large tears this is a very tiring position for the surgeon who has to maintain a Cock-Robin position of his own neck throughout the procedure. It also denies access to the posterior aspect of the scapula. For large and massive tears the surgeon needs to keep his options open. Certainly, he will always need to get right up into the supraspinatus fossa. If the tear is larger than expected a saggital scapular osteotomy may be needed to obtain access to the infraspinatus, or a latissimus dorsi transfer may be required. Neither of these options are open if a supine deckchair position has been used. It is preferable therefore to put the patient in the lateral decubitus position, with the head right up at the top of the table. The surgeon stands at the head of the table and looks straight down into the top of the shoulder. This also allows much better access to the back of the shoulder and is less tiring for the surgeon (Fig. 5.24). The skin flaps need to be more extensive than usual, literally 'scalping' the shoulder. The skin flaps are then sutured to the underlying skin in the retracted position, which rids the surgeon of the necessity of self-retaining retractors for the skin flaps. The Matsen deltoid-on approach is again used and is extended to the acromioclavicular joint. The acromioclavicular joint is excised purely for access to the tear. The joint is excised obliquely, in the direction of the supraspinatus muscle, to give access to the muscle belly. The inferior acromioclavicular ligament is then incised to reveal the tendon of supraspinatus. Trapezius is taken down from the acromion and spine of the scapula, exposing the fat pad overlying supraspinatus. The fat pad is divided, ligating the branch of the suprascapular artery which runs within it. This exposes the muscle belly of supraspinatus in the fossa.

Releases. The releases need to be much greater for the large retracted tear (Table 5.5). The bursa is mobilized. The coracohumeral ligament is divided and the rotator interval released. Bigliani *et al.* (1992) stresses the importance of this release and terms it the 'rotator slide'. An internal release must now be made (Zuckerman 1991) by releasing the shoulder-joint capsule from the glenoid starting at the 9 o'clock position and ending at the 3 o'clock position. The distance of the suprascapular

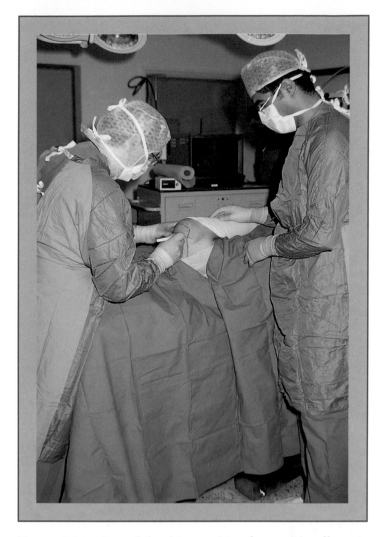

Figure 5.24 – *Lateral decubitus position for rotator-cuff repair. The surgeon stands at the head of the table.*

Table 5.5 The surgical stages in repairing a large rotator-cuff tear.

1 Acromioplasty
2 Acromioclavicular joint excision
3 Rotator-interval slide
4 Spinoglenoid slide
5 Zuckerman internal release

nerve from the edge of the glenoid is 3 cm in the suprascapular fossa and just 2 cm in the infraspinatus fossa. Clearly, any damage to this nerve negates any benefit from the operation. The superior glenohumeral ligament may need to be released to mobilize the anterior slip of the supraspinatus.

Repair. The tendons of the supraspinatus and infraspinatus are mobilized and sequentially released until they can reach the bone trough. Once again the tendon is repaired to bone with intra-osseous sutures, as for a moderate tear. The trough may need to be advanced a few millimetres on to the articular surface itself (Fig. 5.25). Sometimes even this is not enough. Consideration must now be given to tendon transpositions. Once tendon transpositions are needed, the success rate drops off dramatically. They should be avoided if possible. The simplest tendon transposition is that of the anterior supraspinatus to the posterior supraspinatus. In massive tears the head buttonholes upward through the rent, quite literally a boutonnière deformity. The tear occurs 1 cm posterior to the leading edge of the supraspinatus, effectively splitting it in half. Once the tendons have been mobilized as far forwards as possible the anterior strip is released from the tuberosity, forwards to its junction with the subscapularis, and then the release continues into the rotator interval.

The rotator interval is difficult to find because it is contracted and the coracohumeral ligament is contracted, pulling the anterior strip further forwards. The coracohumeral ligament is divided and the whole of the anterior strip is now a rectangular flap. This flap is transposed backward and sutured side to side to the posterior strip. The free end is now sutured into the trough. Sometimes this simple transposition is not enough because the head now tries to buttonhole in front of the anterior strip, through the rotator interval slide. If this occurs then the upper half of subscapularis needs to be advanced and sutured side to side to the anterior strip. Karas and Giachello (1996) caution against the use of such a subscapularis transfer. In his series of 20 patients undergoing subscapularis transfer 19 had an improvement in pain, but concern was centred on the poor postoperative ability to elevate the arm. Two patients had worse elevation after surgery than before. The more demanding transposition is to release the infraspinatus posteriorly and the subscapularis anteriorly, bringing the two together as an inverted T by the method of McLaughlin and Asherman (1951). The results are generally less favourable if a transposition technique has to be used (Ellman, 1993). The long head of the biceps is often hypertrophied and subluxed from its groove. This subluxation reduces the effectiveness of the biceps as a head depressor. It is important to try to replace the biceps in its groove (which may need to be deepened and widened), and to keep it there with a sling of tissue, so that it is still effective and not tenodesed. Occasionally it may appear attractive to use the long head of the biceps in the repair, but this tenodesis restricts the range of postoperative motion. This should be avoided if possible. Other grafts have been used in the past, such as fascia lata (McLaughlin and Asherman1951, Bateman 1972), but most surgeons today prefer advancement techniques, and shun grafts. The need for a graft is a matter of desperation. There is debate over what should be done to the bursa. Some authors recommend excision as it gets in the way. However, Uhtoff *et al.* (1991) stress the importance of the bursa as a source of a blood supply to the repairing cuff. Be as sparing with the bursa as possible.

Closure. Closure is more demanding due to the extensions which have been made. The inferior acromioclavicular ligament is reattached to drill holes on the acromion; the trapezius is reattached to drill holes on the scapular spine and acromion. The clavicle is stabilized, using the coraco-acromial ligament, by way of the Weaver–Dunn technique; finally the superior acromioclavicular ligament and flaps are sutured together. Subcutaneous sutures are placed and then a subcuticular stitch to the skin. Often with such a tear the arm should be rested in a degree of abduction. A true aeroplane splint is very difficult for the patient to manage (have you ever tried to get into a small toilet with your arm in an aeroplane splint, or tried to sleep in one?). A 40° foam-wedge is relatively comfortable, takes the stress off the repair, and warns the physiotherapist that this is a large tear and that they should seek further instructions and protect the repair for a greater length of time.

Massive tears (greater than 5 cm)

Tears greater than 5 cm are often termed irreparable. The indications for repair have to be strict. Such a tear should have recently occurred in a previously normal shoulder; the patient should be active, young (under a physiological age of 60 years) and severely disabled from the tear. The MRI scan should show retraction to the rim of the glenoid, but with a good quality tendon-edge and a bulky, good-quality muscle. This patient only has one chance of surgery for this shoulder, and if you are repairing less than one rotator-cuff per month you should contact your local shoulder specialist. Each

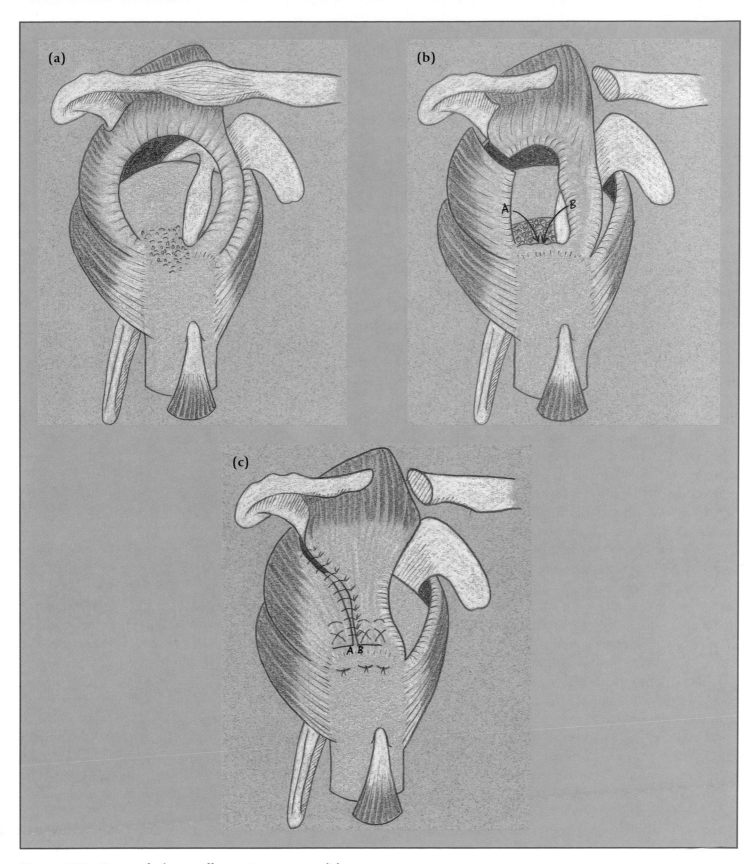

Figure 5.25 – *Repair of a large cuff tear using a rotator slide.*

shoulder specialist will have his or her own tricks of the trade for repair of such a tear. The key to the repair is exposure. Most surgeons would approach such a tear with the patient in the deckchair position. The first debatable point is whether to preserve the coraco-acromial ligament. If there has been any delay in the surgery the head will have migrated upwards, and the only structure preserving the position of the head is the coraco-acromial ligament. If the ligament is sacrificed then there is nothing to prevent further superior migration of the head; if there is any residual cuff dysfunction (and there always is) the patient may be worse than they were prior to surgery. Lazarus *et al.* (1994) have shown how excision of the coraco-acromial ligament, in a laboratory setting, allows the humeral head to escape from the coraco-acromial arch, and stress that the loss of this barrier may have a substantial effect in rotator-cuff surgery. Moorman *et al.* (1996) stress the importance of this ligament and conclude that: far from being a vestigial organ, it is a vital stabilizing structure, which should be judiciously spared. Clearly, the ligament has to be taken down but this should be done in a Z lengthening manner so that, on closure, it can be repaired side to side. For massive tears the oblique excision of the acromioclavicular joint should be performed, as for large tears. The releases have to be extensive. In this situation, not only does the coracohumeral ligament have to be taken down from the coracoid, but a contracture also develops around the spine of the scapula where the spinoglenoid ligament (inferior transverse scapular ligament) attaches to the spine. Release at this point has to be very carefully performed, so as not to damage the suprascapular nerve. Otherwise, the external and internal releases are the same as for large tears. The author prefers to use a scapular osteotomy for exposure of such massive tears (Fig. 5.26). The patient is placed in the lateral decubitus position which allows access to the back as well as the front of the joint. The spine of the scapula is split with a sagittal-saw cut at its junction with the acromion. At the end of the procedure it is replaced with a tension-band technique. In this approach the osteotomy is in the saggital plane which allows access to the infraspinatus, whereas the Kessel approach uses a coronal osteotomy of the acromion, which only allows access to the supraspinous fossa. The sagittal-scapular osteotomy allows an excellent view of infraspinatus and teres minor. The coraco-acromial ligament is not damaged

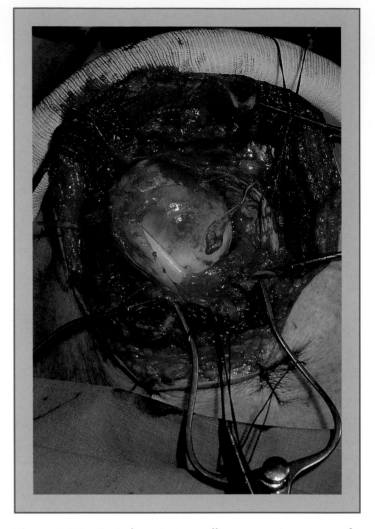

Figure 5.26 – *Scapular osteotomy allows a massive exposure for repair of a massive rotator-cuff tear.*

during this approach but is Z lengthened and repaired side to side in the closure. The acromion with its attached deltoid is folded outward giving a massive exposure.

Repair

Once the three muscle margins have been isolated, released, and advanced on stay-sutures, it is time to consider the repair. If the inferior capsule has tightened, such that it is difficult to depress the head, then the inferior capsule should be stretched or torn with a manipulation.

The long head of biceps is usually found to have subluxed out of its groove, and is defunctioned. The vital first step is to make a new sulcus posterior to the normal sulcus position. The tendon is then pulled into its new groove and held in that position, and transfixed with a temporary stout Kirschner wire. Interosseous sutures are then inserted to hold, but not to tenodese, the tendon into its new sulcus. The shoulder is then held in a position of 70° abduction by an assistant whilst the repair is performed. A trough is made and the repair performed using a combination of interosseous sutures and anchors. If closure is not possible consideration should be given to a latissimus transfer.

Latissimus transfer

Gerber (1988) has described the technique of latissimus-dorsi transfer in the irreparable tear. When there is a massive tear, leading to upward migration of the head on attempted elevation of the arm, and loss of external-rotation control there may be a place for this transfer. The details of this procedure are given in Gerber's original paper. The technique is similar to the L'Episcopo transfer in obstetric brachial-plexus palsy. The latissimus is exposed through a posterior incision. Teres major is retracted so that the insertion of the latissimus can be seen and released from the humerus. The freed tendon is then tunnelled under the deltoid and acromion so that it emerges in the superior cuff-repair incision. The tendon is then sutured to the posterosuperior cuff, in as tight a position as possible, or actually used to bridge the remaining hole in the cuff. (Fig. 5.27). Clearly, this transfer is only used occasionally and, although Gerber reported on the results of the first 4 of his 14 cases as comparing favourably with other techniques, there is no technique which is going to give excellent results in this end-stage massive tear. Massive tears will require some form of abduction brace for 6 weeks postoperatively. Bigliani *et al.* (1992) reported the results of repair in 61 patients with massive tears (over 5 cm in one direction). Overall 85% had satisfactory results. Results varied according to the size of the tear and the age of the patient. Tears of all four tendons were satisfactory in only 50% of cases, whereas tears involving the supraspinatus and the anterior edge of the infraspinatus were all satisfactory. Patients under 60 years of age had results which were satisfactory in 89% of cases, but patients over 60 were satisfactory in 82% of cases. These results are from one of the best shoulder units in the world, the unit founded by Neer, and it is unlikely that the occasional surgeon would get results anything like as good as those of Bigliani. These tears should only be repaired by an experienced surgeon working in a good unit.

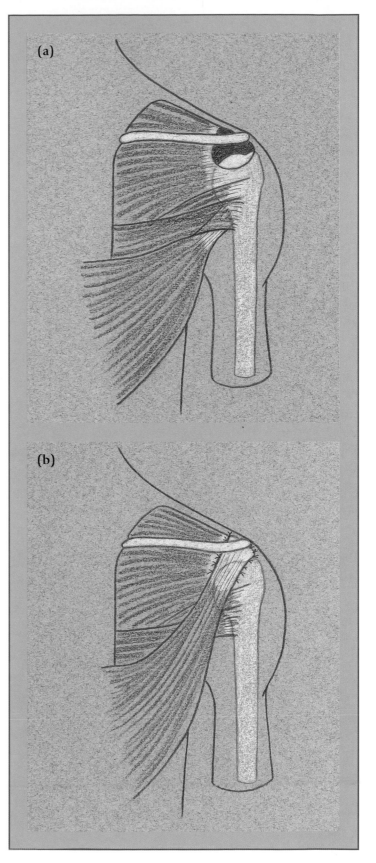

Figure 5.27 – *Latissimus dorsi transfer for massive tear of the rotator cuff.*

Complications

Deep infection

Deep infection is fortunately rare, but when it occurs is a major disaster. The patient must be returned to theatre immediately and the cuff repair exposed. Usually it will have come apart and the whole area will need swabbing, debridement, thorough lavage, immediate re-repair and closure over drains with antibiotic control and splintage. Many surgeons give prophylactic antibiotics on induction for rotator-cuff repairs. Whilst this is not strictly necessary for small and moderate tears, any patient undergoing cuff repair and requiring over 1 hour in surgery should be given prophylactic intravenous antibiotics.

Deltoid detachment

This is a rare complication (Fig. 5.28). Some authors feel that the Matsen deltoid-on approach gives a weak closure and may lead to detachment. Using the medial modification we have not found this to be a problem. In some small ladies the flap may become exremely thin and if this is the case then either a purse string around this weak area or an intra-osseous suture through the anterior acromion needs to be employed. Ideally, this complication should not be allowed to occur in the first place and closure of the deltoid should be conducted with meticulous care.

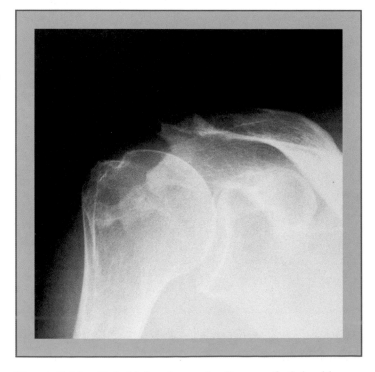

Figure 5.28 – *Deltoid detachment leading to a flail shoulder.*

Failure of the repair

Bigliani looked at the causes of failure in 31 patients who had undergone a previous repair. Ninety-seven percent had a massive tear and 90% were still impinging. The poor prognostic features were lateral acromionectomy, deltoid detachment and poor-quality cuff.

Postoperative protocols

There are three phases to the rehabilitation protocol. The first phase is protective. The goals of the protective phase are to regain movement and prevent muscle wasting, whilst protecting the rotator-cuff repair and the deltoid closure. The amount and duration of protection are dependent upon the size of the repair. For a small tear (less than 1 cm), the tear can be ignored and the patient follows a routine acromioplasty regime, as in the previous chapter. For a moderate tear (1–3 cm) the supraspinatus has to be protected until it is repaired to bone, a process that takes 6 weeks. The other muscles of the cuff are unaffected and can be used straight away, even using resisted TheraBand exercises. A large tear (3–5 cm) will usually affect the infraspinatus as well as the supraspinatus; protection will have to be greater, and for a judicious 8 weeks rather than 6 weeks. Massive tears are one-offs. The treatment really has to be tailored individually to the tear and the patient, but the protective phase will often stretch out to 12 weeks. Remember that the protocols are guidelines for patient, surgeon and physiotherapist. If the patient is clearly able to cope with the current protocol, don't let it hold them up. If they are having difficult with the protocol, look for a reason; and only if there is no apparent reason push them up to speed.

Protective phase rehabilitation (Phase 1)

Moderate tears (1–3 cm)
The protective phase lasts up to 6 weeks. The sling is worn by day and night for 3 weeks.

Home exercises
(i) Elbow-extension exercises, from day one, 20 repetitions three times a day.
(ii) Pendulum exercises, from day one, gentle, starting with inner range only (arc 30° building under physiotherapist control to 150° by 6 weeks).
(iii) Rotation exercises. Since infraspinatus and subscapularis have not been interfered with these can start immediately.

(iv) Forearm fist, wrist, twist exercises to 3 weeks, whilst in sling.

(v) Shoulder shrug and bracing exercises.

Supervised exercises. Closed-chain only. The concept of closed-chain exercises in the arm requires explanation. Closed chain is usually applied to lower limb exercises, where the foot is in contact with the ground, or fixed. This is, of course, the usual function of the leg. The usual mode of action of the upper limb in contrast is open-chain, the hand moving through space unsupported. If one took the strict definition of closed-chain and applied it to the arm it would mean exercises where the hand is fixed to the ground, such as a press up. This strict definition is not applicable to rotator-cuff exercises, what we mean here is the avoidance of open-chain movement, the hand must always be supported, either by the physiotherapist, the patient, a pulley or the wall. (i) Assisted elevation. (ii) Pulley exercises. (iii) TheraBand resisted internal- and external-rotation exercises. Make sure that a book is held clamped under the armpit to ensure that the deltoid and supraspinatus are relaxed.

Large tears (3–5 cm)
The protective phase should last for 8 weeks. Smaller tears of 3 cm may be treated in a sling for the first 3 weeks by day and night. Larger tears up to 5 cm will need to be in an abduction brace for the first 3 weeks, then weaning in and out of sling over the next 2 weeks.

Home exercises. Home exercises are consequently very restricted. (i) Forearm exercises, fist, wrist, twist. (ii) Shoulder shrugs and bracing.

Physiotherapist supervised exercises. These should be started under supervision of a physiotherapist and then performed at home when the physiotherapist allows. (i) Elbow-extension exercises; depends upon whether the biceps has been relocated in its sulcus, if so then elbow extension should be avoided for the first 3 weeks and then started under a physiotherapist's supervision. (ii) Pendulum exercises should be avoided for first 3 weeks, then start gentle supervised inner-arc regime. (iii) Active-rotation exercise should be avoided for 6 weeks. The physiotherapist may have the patient do passive inner range rotation. (iv) Closed-chain assisted elevation from 6 weeks. (v) Pulley work starts at 6 weeks. (vi) TheraBand internal

rotation may start at 6 weeks, external rotation should be protected throughout Phase 1 and should only start at 8 weeks.

Massive tears
The protective phase lasts up to 12 weeks. The arm is protected in an aeroplane splint or foam-wedge for the first 6 weeks. During this time forearm exercises, shoulder shrugs and bracing should be performed. At 6 weeks elbow extensions, pendulums and passive rotations are started. Closed-chain exercise begins at 8 weeks under a physiotherapist's control.

Strengthening (Phase 2)

The goals of Phase 2 are to regain and improve strength around the shoulder and to improve neuromuscular control. Entry criteria to this level are a passive range of two-thirds normal in every direction, and secure healing of the cuff to the tuberosities, which should have occurred by 6 weeks in moderate tears, 8 weeks in large tears and 12 weeks in massive tears. Closed-chain exercises are continued. The requirement for starting open-chain exercises is that the head remains centred on the glenoid on elevation. If the head is still subluxing superiorly then open chain exercises should not be started, as they are only provocative and will increase pain. Clearly patients with a moderate tear will enter phase 2 at around 6 weeks, patients with large tears at 8–10 weeks and patients with massive tears at 12–14 weeks. However, when they enter this phase the cuff is at the same level of functional recovery and now the exercise regime unites. The following exercises are added to those used in Phase 1: (i) TheraBand isotonic strengthening exercises to the subscapularis, infraspinatus, supraspinatus/deltoid and biceps. (ii) Scapular-strengthening exercises. Corner pushups and then progress to floor pushups. (iii) Dumbbells, starting at 3 lbs, depending on patient's build. External rotation in lateral decubitus. Internal rotation whilst supine. Prone elevation and abduction Forward elevation whilst sitting. Isolated biceps curls. (iv) Isometric TheraBand (black/silver strong). (v) Proprioceptive neuromuscular facilitation. This form of exercise uses specific skilled sensory input from the clinician to facilitate certain patterns of movement. The common pattern used in the shoulder is the D2 flexion–extension pattern. These techniques are very hands on and require great physiotherapeutic skills.

Return to work and sport (Phase 3)

The goals of this phase are return to work. Full activities of daily living and sport. Entry requirements to this level are: full range of movement, no pain or tenderness, and the blessing of both physiotherapist and surgeon. Entry to this level will commonly be 20 weeks for moderate tears, 32 weeks for large tears and 40–52 weeks for massive tears. (i) Capsular stretching. (ii) Aggressive strengthening. (iii) High-speed, high-energy strengthening exercises are added to the Phase 2 regime under physiotherapy supervision. (iv) Return to recreational sport (golf, breast-stroke swimming, cycling, underhand raquet sports). Remember that the average age of these patients is 60–65 years and their need for sport is recreational alone.

The concept of partial repair and debridement for massive irreparable tears

What can be done for the patient of 70 who has an old massive rotator-cuff tear with tendon retraction and severe muscle wasting? The first thing to realize is that any form of surgery will have imperfect results. It may be better to treat the patient conservatively. This does not mean neglecting the patient, but there are several simple ways in which the patient can help themselves, or can be helped by an occupational therapist. Patients tend to need help in four critical areas.

Dressing

Patients with massive-cuff tears can not pull clothing over their heads. The solution is for them to wear loose-fitting clothes with front fastenings. Many patients have already worked this out and attend the shoulder clinic with button-up shirts and cardigans. Loops sewn into the clothes, or the use of a dressing stick may help. Secondly, they are unable to pull up pants, tights or trousers. These movements can be achieved with the arms adducted or by pulling up the other side. Loops sewn into the clothes are again helpful. Putting on a coat is always difficult. This may be made easier by using a dressing stick or hanging the coat on a low small hook, dressing the arms first and then bending the head and shoulders to place the jacket on the back.

Personal care

Wiping the bottom can be made easier by the use of a washer wiper, or installing a bidet with drier. Washing under the arms can be helped with an angled sponge. Drying the arms and back can be eased with a body drier. A bracket to hold a hair drier on the wall can be used to dry the hair.

Domestic activities

All equipment in the kitchen should be rearranged at bench level, or brought down out of the wall cupboards. High electric sockets should be re-sited at bench level. Saucepans should only be filled a little way and saucepans with two handles should be bought. Lever taps may be fitted. A small lightweight jug should be used to fill the kettle instead of filling the kettle itself. A kettle or teapot tipper should be used to pour boiling water or tea. A lightweight iron should be used and old fashioned pull-up washing lines installed, otherwise a static low line with washing post should be used. Newspapers should be read by placing them on the kitchen table instead of trying to hold them up at eye level. A wooden bookrest can be used for books.

Driving

Patients should be advised to change their car for one with power steering and an automatic gearbox.

These are just a few suggestions and patients may need to be assessed individually by an occupational therapist. Surgery is then reserved for patients in severe pain who can not cope with analgesia, steroid injection and adaptations to the home. For these patients consideration should be given to debridement or partial repair or else they should be treated as a patient with cuff arthropathy.

The concept of debridement came about when a series of patients in whom the shoulder had been explored, but the tear found to be irrepairable were reviewed. A debridement was carried out, and to the surgeon's and patient's surprise pain was markedly reduced. The theoretical basis of this effect is that it is not the tear that causes the pain, because a tear is only a hole, it is an empty space, it is thin air, it has no nerves and therefore can not cause pain. Theoretically, then, it must be the edges of the tear that cause the pain, either due to entrapment of the edges, or due to inflammation, or synovitis. Thus if the edges are debrided so that they can not impinge, get caught, or become inflamed the pain may be reduced. However, a word of warning. There have now been several prospective studies of debridement versus repair, and repair wins out every time. The message therefore is to repair the tear and only if this is totally impossible to consider debridement. A second word of warning. The coraco-acromial ligament may be the only structure holding the humeral head under the coraco-acromial arch and you dispense with it at your peril. Patients may be made far worse if the coraco-acromial ligament is removed because the head may sublux out of the orbit of the coraco-acromial arch and end up under the skin, leaving the patient severely disabled and with a flail arm. If debridement is to be carried out, Z-tenotomize the coraco-acromial ligament and repair it during surgical closure. Some surgeons advocate partial repair of the cuff. This means repairing a bit of the cuff at the front or the back, so that the forces across the joint are balanced and act to centre the head on the glenoid, rather than sublux the head either anteriorly or posteriorly. This method remains unproven.

Cuff-tear arthropathy

The end-stage of the spectrum of rotator-cuff disease is cuff-tear arthropathy. In this disease the rotator-cuff is massively torn, the humeral head and glenoid are arthritic (Fig. 5.29), the head is subluxed upward to articulate with the undersurface of the acromion, and there are secondary erosive changes to the humeral head and to the glenoid. Fortunately only 4% of patients with

cuff tears go on to develop cuff-tear arthropathy. What can be done for these patients? Unfortunately we do not know the answer to this question. Sit 10 shoulder surgeons in a room and they will all give a different answer. So what are the options?

Conservative treatment

This is the most sensible option. Explain the situation to the patient, and let them know that we do not have all the answers and that treatment may make them worse, rather than better. Once again analgesics, steroid injections and adaptations to aid dressing, personal care, cooking, cleaning and driving may improve the patients situation.

Hemiarthroplasty

This is favoured by some. A large humeral head is inserted which articulates with the undersurface of the acromion (Fig. 5.30). The coraco-acromial ligament

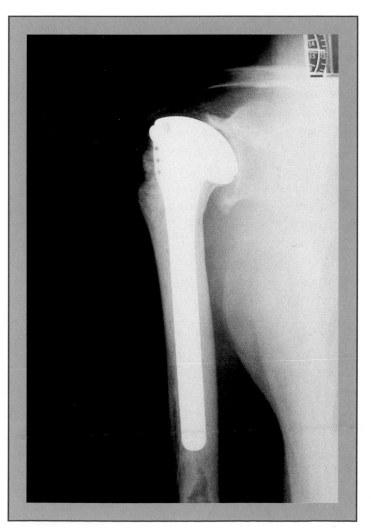

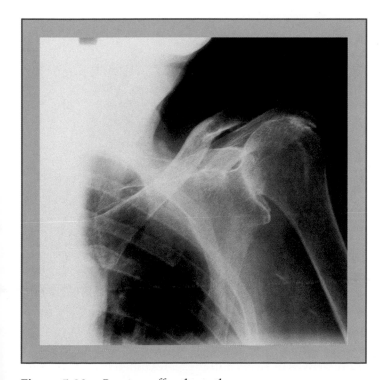

Figure 5.29 – *Rotator-cuff arthropathy.*

Figure 5.30 – *Hemiarthroplasty for cuff-tear arthropathy.*

must not be excised. Results are poor but with the occasional patient who is improved from the point of view of pain. Function is not improved.

Bipolar hemiarthroplasty

This is a variation on the hemiarthroplasty theme. The aim is to have a hemiarthroplasty which moves somewhat better.

Constrained total shoulder replacement

The old lady, aged over 80, with low demands and cuff-tear arthropathy, who has severe pain, may be one of the very few indications for considering a constrained prosthesis (Fig. 5.31). Function should be better than with a hemiarthroplasty. The down-side is that a cuff-deficient shoulder will impose massive forces upon the glenoid and lead to early loosening. The surgeon employing this technique should realize that, from the day of implantation, a race starts as to which should expire first, the patient or the prosthesis.

Fusion

Shoulder fusion is not easy in the frail, octogenarian lady with osteopenic bone. The main worry is that the implants inserted to stabilize the fusion — the plates and screws — may cut out of the soft bone before union has been achieved. Because of this worry a plaster spica is used as an adjunct to the internal fixation; however, octogenarians and plaster spicas for the shoulder do not get on well together. However, if fusion is achieved then pain relief is predictable. The patient remains at risk of fracture at the end of the plate on the humerus (Fig. 5.32), which is a stress riser, between the strong plate and the osteoporotic humeral bone.

Summary

There is a definite and specific pattern of rotator cuff tearing. The tear always starts at the insertion of the supraspinatus tendon, 7 mm behind its strong anterior leading edge where the strong fibres of the central bipennate tendon meet the weaker fibres of its posterior tendon sheet.

As the tear progresses the humeral head boutonnieres upwards through the rent in supraspinatus and the anterior and posterior borders of the tear are stretched out and contract up. The strong anterior tendon band of

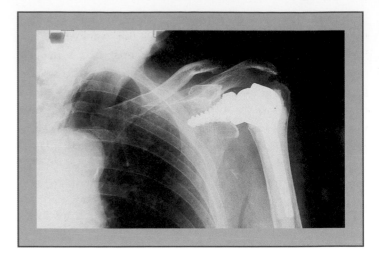

Figure 5.31 – *Constrained shoulder replacement for a cuff-deficient shoulder.*

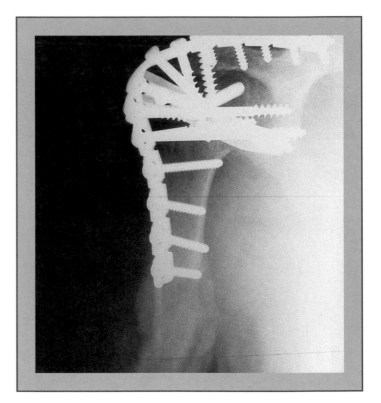

Figure 5.32 – *A fracture has occurred below the plate following shoulder fusion for cuff arthropathy.*

supraspinatus is pushed forwards by the head and pulled forward by the contracture of the coracohumeral ligament. The pulley of long head of biceps may tear (the hidden lesion of Walch), allowing long head of biceps tendon to sublux, and tears to occur in the superior fibres of supscapularis as they enter the lesser tuberosity.

The posterior rim of the tear is pushed backwards by the ascending humeral head, and pulled backwards by infraspinatus and the spinoglenoid ligament.

Repair of the tear needs a sequence of manoeuvres starting with an adequate exposure, then inspection of the tear, followed by mobilization of the cuff edges, release of the contractures, preparation of the bone, reattachment of the tendon using bone tunnels and suture anchor systems and finally a closure which allows early rehabilitation.

The surgery of large cuff tears is one of the most demanding areas of shoulder surgery. There is a massive body of ongoing research in this area and significant advances are sure to be seen over the next decade both in the engineering and biology of repair.

CHAPTER 6

The young sportsman with traumatic recurrent dislocation

T. Bunker

Introduction

The remarkable thing about the shoulder is not that it should dislocate but that it should ever remain located!

The shoulder is the most mobile joint in the body, yet it can toss a caber, lift a small car, accelerate a ball from nought to one hundred miles an hour and then decelerate to zero, and usually it remains located. Quite a feat for a joint that has minimal bony constraint and somewhat flimsy ligaments.

Classification

There is some confusion over the classification of shoulder dislocation. Any classification is only a method of transferring information from one surgeon to another in the most concise, precise and practical way. In terms of dislocation, the surgeon needs the answers to five questions: (1) When did the dislocation occur?, (2) How did it occur?, (3) Which way did it dislocate?, (4) Why did it dislocate?, and (5) How far does it dislocate? (Table 6.1).

When did the dislocation occur?

If the shoulder has just dislocated, then clearly this is an acute dislocation. If the dislocation occurred more than 48 hours before, and remains dislocated, it is termed a neglected or locked dislocation. If the shoulder has dislocated and been reduced on a number of occasions this is termed recurrent dislocation.

How did it occur?

Most dislocations are the result of trauma — a heavy tackle during contact sports, or a heavy fall. These

Table 6.1 Classification of instability.		
When?	Onset	Acute
		Neglected or locked
		Recurrent
How?	Onset	Traumatic
		Atraumatic
		Voluntary
Where?	Direction	Anterior
		Posterior
		Multidirection
Why?	Pathology	Torn loose
		Born loose
How far?		Dislocation
		Subluxation

shoulders are literally torn loose. This is a traumatic dislocation. If the shoulder has pre-existing disease (commonly abnormal ligamentous laxity which may be associated with generalized laxity, more rarely abnormalities of version, and extremely rarely primary glenoid dysplasia) then it may dislocate for the first time with minimal trauma. These shoulders are born loose (Fig. 6.1). This is termed atraumatic dislocation. Often loose shoulders will reduce of their own accord, quite unlike the acute traumatic dislocation, which nearly always needs to be reduced under sedation or anaesthetic. It is essential that the surgeon recognizes that there is a very important difference in the

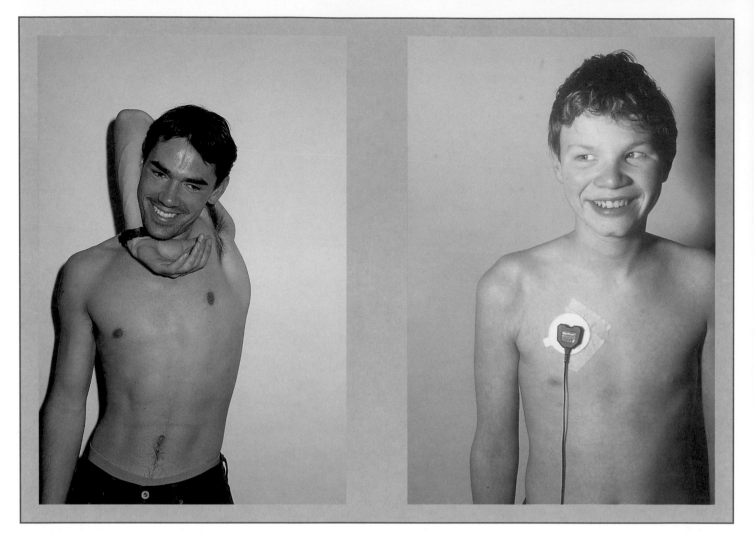

Figure 6.1 – *The 'orang-utan' sign of shoulder instability. The patient is able to touch his ipsilateral ear with his hand. This demonstrates that the shoulder is lax.*

Figure 6.2 – *Voluntary dislocation. This patient is able to use his latissimus dorsi to inferiorly dislocate the shoulder at will.*

presentation, pathology and associations of traumatic and atraumatic dislocation.

There is a very special group of dislocations which occur without any trauma at all and these are the voluntary dislocations, sometimes called the habitual dislocations. Voluntary dislocation occurs in a child who has a loose shoulder joint and learns that they can use their own muscles to pull the shoulder joint out of its socket for secondary gain (Fig. 6.2). Usually this starts as a party trick to frighten their peers, thus gaining power over them. It may be used to gain power over parents who fuss around when the shoulder dislocates. It may even be used to gain power over the medical profession, who even give anaesthetics to reduce the shoulder. Beware of the voluntary dislocator!

Patients with recurrent voluntary dislocation can dislocate at will by using pectoralis major or latissimus dorsi muscles. These muscles can be felt to power-up, when the examiner feels the anterior or posterior axillary folds, as the patient dislocates the shoulder.

Which way did it dislocate?

The vast majority (97%) of shoulder dislocations occur in an anterior direction. This is recognized both clinically, because the humeral head is medialized, and can be seen and felt in front of the scapula, and because radiographs are easy to interpret showing the dislocation. In 2% of dislocations the humeral head dislocates in a posterior direction. It is less easily detected clinically than are dislocations occurring in an anterior direction because the head is not medialized, the deformity is not as noticeable, and the clinical signs of a fullness behind the shoulder are more subtle, particularly if the patient is obese or very muscular. In addition to this, the anteroposterior (AP) radiograph may be interpreted incorrectly, and if a lateral radiograph is not taken the dislocation may be missed. Such dislocations may occur during epileptic seizures. Unfortunately, such dislocations are all too often missed. It should be hospital policy throughout the world that every patient with a suspected dislocation must have a lateral radiograph as well as an AP radiograph taken, even if it is not requested. This is a classic diagnostic trap which causes untold misery, not only to the poor patient, but also to the unwary junior doctor and their insurance company.

Even rarer is the inferior dislocation, the so-called subluxio erecta (Fig. 6.3). It is unlikely that the reader will ever witness a superior dislocation, which always involves a fracture of the acromion, but a few cases have been reported in the world literature.

Why does the shoulder dislocate?

This question really applies to recurrent dislocation. In the acute episode it is clearly the force applied to the shoulder which makes it dislocate, but in the recurrent situation the surgeon wants to know what has weakened the shoulder and so made it prone to dislocation with minor force. This involves understanding the pathology of recurrent dislocation; if the shoulder surgeon can identify the essential lesion that has weakened the shoulder, and consequently made it prone to recurrent dislocation, he or she is in a position to repair that lesion.

Matsen has applied acronyms to the two most common forms of recurrent dislocations, the traumatic form TUBS and the atraumatic form AMBRI. The acronym TUBS means that the dislocation was caused by *Trauma*, occurs in only one direction (*Unidirectional*) which is normally anterior, the pathology is a *Bankart* lesion, and the patient requires *Surgery* in the form of a Bankart repair. These patients are 'torn loose.'

Conversely AMBRI means that the dislocation occurred with only minor trauma *(Atraumatic)*, that because the shoulder is so loose it may dislocate from the socket in any direction (*Multidirectional*), that often the asymptomatic shoulder is also loose *(Bilateral)*, that the treatment of choice is *Rehabilitation*, and that only if rehabilitation fails to cure the patient should surgery be considered in the form of an *Inferior capsular shift*. These patients are 'born loose'.

TUBS and AMBRI (torn loose and born loose) are the two ends of the spectrum of antero inferior dislocation and many people will have an element of each (Fig. 6.4). Patients with recurrent posterior dislocation will drop out of joint posteriorly if the arm is internally rotated and elevated. By 30° of elevation the shoulder is already dislocated and can be reduced with a 'clonk', the shoulder equivalent of Ortolani's sign.

How far does the shoulder dislocate?

The final piece of information we need is how far the shoulder dislocates. Is this a full dislocation or is it almost a dislocation, in other words is the shoulder subluxing? These patients never dislocate fully, but they do experience shoulder pain, often a feeling of insecurity and neurological symptoms such as the arm feeling heavy or 'dead'. Subluxation is sometimes referred to as 'dead-arm syndrome'.

This chapter is dedicated to the young sportsman with traumatic recurrent dislocation (TUBS) and the following chapter by Professor Wallace will be dedicated to the young girl with atraumatic dislocation.

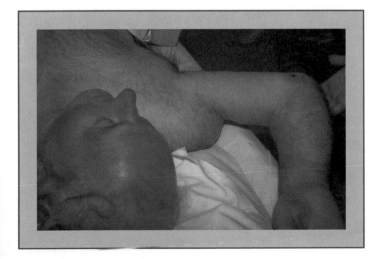

Figure 6.3 – *Subluxio erecta. This is a true inferior dislocation of the joint.*

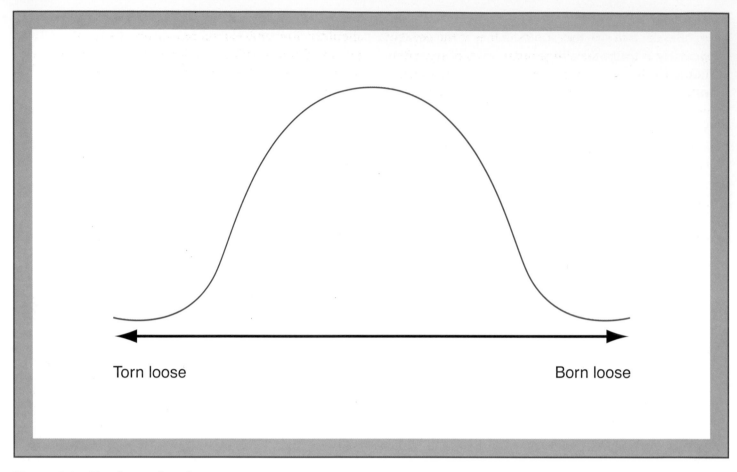

Figure 6.4 – *Torn loose to born loose.*

The essential lesion of recurrent dislocation

The essential lesion — the cause of recurrence — was the 'Holy Grail' sought by many surgeons during the late 19th century and the first half of the 20th century. Broca and Hartmann (1890), and Perthes (1906), recognized that detachment of the anterior capsule from the glenoid was found in association with dislocation of the shoulder. It was Bankart who popularized this concept, and the lesion has come to be known as the Bankart lesion. Bankart suggested that the detachment of the anterior capsule from the glenoid, with or without detachment of the glenoid labrum, was the essential lesion of recurrent shoulder dislocation. However, we now understand that the Bankart lesion is not a single lesion, but that there are a cluster of similar lesions. We also understand that the Bankart lesion is not the only lesion, but just the commonest lesion associated with recurrent dislocation (Table 6.2). Congenital laxity,

Table 6.2 The pathology of dislocation.

Capsule	Bankart lesions
	Stretch in continuity
	Congenital laxity
	Wide rotator interval
Glenoid	Bony Bankart
	Ideburg-I fracture
	Crevassing
LHB	SLAP tear
Labrum	Bankart tear
	Posterior labral tear
Humerus	Tear ligament insertion
	Fractured greater tuberosity
	Hill–Sachs lesion
Rotator cuff	Tear supraspinatus
	Subscapularis avulsion

traumatic stretching of the capsule, osseous lesions, avulsion at the point of insertion as well as at the point of origin of the glenohumeral ligaments, tears of secondary restraints and associated superior labrum anteroposterior (SLAP) lesions are all found with recurrent dislocation. There is no essential lesion for dislocating shoulders but there are several factors that may lead to recurrence. Not all shoulder dislocations are due to an identical cause, nor should they be treated identically.

The essential lesions: theory and fact

Many factors contribute to the stability of the shoulder. These can be classified as physical restraints, dynamic restraints and static restraints.

Physical restraints

The physical restraints act to keep the shoulder located when at rest. They are the reason why, even under anaesthetic, the joint does not fall apart until the capsule is opened or great force is applied.

Atmospheric pressure

We take atmospheric pressure for granted but it is a very powerful force, a force so strong that it powered the industrial revolution. The forerunner of James Watt's steam engine was Newcomen's atmospheric engine of 1705. Newcomen's engine had a vertical cylinder containing a piston, which was counterbalanced by a weight. Steam was introduced into the cylinder below the piston, which then rose to the top of the cylinder on its counterweight. When the piston reached the top of the cylinder it tripped a valve, which sprayed a jet of cold water into the cylinder. This condensed the steam, creating a partial vacuum below the piston, and atmospheric pressure, acting on the top surface of the piston, powered it back down, creating the power-stroke of the engine.

Humphrey in 1858 described an experiment on the hip joint to show how atmospheric pressure held it together. He stated 'The articular surfaces cannot be held in apposition by the ligaments, in as much as they must be loose...to permit the movement of the joint...Atmospheric pressure is the real power...One convincing experiment...bore a hole in the acetabulum... and the joint drops apart by half an inch'.

The same experiment has been performed on the shoulder (Kumar & Balasubramaniam 1985) who showed that the shoulder subluxed after percutaneous puncture of the capsule (Fig. 6.5). Of course these experiments were performed in the cadaver and the conditions used do not occur in reality. Air arthrograms do not lead to subluxation in the conscious patient, showing that the most important stabilizers are the muscles — the dynamic stabilizers — which we will consider later.

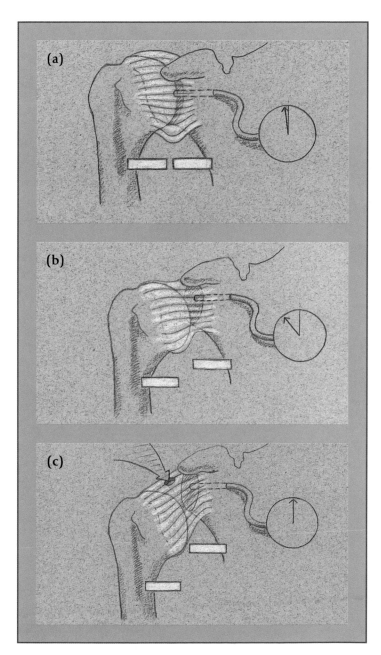

Figure 6.5 – *The effects of atmosphere. Balasubramanium's experiment: when the cadaver capsule is intact the shoulder is located by atmospheric pressure alone (a); however, when the capsule is vented the shoulder drops out of joint (c).*

Suction effect

The labrum acts like a plunger which has a suction effect upon the head. This acts in a similar way to a plumber's plunger which he uses to clear a blocked sink.

Adhesion–cohesion

Adhesion–cohesion is the term given for the forces which act between two smooth surfaces with a liquid film between them. Dry glass-slides are easy to separate, but wet glass-slides are vey difficult to separate. All synovial joints are held together by the physical restraint of adhesion–cohesion.

Glenoid version

There is great controversy as to whether abnormal glenoid version is associated with instability. Some studies suggest that it is whereas others suggest that it is not. Measuring glenoid version from plain radiographs is highly inaccurate, and may even be confusing on CT scans, because the version measured at the top of the glenoid may be very different from the measurement at the bottom of the glenoid. Abnormal glenoid version may have a bearing on a few cases with recurrent posterior dislocation, but its general effect is small. The exception is the patient with congenital-glenoid dysplasia.

Humeral retroversion

This usually measures 21°. Some studies have shown a significant reduction in humeral retroversion in patients with recurrent anterior dislocation (Kronberg *et al.*, 1990). This lends scientific credibility to the operation of rotational osteotomy for this condition, as practiced in continental Europe.

Dynamic restraints

The dynamic restraints are the most important restraints during activity. It is the muscles, acting in a coordinated manner, under the control of proprioceptive feedback, that keep the shoulder located. It is only when the shoulder passes outside its normal range that the static restraints — the labrum and ligaments — are called into play, and in collisions may be strained to failure.

The rotator cuff

The four muscles of the rotator cuff provide most of the stability of the shoulder. During shoulder movement the rotator cuff controls the position of the humeral head and makes sure that it remains centred on the glenoid. If the cuff is torn then the shoulder will sublux.

Proprioception

Recent investigations have demonstrated the importance of proprioception in the normal shoulder. Anatomic studies have revealed mechanoreceptors within the shoulder joint capsule. Pacinian corpuscles are rapidly adapting mechanoreceptors that act as receptors for rapid acceleration and deceleration. Ruffini endings and Golgi tendon organ-like endings are slow reacting and convey information on joint position sense.

Lephart *et al.* (1994) studied joint position sense by reproducing a shoulder position, set using a test apparatus. They then studied proprioception by marking the speed with which the subject recognized a random initiation of shoulder movement, brought about by the test apparatus.

Three groups were studied, normal shoulders, unstable shoulders and reconstructed shoulders. They found that proprioception was significantly reduced in the unstable shoulders, but returned to near normal in the operated group.

This study is fascinating because it was the first to demonstrate the effect of proprioception in shoulder instability, and leads us to ask further questions. Does the Bankart lesion damage the proprioceptive input to shoulder control? Does the operation of repair actually work by resetting proprioception around the shoulder? Does reconstruction work by allowing proprioceptive rehabilitation to the shoulder?

Long head of biceps

Glousman *et al.* (1988) were the first to consider the long head of biceps as a dynamic stabilizer. Using electromyograph (EMG) studies they found that the biceps was more active in patients with recurrent dislocation than normal volunteers.

Several cadaver studies have backed up these findings. Itoi *et al.* (1993) showed, in the cadaver model, that anterior translation of the humeral head was significantly reduced by loading both the short and long heads of the biceps in all capsular conditions. They suggested that strengthening the biceps should be included in all physiotherapy rehabilitation protocols following dislocation or repair.

Static restraints

We have seen how physical restraints act to locate the shoulder at rest, and how dynamic restraints locate the shoulder during movement, but the final restraints are those that locate the shoulder at the extremes, and during collisions. These are the labrum and the ligaments. It is these structures that eventually fail, leading to traumatic dislocation in the young sportsman.

The labrum

The labrum acts to deepen the glenoid, loss of the labrum can decrease the socket depth by 50%. The labrum also acts as a chock block (Fig. 6.6), and also acts as the origin for the glenohumeral ligaments.

The ligaments (Fig. 6.7)

The ligaments are thickenings within the capsule of the shoulder joint. They are best seen from inside the shoulder joint by arthroscopy.

At the top of the shoulder are the coracohumeral ligament and the superior glenohumeral ligament. These two ligaments are closely connected, indeed they merge to insert in a common insertion into the humerus, forming the pulley for the long head of the biceps (Walch *et al.*, 1994) (Fig. 6.8). The coracohumeral ligament is very powerful and selective cutting studies have shown that it is the primary restraint against posterior dislocation.

The middle glenohumeral ligament is a condensation in the capsule which runs obliquely from the 2 o'clock

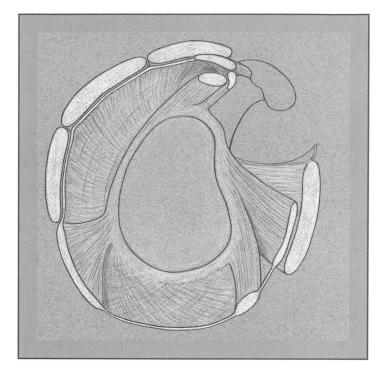

Figure 6.7 – *The ligaments of the shoulder (see text).*

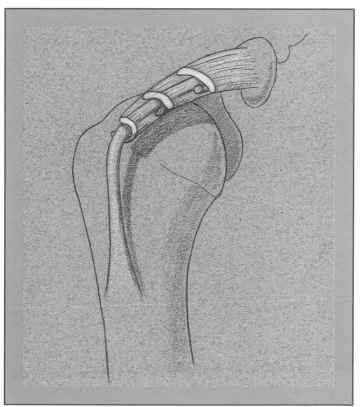

Figure 6.8 – *The relationship between the long head of the biceps, the coraco-humeral ligament and the superior glenohumeral ligaments. The coraco-humeral ligament and the superior glenohumeral ligament merge to form the pulley for the long head of the biceps.*

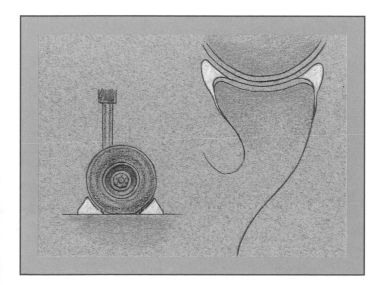

Figure 6.6 – *The labrum acts like a chock block to prevent dislocation.*

position on the glenoid to insert at the 5 o'clock position on the humerus. The middle glenohumeral ligament is best seen arthroscopically (Fig. 6.9) and is very variable in its thickness. Sometimes it is substantial; at other times it appears as a whispy, flimsy veil. It runs obliquely across the superior edge of subscapularis tendon, which allows it to be easily identified during shoulder arthroscopy.

Shoulder surgeons talk not of the inferior glenohumeral ligament but of the inferior glenohumeral ligament complex (IGHLC), which reinforces the joint capsule from the 4 o'clock position right around to the 8 o'clock.

The IGHLC consists of an anterior band, then the sheet of tissue that makes up the infraglenoid recess, and then the posterior band. Warren's group in New York have studied the IGHLC in fine detail — histologically as well as in various selective cutting experiments. They liken the IGHLC to a hammock supporting the head. The hammock is slung from its guy ropes at the front and back — the anterior and posterior bands (Fig 6.10).

The posterosuperior capsule possesses no thickenings.

Most of the experimental work on the function of the glenohumeral ligaments has been conducted by undertaking selective-cutting experiments to simulate

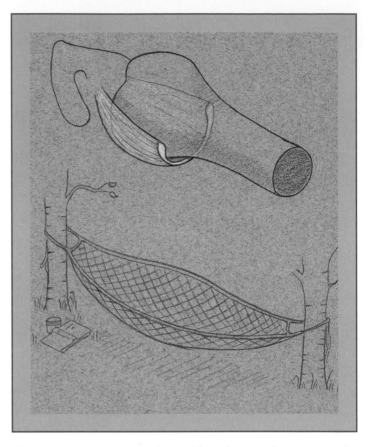

Figure 6.10 – *The IGHLC acts like a hammock to support the humerus. Should one of its guy ropes be damaged then the head will fall out of bed.*

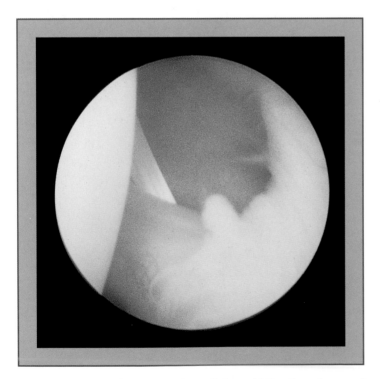

Figure 6.9 – *Arthroscopic view of the middle gleno-humeral ligament. The ligament is seen to cross the subscapularis tendon obliquely.*

Bankart lesions. However, in one in five patients at surgery the capsule is found to be pouched and redundant, rather than torn. This raises the question as to whether this redundancy is congenital or traumatic in origin.

Uhtoff and Picopo (1985) studied the capsule in embryonic and foetal shoulders and found that the capsule originated from the labrum in 77% of cases, but in the remaining 23% of cases originated from the neck of the scapula, so creating a pouch.

O'Driscoll and Evans (1991) found a high incidence of bilateral shoulder instability (24% in 188 shoulders followed for 9 years), and suggested that an intrinsic abnormality, such as capsular laxity or muscle imbalance, may be involved. He then looked at family history and found a 24% incidence of shoulder instability in first degree relatives.

The first selective-cutting experiment was that of Turkel *et al.* (1981), a paper which should be read by all aspiring shoulder surgeons. They showed that with the arm at the side the major restraint to anterior translation was the subscapularis, but as the shoulder is elevated towards the position of apprehension (90° abduction and external rotation) the main, and indeed only, restraint is the IGHLC. These selective-cutting experiments have been repeated using more and more elaborate tracking devices and the results of previous experiments have been confirmed.

Having discussed the theory of dislocation in detail, and the experiments (mainly on cadaver shoulders) that have been conducted to validate these assumptions, the question arises as to what happens in reality?

The essential lesions

Baker (1990) examined 45 acute traumatic shoulder dislocations arthroscopically. He found three groups of lesions (Fig. 6.11).

Group I

The capsule was torn without labral pathology. These patients (6 of 45) were stable under anaesthesia, there was a minimal haemarthrosis, with some haemorrhage between the middle and inferior glenohumeral ligaments. This was the smallest group.

Group II

These patients (11 of 45) had a partial-labral tear, anterior subluxation under anaesthesia, varied instability, and a moderate haemarthrosis.

Group III

This was the largest group of patients by far (28 of 45). In these patients there was complete disruption of the anterior labrum, frank dislocation under anaesthesia, a large haemarthrosis and 18 of 28 shoulders had a Hill–Sachs lesion.

Clinical presentation

The patient with recurrent traumatic dislocation will present to the orthopaedic surgeon in one of three ways.

Firstly, the patient may present to the shoulder clinic, referred from a general practitioner, with a history of more than one dislocation of the shoulder.

Secondly, the patient may present in the fracture service with his second dislocation.

The third method is rather novel. This is the young sportsman presenting with his first dislocation, in which a

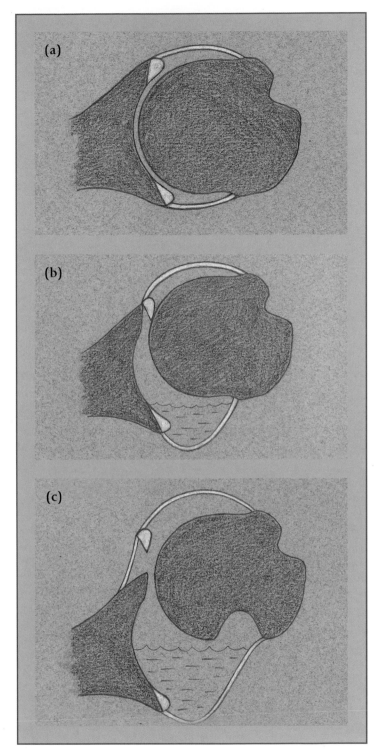

Figure 6.11 – *Baker classification of acute dislocations (see text).*

recurrence can be predicted, and in whom a repair should be performed before the dislocation recurs. In other words a prophylactic repair! Jakobsen and Sjobjerg (1996) arthroscoped 76 patients following a primary traumatic dislocation. Fifty-one percent redislocated within 3 years. Eighty percent of those who redislocated had an extensive detachment and Hill-Sachs lesion (Baker Group III Lesion). Caution should be used in this interpretation because Hovelius (1987,1996) states that there is still no valid reason to recommend routine primary prophylactic operative procedures for patients in the youngest age group. Moreover, patients who do not redislocate for 5 years will probably never need an operation.

Presentation to the shoulder clinic

Presently the commonest mode of presentation to the shoulder surgeon will be the referral of a patient from a colleague.

The history follows the pattern shown in chapter one, and is recorded on the modified American Shoulder and Elbow Surgeons (ASES) assessment form. The patient is usually a well muscled, sports-playing, young man. The great majority of traumatic dislocations are sustained playing contact sports. The usual method of injury is a collision. It is important to gain some idea of where the hand was at the time of the dislocation, and in which direction the collision force was applied. Often the arm will have been in the 'position of apprehension', which is with the arm abducted to 90° and fully externally rotated.

It is important to note how easy, or difficult, the shoulder was to relocate, and whether this was done under sedation or anaesthesia. How many recurrences have occurred, how did these occur, and how were they reduced?

Ask how the shoulder is between episodes of dislocation. Is the shoulder predictable? Does the shoulder sublux? Does it click? Does the arm go dead? What activities are affected? Which positions of the arm lead to apprehension or subluxation? How often does this occur? All these questions are important in building a picture of how the episodes of subluxation and dislocation affect your patient.

Examination follows the normal pattern using the ASES format, as shown in chapter one. Clearly great attention is paid to stability testing of both the dislocating and normal shoulders.

Instability testing

The reader is referred to the section on instability testing in Chapter 1.

The apprehension test

This is the classic test for anterior instability. This test can be performed with the patient either sitting or standing. To test the right arm the examiner stands to the right and just behind the patient. The examiner bends the patient's elbow to 90° and holds the elbow in his/her right hand. The examiner places his/her hand over the patient's shoulder, with the thumb on the back of the humeral head. The affected arm is fully externally rotated at 45°, then at 90° and finally at 135°. As the arm is externally rotated the patient realizes that the shoulder is about to 'slip out'. At this point the patient winces and involuntarily resists any further movement (Fig. 6.12).

The crank test

This is a continuation of the apprehension test. If the patient does not wince at full external rotation then overpressure is applied, or the shoulder is cranked out. Again the end-point is apprehension (Fig. 6.13).

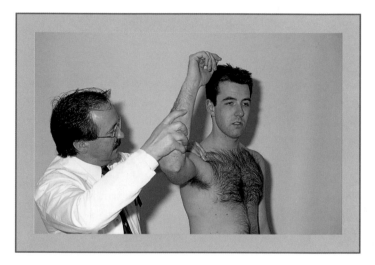

Figure 6.12 – *The apprehension test. As the arm is brought into 90° of abduction and full external rotation the patient starts to grimace and the muscles go into protective spasm.*

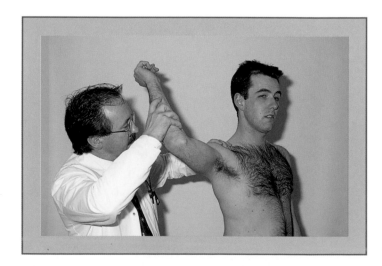

Figure 6.13 – *The crank test. Once the arm is in the position of apprehension the surgeon applies overpressure.*

The relocation test

This is the third part of the apprehension test. When the patient starts to feel the joint slipping out the examiner presses backwards on the humeral head, thereby relocating it. The patient's wince disappears and the muscles relax, the patient once again becomes comfortable with the examination (Fig. 6.14).

The anterior drawer test

This test is analogous to the anterior drawer test of the knee. The test was first described by Gerber and Ganz (1984) and their description of the test is very precise, but has been incorrectly copied into major text-books.

This test must be performed with the patient supine, it can not be performed with the patient sitting or standing, as this makes the test unreliable. The shoulder is held in 80–120° of abduction, 10° of forward flexion and neutral rotation. To examine the right arm the patient's wrist is gripped in the surgeon's axilla, and the elbow held by the examiner's right hand. The examiner's left hand stabilizes the scapula. With the patient fully relaxed, the humerus is drawn forwards and back with a force comparable to that in the Lachman test.

The key elements to this test are that the patient is supine, the arm abducted and the patient relaxed (Fig. 6.15).

Some authorities suggest that the test be performed with the patient seated and with no abduction. In this position subscapularis protects the front of the shoulder and the test is unreliable at best.

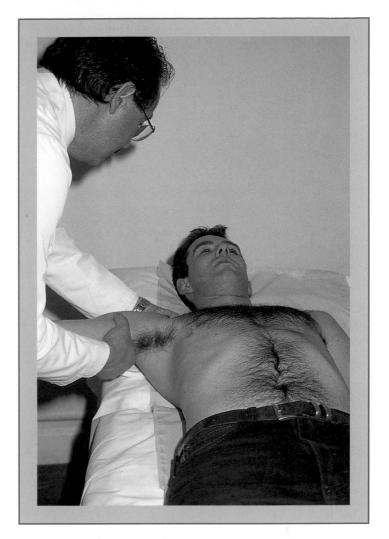

Figure 6.15 *The anterior drawer test.*

The load and shift test

This test can be performed in the clinic but caution must be exercised as it can provoke a true dislocation. There are recorded episodes of such a dislocation being irreducible, and the patient requiring a general anaesthetic for reduction! This is a provocative test, being the shoulder equivalent of the Barlow and Ortolani test of the hip, or the pivot shift in the knee. Every opportunity should be taken to practise this test on the anaesthetized patient, prior to every surgical repair.

The patient is positioned supine or semirecumbent. For the right shoulder the surgeon stands at the side of the couch and stabilizes the scapula with his/her left hand. The patient's elbow is flexed and held in the surgeon's right hand. The shoulder is then abducted to 100° and externally rotated to just below the apprehension threshold. Pressure is then applied to the arm compressing the joint surfaces (as in the pivot shift).

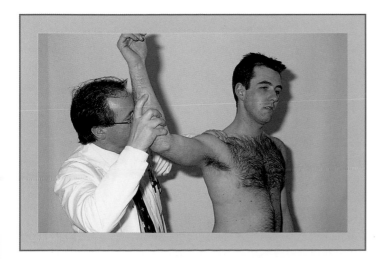

Figure 6.14 – *The relocation test. Pressure is applied on the humeral head to relocate it from the position of apprehension.*

With the shoulder loaded the humeral head is shifted forwards, the surgeon taking the attitude that he/she is going to dislocate the shoulder! The resulting shift is graded. Grade 0 is normal; Grade 1 is anterior translation to the edge of the glenoid; Grade 2 is subluxation over the front of the glenoid, easily reduced; Grade 3 is the full clunk of dislocation, and the clunk of relocation.

Having completed the tests for anterior instability the surgeon must see if there is an element of inferior, posterior or generalized laxity.

Sulcus sign

The clinical diagnosis of inferior instability is made by gentle downward traction on the relaxed upper arm (Neer & Foster, 1980). This produces a sulcus between the lateral acromion and the humeral head (Fig. 6.16). The test is conducted with the patient upright. The sulcus sign is the hallmark of multidirectional instability.

Posterior jerk test

Tests for posterior instability are poorly covered in the literature. The key to posterior subluxation and dislocation is that it occurs with the arm in internal rotation, that is then elevated in the plane of flexion and not in the plane of abduction.

To test the right arm the surgeon stands behind and to the right of the patient. The surgeon's hand is placed over the scapula with the thumb on the back of the humeral head. This is very important because it is the surgeon's thumb that detects the subtle posterior translation in subluxation. The surgeon takes the patient's elbow in his/her right hand and fully internally rotates the humerus. The shoulder is then slowly elevated in the plane of flexion. Almost immediately (30° of flexion) the humeral head is felt to sublux and then to dislocate. Often the patient is not aware of the subluxation, but may be aware of full dislocation. The arm is further elevated to 100°, at this point the arm is moved from the plane of flexion to the plane of abduction, and the humeral head relocates with a jerk, the patient experiences brief pain and then relief from pain (Fig. 6.17).

Once again every sentence of this description must be followed precisely. If the test is performed in neutral, or external rotation the patient will not dislocate. If the test is conducted in the plane of abduction, and not the plane of flexion, the patient will not dislocate.

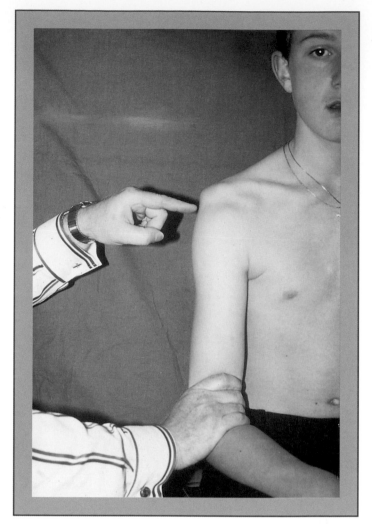

Figure 6.16 – *The sulcus sign. Gentle traction on the arm causes inferior subluxation which is shown by a sulcus forming between the humeral head and the acromion (with permission from Bunker and Wallace, Shoulder Arthroscopy, Dunitz).*

The posterior drawer test

The patient must be supine. To examine the right shoulder the surgeon stands level with the shoulder (Gerber & Ganz, 1984). The patient's elbow is flexed to 120° and supported by the surgeon's right hand. The shoulder is held abducted by 80°–120° and slightly flexed. The surgeon places his/her left hand over the shoulder with the fingers on the scapular spine and the thumb just lateral to, but still in contact with, the coracoid process.

The shoulder is internally rotated and flexed to 80°, and at the same time the thumb of the left hand presses back upon the humeral head. The amount of posterior displacement of the head, relative to the coracoid and the spine of the scapula, can be felt and graded.

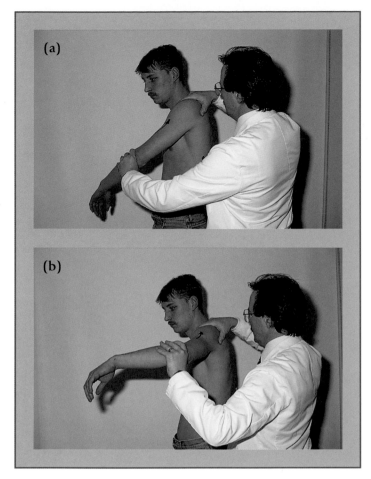

Figure 6.17 – *The posterior jerk test. The arm is elevated in internal rotation and a degree of adduction. The head subluxes posteriorly out of the glenoid. The arm is then brought into the plane of abduction and relocates with a jerk.*

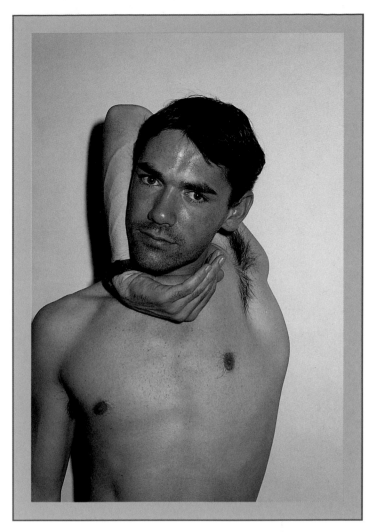

Figure 6.18 – *The 'orang-utan' sign. A demonstration of capsular laxity.*

Generalized joint laxity

The patient must be examined for generalized laxity. Generalized laxity is graded 0–9. Points are scored for wrist flexion (thumb to forearm), finger extension (little finger and wrist extend so that the little finger is parallel with the forearm), recurvatum at elbow and recurvatum at knee. Both sides are tested giving a potential score of 8. Finally spinal flexion, so that the patient can place the palms of the hand on the ground, scores the ninth point.

Shoulder laxity may be isolated and is characterized by excessive movement, external rotation to 95°, internal rotation to a T5 vertebral level and a positive 'Orang-utan' sign (Fig. 6.18).

Finally a word of caution about applying these tests to children and adolescents. Emery (1991), using the drawer tests, found positive results in 57% of boys and 48% of girls, all of whom had asymptomatic shoulders.

Further investigations

Having taken a full history and performed an examination, the diagnosis of traumatic anterior dislocation should now be confirmed. However, there will be a small group of patients in whom the diagnosis remains in doubt. These patients will need further investigation with plain radiology, arthroscopy and an examination under anaesthetic. Computerized tomography (CT) and magnetic resonance imaging (MRI) scanning are favoured by some, but like all investigations can be misinterpreted.

Radiology
Plain films
The Stryker-notch view is used to show a Hill–Sachs lesion (Fig. 6.19). The presence of a posterolateral humeral-head

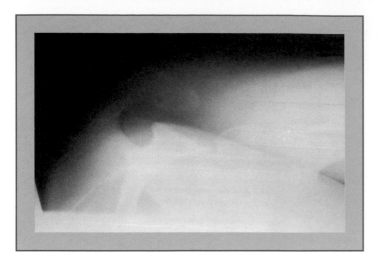

Figure 6.19 – *The Hill–Sachs lesion. The impaction fracture of the posterior humeral head caused by impaction on the anterior rim of the glenoid during traumatic anterior dislocation.*

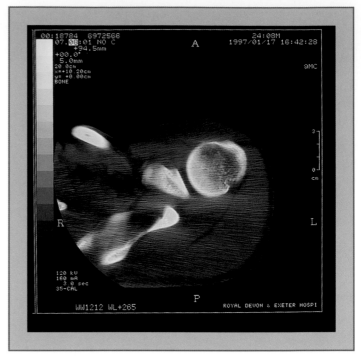

Figure 6.20 – *A CT scan of the Hill–Sachs lesion on the posterior aspect of the humeral head.*

defect (the Hill–Sachs lesion) confirms the diagnosis of a previous traumatic anterior dislocation. The presence of a Hill–Sachs lesion is associated with a higher recurrence rate.

Computerized arthrotomography

Double-contrast CT scans can be used to demonstrate the essential lesions. Ribbans *et al.* (1990) scanned 33 consecutive patients presenting with a primary anterior dislocation. Damage to the anterior glenoid labrum was seen in all the younger patients and 75% of the older patients. A redundant anterior capsular pouch was seen in most of the elderly patients and 35% of the young patients. A Hill–Sachs lesion was seen in 82% of the younger and 50% of the older patients (Fig. 6.20). Associated fractures were seen in almost one-third of patients, and rotator-cuff tears were observed in 63% of the older group of patients; however, no rotator-cuff tears were seen in the younger group of patients.

The authors state that computerized arthrotomography should not be used in all dislocations, but that it can be helpful in difficult diagnostic groups.

Magnetic resonance imaging

Magnetic resonance imaging is non invasive and can be used to investigate labral pathology in patients with a difficult diagnosis. The findings are very similar to CT scanning.

Both of these scanning techniques need to be interpreted with caution. In particular the normal labral variants at the 2 o'clock position — the Detrisac type — II labrum and the Buford complex — can be misinterpreted as a Bankart lesion.

Arthroscopy and examination under anaesthetic

Arthroscopy and examination under anaesthetic (EUA) should be considered as one because they are complimentary and if a general anaesthetic is being given the opportunity must be taken to perform both investigations. Together they are the gold standard investigation.

The examination under anaesthetic should be performed first. This consists of the drawer tests, sulcus sign and load and shift tests, as already described in chapter one. Often these tests are conclusive.

Shoulder arthroscopy is performed as described by Professor Ogilvie-Harris in his chapter on arthroscopy (see Chapter 3).

Bayley (1990) looked at the value of arthroscopy in a consecutive series of 166 patients with symptoms of subluxation but no clear-cut clinical diagnosis. Arthroscopy confirmed the working diagnosis in 80%, but changed it in 20%.

Ellman and Gartsman (1993) contrasted the arthroscopic findings in TUBS as opposed to AMBRI. In

TUBS the following may be found: biceps a SLAP tear; the cuff a posterosuperior partial tear; loose bodies; a frayed, detached or torn labrum; a normal or torn middle glenohumeral ligament; a Bankart tear of the IGHLC; and a Hill–Sach's lesion (Fig. 6.21).

In contrast, in AMBRI the following will commonly be found; normal biceps; normal cuff; no loose bodies; normal, atrophic or 'over the top' labrum; an attenuated middle glenohumeral ligament; a normal IGHLC; and no Hill–Sach's lesion.

In patients with a normal shoulder, or with TUBS, resistance is felt against the scope as it is manoeuvred from the superior part of the joint into the infraglenoid recess. In AMBRI there is little or no resistance, this is termed the positive 'drive thru' sign. In patients who are extremely lax there may not only be no resistance to the arthroscope, but a good view of the anterior structures from the back all the way down may be obtained, this is called the positive 'see through' sign (Copeland 1995. Note the different spelling of these signs which originate from different sides of the Atlantic!) (Fig. 6.22).

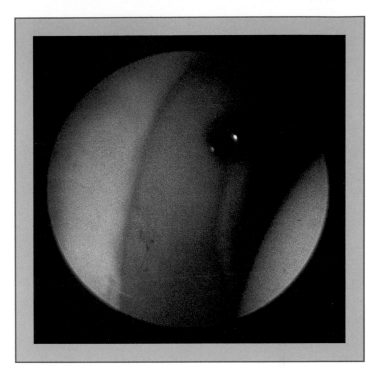

Figure 6.22 – *Positive 'see-through' sign. The whole of the anterior rim of the glenoid can be seen in this overly lax joint.*

Indications for surgery

Following the history, examination and investigation (if necessary) the diagnosis of traumatic anterior dislocation has been established. The next question to ask is 'who is in need of repair?'

There is no doubt about young patients (under the age of 30) who have had a recurrence within 2 years of the original episode; these patients need surgical repair. However, the 50-year old non-athletic man who has his second dislocation after a gap of 16 years should clearly not undergo surgery. Between these extremes the surgeon must display a degree of wisdom based upon titrating the age of the patient, the time between recurrences, the sporting and professional needs of the patient, dominance, the ease of redislocation, the ease of relocation, clinical stability on testing, degree of apprehension and the frequency of subluxation symptoms between the two dislocations.

Method of surgical repair

The surgical approach

Prior to surgery it is essential that certain vital items of equipment and instruments are present. Firstly, a second

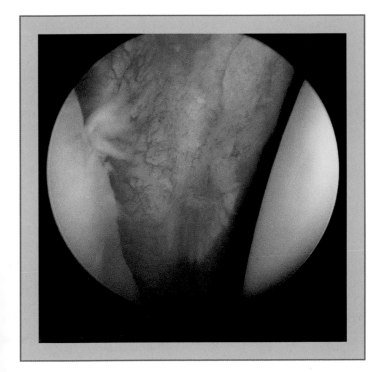

Figure 6.21 – *An arthroscopic view of the Bankart tear. A defect can be seen between the labrum and the glenoid. The labrum is inflamed.*

Mayo stand should be padded-up and sterile draped so that the arm can be rested upon it. The operation is transformed by using the Link instruments for the shoulder, and in particular the Link-Kölbel shoulder self-retaining retractor with interchangeable blades, the Fukuda retractor, and the Link-spiked retractors (Fig. 6.23). A suture-anchor system must be available for this operation. There are many different types on the market.

The fully consented and prepared patient is anaesthetized with a general anaesthetic and endotracheal intubation. If suture anchors are to be used then prophylactic antibiotics should be administered upon induction. The patient is placed supine on the operating table, with an anaesthetic circuit which allows the anaesthetist to be at the foot-end of the table, and allows the surgeon uninterrupted access to the head-end of the table.

The head is placed on a head ring, and a sand bag, or equivalent, is placed under the medial border of the scapula in order to allow freer access to the shoulder. The skin in the line of the incision is injected with adrenaline solution (1:200 000).

The skin is then prepared from nipple to neck, and from table to midline. The patient is draped with adhesive sealing drapes and with the arm free draped. The outline of the clavicle, acromion and coracoid are marked with a skin-marker pen and the line of the incision is planned and marked, choosing one of the skin creases that run up from the armpit, aiming towards the coracoid (Fig. 6.24).

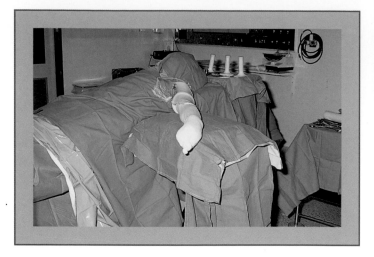

Figure 6.24 – *The patient is draped with the arm free and the arm is supported on a Mayo stand.*

The incision depends upon the sex and build of the patient. A cosmetic axillary approach should be used in a young girl (Fig. 6.25), but this requires a lot of skin undermining and adds some 10 minutes to the procedure. On the other hand, such an approach should not be used in a strongly muscled man; here the standard deltopectoral approach from the coracoid tip to the armpit should be used. Finally, an adhesive drape is placed over the skin.

The surgeon stands in the axilla, the arm is placed on the padded Mayo stand, and the assistant stands on the same side as the surgeon, cephalad to the Mayo table. The reason the assistant stands there is that a better view is obtained and the assistant does not have to stretch across the table, which inevitably leads to backache! The scrub nurse stands opposite the surgeon.

The incision is made through skin and fat down on to the fascia overlying the deltoid and pectoralis major. The cephalic vein is identified within the deltopectoral groove. The cephalic vein should be preserved during this operation, which means that the dissection proceeds to the medial side of the vein and the vein is left on the deltoid. Why is this? Simply, the vein has many tributaries entering it from the deltoid and none from the pectoralis major muscle, so if the vein is left on the deltoid no damage will be incurred. If the surgeon tries to dissect the vein off the deltoid it will result in immeasurable damage to the vein, and the operation will take considerably longer.

There is only one structure which crosses the deltopectoral groove below the cephalic vein. This is the deltoid artery and its venae comitantes which originate

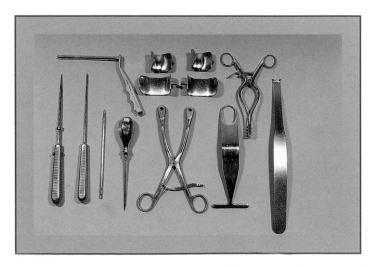

Figure 6.23 – *Instruments needed for surgical repair of dislocation. The Kölbel self-retaining retractor with interchangeable blades; the Fukuda-humeral head retractor; the anterior-spiked retractor and a suture-anchor set.*

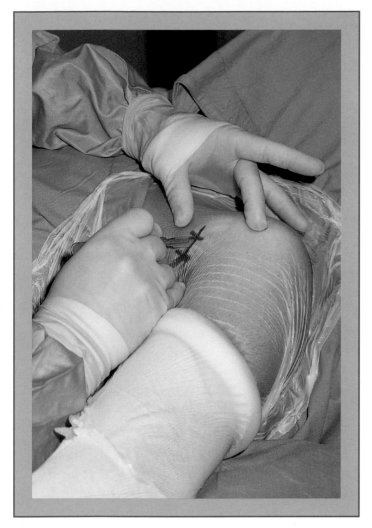

Figure 6.25 – *A cosmetic incision should be performed in the young girl.*

head?' Firstly it is necessary in order to expose the glenoid from the 4 to 6 o'clock position, and the inferior capsule which is often stretched. It does not damage the blood supply to the head because it anastomoses with the posterior circumflex artery via its descending branch. You can prove this to yourself by releasing the clamp from its divided distal end!

If you plan to do an inferior capsular shift then the axillary nerve should be exposed and protected. This requires exposure of the quadrilateral space, within which is found the posterior humeral circumflex artery and vein; the axillary nerve is located directly behind them.

Two stay-sutures should be placed in the subscapularis. These should be fairly superficial so they do not go into the capsule as well. A Trethowan spike is inserted into the rotator interval to mark the top of the subscapularis. The arm is now taken into full external rotation, with the elbow at the side, so that extreme tension is placed on the subscapularis. Using cutting diathermy, a vertical capsulotomy is now made in the subscapularis. The subscapularis tendon has transverse fibres which are under tension and spring apart under the tip of the diathermy, much the same as the fibres of the transverse carpal ligament 'give' during a carpal-tunnel release. The capsule is much more amorphous and is not under such tension. It is also easier to distinguish between the two at the lower-muscular third of the subscapularis than in the tendinous upper-third.

The repair
The repair depends upon the pathological findings. As already stated, the two main elements that need to be considered are the detachment of the anterior capsule from the glenoid (the Bankart lesion) and the degree of capsular stretching. Additionally, the surgeon must consider if there is an element of congenital capsular laxity (a loose inferior recess), any weakening of the rotator interval, any damage to the biceps insertion (SLAP tear), any tearing of the capsule from the humerus (rare), and any bony damage to the glenoid rim. Let us first look in detail at the two commonest lesions — the Bankart tear and the capsular-stretch lesion.

In order to define pathology the capsule has to be opened. Most surgeons prefer to open the capsule with a vertical incision from the rotator interval about 7 mm from the capsular insertion to the humerus. The rotator interval is then incised down to the glenoid rim. Often this is enough for good access to the Bankart lesion. If

from the acromiothoracic trunk and enter the deltoid. It is often best to ligate and divide the deltoid artery at this juncture.

Having spread open the deltopectoral groove the clavipectoral fascia is incised on the lateral border of the conjoined tendon. The arm is now placed in 90° of abduction and the deltoid is mobilized upward. The Kölbel self-retaining retractor is then inserted, with the lateral long-blade between the deltoid and the humerus, and the medial long blade under the conjoined tendon. A small (1.5 cm) tenotomy may be made in the upper border of the pectoralis major tendon. An excellent view of the subscapularis with the anterior circumflex humeral artery and its venae comitantes is now achieved. The anterior circumflex humeral artery is ligated and divided. The question which should be asked is 'is this necessary, and does it damage the blood supply to the

the inferior capsule is very loose then a further 'T' incision will be required in the capsule from half way along the vertical limb of the capsulotomy to the 4 o'clock on the glenoid rim. Stay-sutures are inserted in order to control these flaps (Fig. 6.26).

In the normal shoulder the glenoid labrum should be firmly attached to the glenoid. The exception to this is at the 2 o'clock position where various abnormalities can be found. The first is the Detrisac Type-II defect, here there is a straightforward detachment of the labrum at the 2 o'clock position; this is a normal variant. The second is the Buford complex. The Buford complex is a high take-off of a cord-shaped middle glenohumeral ligament, from the long head of biceps, with an accompanying detachment of the labrum at the 2 o'clock position, again this is also a normal variant. The key point with both of these normal variants is that the glenoid is firmly attached from the 3 o'clock position downward, whereas a Bankart lesion has detachment of the labrum which extends down to the 5, 6, or 7 o'clock position.

The Bankart lesion may be represented by a small cleft to a massive detachment with the labrum and ligaments wafting around in the breeze. Often the labrum is abraded or torn, and there may be cartilage scuffing at the anterior edge of the glenoid.

If a Bankart lesion is present it should be reattached to the bone, this requires two steps: preparation of the bony bed, followed by re-attachment. The bony bed must be prepared, such that there is an area of bleeding cancellous bone, and this can be done either with Stille osteotomes, or with a dental-type burr. The re-attachment can be performed in the traditional manner with interosseous sutures, but this damages the articular surface of the glenoid, requires specialized instruments, is tedious to the surgeon, and is time consuming. Most shoulder surgeons will now use a suture anchor for reattachment.

The suture anchors

There are a whole host of proprietary suture anchors on the market, each with its own advantages and problems. Barber (1995) tested the pull out strengths of 23 different suture anchors. The suture anchors were tested in diaphyseal bone, metaphyseal bone and in cancellous troughs. Four of the more commonly used anchors were implanted to see if the fixation strength fell off with time; the metal anchors stayed at 100% strength

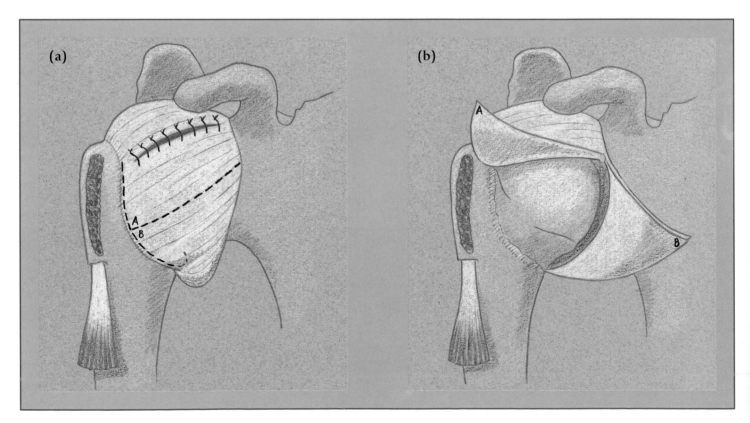

Figure 6.26 – *A T-capsulotomy is made in the anterior capsule.*

throughout the 12-week test period, whereas the plastic anchors started weaker but by 3 weeks were as strong as the metal anchors. This study concluded that all the anchors tested were stronger than the suture, and that the weakest link in the repair is always the suture-soft tissue interface. All the absorbable sutures tested *in vivo* had lost all their strength by 3 weeks, with the exception of polydioxanone (PDS) which lasted to 5 weeks, beyond this a non-absorbable suture is needed.

The most important features when choosing a suture anchor are the surgeon's familiarity and comfort-level with the anchor and its instrumentation. What is important is to place the anchor in the correct position, which is as close to the glenoid rim as possible, without damaging the articular surface. This re-establishes the labrum right up on the edge of the glenoid so that it can act as a labral bump, i.e as a chock block, and so that the labral-suction effect upon the head can be effective. The anchors must be placed around the face of the glenoid so that the whole of the Bankart lesion is re-attached; this means getting one anchor right down at the 5 o'clock position. Usually two to three anchors are all that is needed.

Capsular tensioning

Once the attachment of the capsule to the glenoid has been re-established, then the capsule needs to be re-tensioned. This is perhaps the most difficult part of the operation for the inexperienced surgeon. The capsule has to be re-tensioned so that the shoulder is tight enough so as not to re-dislocate, but not over-tight, such that movement will be restricted, or so tight that arthritis of dislocation will ensue. Essentially, the capsule should be repaired with the forearm in neutral, at 30° of abduction; this should allow a good range of movement. The rotator interval should be repaired, and the slack should be taken out of the capsule globally, that is from the inferior capsule as well as the anterior capsule. Effectively this means performing a Neer-capsular shift.

In order to perform the Neer-capsular shift the rotator interval is carefully closed with two sutures. A 'T' capsulotomy is performed by incising the capsule from half way down the vertical limb to the 4 o'clock position on the glenoid. This gives the surgeon two triangular flaps based upon the reconstructed labrum. The free corner of the upper flap is then grasped with a toothed forceps and stretched until it is under sufficient tension, it is then sewn to the humeral stump of capsule in a

lower, and more lateral position than it started. Further sutures are then placed to repair the lateral edge of this flap to the stump of the humeral capsule.

The free corner of the lower triangular flap is now grasped and pulled upwards, superficial to the first flap, until it is under sufficient tension, at which point it is sewn to the humeral stump, as close to the rotator interval as possible. The lateral border is then sewn to the humeral stump, finally one stitch is inserted to sew the two flaps together (Fig. 6.27).

If the inferior capsule is not lax, and a 'T' capsulotomy is not necessary for exposure of the Bankart lesion, the re-tensioning repair does not need to be so extensive. In this case the capsulotomy has two limbs, the vertical limb and the incised rotator interval, so that it has the appearance of an inverted 'L'. The apex of the flap is pulled laterally and superiorly, until it is under sufficient tension, and sewn to the humeral stump and the rotator interval.

Some surgeons advocate a reversed-T capsulotomy, with the vertical limb close to the glenoid, but there is

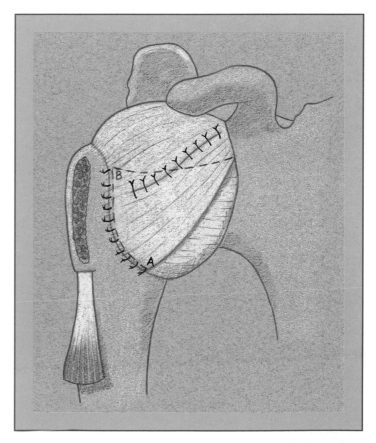

Figure 6.27 – *The capsular shift is completed. Note that the rotator interval is sutured, the flaps are overlapped, the inferior capsule is tight, and the flaps are sutured to each other.*

recent experimental work to add a note of caution to such an approach. Solomonow *et al.* (1996) have demonstrated a protective reflex arc between capsular mechanoreceptors and the rotator-cuff muscles. This reflex arc is actioned by articular branches from the suprascapular and subscapular nerves, which enter the capsule from the medial side. A vertical capsulotomy of the medial capsule may well damage these nerves and lead to a further loss of dynamic stability to the joint. This protective reflex arc must be preserved at all costs.

Associated lesions

The main lesions are the Bankart defect and the capsular-stretch lesion, but occasionally there may be a SLAP lesion, disinsertion of the humeral end of the capsule, loose bodies and bony damage to the glenoid rim.

If a SLAP lesion is present it can be repaired to the glenoid with a suture anchor in the 1 o'clock position. If the humeral end of the ligament is disinserted it should be re-attached to bone with suture anchors. Loose bodies should be removed. If there is bony erosion of the anterior glenoid it should be noted, because recurrence is more common if there is severe erosion, and this is one indication for a bone-block technique such as the Bristow procedure. If there is a bony Bankart lesion it should be repaired using internal fixation with interfragmentary screws (Fig. 6.28).

Closure

Subscapularis is closed, without shortening, to prevent limitation of external rotation. Limitation of external rotation was common with the old Putti–Platt operations, but modern anatomical reconstructions allow for a near-normal range of motion. The wound is washed out, local anaesthetic is instilled, the deltopectoral interval is allowed to fall back together, and the subcutaneous tissues and skin are closed using a subcuticular stich to the skin. The arm is placed in a sling, with body band, overnight. The band is then removed and the rehabilitation programme started. The patient usually leaves the hospital on the morning after surgery. Although this is not day-case surgery, hospital stay is often less than 1 day.

Rehabilitation

The sling is worn by day and night for the first 3 weeks following surgery, except when doing the rehabilitation exercises.

There is one golden rule to remember following shoulder repair, that is that the shoulder should not be externally rotated beyond neutral for the first 3 weeks after surgery; this is to protect the Bankart and capsular repair.

From day one elbow-extension exercises, gentle pendulums and external rotation to neutral are performed. Submaximal isometric exercises to the external rotators and the deltoid (but not to the subscapularis) may be started on day 2, along with scapular shrugs. The strongest TheraBand can be used for submaximal isometric exercises. From week 3 the patient is weaned off the sling. Passive flexion is started, building up to 140° by week 5 and 180° by week 6. External rotation is initiated building up slowly to 30°

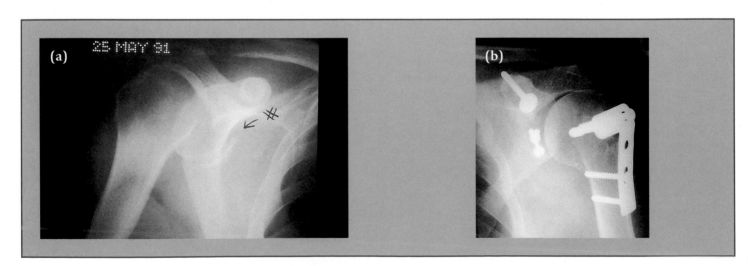

Figure 6.28 – *A bony fragment from the anterior capsule (a) is fixed with an AO screw (b).*

by week 6. Isotonic exercises against weaker TheraBand resistance can be undertaken gradually, allowing external rotation to 30° by 6 weeks. Continue scapular stabilizing exercises and isometrics as above.

At 6 weeks the repair should be healed well enough to allow both some stretching and the ability to power-up the subscapularis. Passive external rotation may slowly build up to 60° by 12 weeks. Active flexion, abduction and internal rotation exercises are performed. TheraBand isotonic exercises, only limiting external rotation to the physiotherapists passive range. Isometric exercises may continue, now allowing submaximal internal rotation. Proprioceptive retraining using closed kinetic chain exercises, kneeling using a wobble board on the operated arm, are commenced. This continues up to 3 months.

At 3 months non-contact sport may be resumed, breast-stroke swimming, jogging, and bicycle riding. A full range of motion should now be achieved, restricting external rotation to 60°. Isotonics are gradually increased by using stronger TheraBand, and then light weights (dumbbells). Proprioceptive retraining using closed-chain exercises, continues, moving on to proprioceptive neuromuscular facilitation pattern exercises. If Cybex is available submaximal isokinetic (60° to 90° per second) limited-arc exercises can be started.

Power and endurance exercises may be started at 4 months. No contact sports are allowed until 6 to 8 months. No overhead sport is allowed until 12 months.

Complications

Nerve injuries

Musculocutaneous nerve

Injury to the musculocutaneous nerve is rare. Neuropraxia can occur from pressure of the Kölbel self-retaining retractor blade under the conjoined tendon. This is exhibited after surgery by dysaesthesia over the radial border of the forearm (lateral cutaneous nerve of forearm). Later evidence of weakness of the biceps can be shown. The nerve usually recovers rapidly from such a neuropraxia.

The nerve is at greater risk if the coracoid process is osteotomized and moved, for instance in the Bristow and Boychev repairs. The nerve enters the conjoined tendons at a variable point 3–4 cm below the coracoid and great care must be taken not to apply traction to the nerve during the transfer.

Patients with a persistent musculocutaneous palsy are still able to flex the elbow using brachioradialis muscle, but are severely weakened by the palsy of the biceps and brachialis.

Axillary nerve

The axillary nerve is more difficult to injure, despite passing closer to the joint. The nerve leaves the posterior cord of the brachial plexus and travels along with, and behind, the posterior circumflex artery and vein. The nerve can be damaged by a spike-retractor inserted into the quadralateral space, and during mobilization of the inferior capsule for a capsular shift. The nerve can be caught by sutures, placed in the capsule at the 6 o'clock position, close to the glenoid, so great care must be exercised at this point. If necessary the quadralateral space must be dissected to display the nerve. The insertion of the latissimus dorsi and teres major to the humerus is tenotomized for 1 cm and these two muscles are then drawn down with a Langenbeck retractor, thus opening the quadralateral space, to allow identification of the posterior circumflex artery and vein, and the axillary nerve.

Limited motion

Limitation of motion is rare after anatomical repair. Patients with dislocation often have an element of 'born loose', and should be told that the effect of the operation is to return the range of motion to that normally found in the rest of the population. This means that excessive external rotation of 90° will be reduced to about 75° following surgery. The majority of patients are delighted with the outcome, but the elite sportsman is a different matter. Many elite throwers are elite because they have excessive external rotation and are therefore able to wind-up further, and accelerate the ball more than the average person. Limiting external rotation in such an athlete may end their career. Great judgement and experience are required in such cases and the elite sportsman should be counselled, before undertaking any such repair.

Limitation of movement is caused by making the capsular repair too tight, and this is where an apprenticeship under the wing of a shoulder surgeon is invaluable during surgical training. The correct degree of tension is something which can only be felt, it can not be conveyed in writing.

Recurrence

A meta-analysis of 53 papers following surgical repair of dislocation in 3187 patients showed an average redislocation rate of 3% (Rockwood & Green, 1996). Many of these studies were small; only 11 of the 53 studies had more than 100 recruits. Of the 11 studies which purported to show a 3% re-dislocation rate, some only followed-up 50% of the participating patients.

Because the recurrence rate is low there are few papers on revision surgery for failed primary repair. McAuliffe *et al.* (1984) reviewed 36 such patients and found that recurrence could have been avoided in the majority of patients by correct preoperative diagnosis, selection of the correct procedure to effect repair, and the proper execution of the elected surgery.

Damage caused by screws and anchors

Metal implants, staples and screws can loosen around the shoulder and lead to damage to the joint from third-body wear. Incorrect placement, loosening, and migration of metalwork all cause problems around the shoulder.

Even dissolving implants can cause problems around the shoulder. The Suretac implant has been shown to cause synovitis of the shoulder and giant-cell reaction around the implant, leading to postoperative shoulder pain in some patients.

Infection

Infection is rare following surgical repair. Cosmetic approaches within the axilla can result in mild superficial wound infection because the area is difficult to dress and is also humid. Great care should be taken with the postoperative care of these wounds.

If implants, such as suture anchors, are being used, prophylactic antibiotics should be administered at the time of surgery. Careful surgery, maintenance of aseptic conditions, lavage prior to closure and avoidance of haematomas, all act to keep the incidence of infection low.

Arthritis

Arthritis of dislocation can occur after too tight a closure of the subscapularis, such as in a too tight a Putti–Platt operation. It is to be hoped that modern anatomical repairs, which do not restrict movement, will show a low incidence of arthritis of dislocation.

Hovelius (1996) examined the incidence of arthritic change in patients, following traumatic dislocation, 10 years after their initial dislocation. twenty percent had radiographic evidence of arthritis at 10 years. This was moderate or severe in 9% of patients, and mild in the remaining patients. Interestingly, the incidence of arthritis was not associated with the number of recurrent dislocations, which means that the likelihood of arthritis is probably determined by the damage to the cartilage at the initial dislocation.

Summary

The shoulder is the most commonly dislocated major joint. There is a hierarchy of restraints to dislocation. The history is usually conclusive in the young sportsman with traumatic dislocation. Clinical examination will usually determine the direction of dislocation. Subluxation is more difficult to diagnose. Surgery has been transformed by the use of suture anchors. The capsule needs to be re-tensioned, which usually means performing a Neer shift, after the labrum has been repaired. The patient must undergo a strict rehabilitation programme in order to recover rapidly, and to best effect.

CHAPTER 7

The teenager with atraumatic shoulder instability

J. Kiss and W.A. Wallace

Introduction

Orthopaedic surgeons regularly see patients with traumatic shoulder dislocation and their management is usually straightforward. However, the management of the young teenager with shoulder instability can be very difficult. This group of young patients (children, teenagers, or young adults) may, or may not, have suffered a significant shoulder injury and have either a momentary shoulder dislocation, often with a spontaneous reduction, or complain of pain, clicking and occasional numbness in the upper arm. Most of these patients present to their primary-care physician and are subsequently referred to an orthopaedic surgeon for further management.

Establishing a diagnosis in these teenage patients, and young adults, may be very difficult. The diagnosis depends on taking a careful history and performing a thorough physical examination, sometimes with repeated clinical reviews by differing members of a multiskilled team, including a physiotherapist and a psychologist. A variety of investigations, including radiographs, computerized tomography (CT) scanning, gadolinium-enhanced magnetic resonance imaging (MRI), and dynamic Moire topography, may be needed to establish the diagnosis of multidirectional shoulder instability (MDI).

Multidirectional shoulder instability

Definition

Laxity of the shoulder is present when there is an abnormal amount of excursion (slide) of the humeral head on the glenoid, forwards, backwards, downwards or even upwards. Laxity is typically bilateral. Instability is present if this laxity is associated with symptoms.

Instability of the glenohumeral joint in more than one direction is considered to be MDI. The condition is often bilateral, but with a different severity of instability of the two shoulders.

Although the diagnosis of MDI did not exist before Neer and Foster (1980) published their paper on the condition, and on the preliminary results of the inferior capsular-shift operation, there have been several other publications that have described similar disease characteristics and their management. Most of these earlier reports described cases with bilateral, mostly posterior, dislocations, often with a voluntary element. The first such case was described in 1722 by Portal and Parona; this was also the first study to differentiate between ordinary recurrent and voluntary dislocation.

Classification of multidirectional shoulder instability

MDI presents with a primary instability which is most obvious in only one direction. Neer and Foster (1980) described three subgroups (Table 7.1).

Table 7.1 The classification of MDI.		
Neer	Group 1	Antero-inferior dislocation
		Posterior subluxation
	Group 2	Postero-inferior dislocation
		Anterior subluxation
	Group 3	Global dislocation

Matsen *et al.* (1990) established two main categories (TUBS and AMBRI) of shoulder instability as described in the previous chapter. AMBRI covers those patients whose instability is *Atraumatic* in onset, often *Multidirectional*, commonly *Bilateral*, and who often respond to a *Rehabilitation* programme. However, if surgical treatment is needed it should involve some form of inferior-capsular shift.

Wallace (1993) identified six main groups of patients, with shoulder instability, based on the four criteria indicative of the AMBRI category shoulder:

(1) traumatic involuntary anterior instability
(2) atraumatic involuntary anterior instability
(3) traumatic involuntary posterior instability
(4) atraumatic involuntary posterior instability
(5) MDI
(6) voluntary instability

More recently Maruyama *et al.* (1995) used the level of trauma, the direction of the instability, and the degree of voluntarism and recorded each using the letters ('T', 'I', 'V') and recorded stages in lower-case letters. The trauma level is recorded as T with four stages. T0 is nontrauma, T1 is mild trauma (repetitive forceful movements), T2 is moderate trauma (dislocation during skiing), T3 is severe trauma (road-traffic accident). There are four special additional cases of trauma, Tc represents convulsion in history, Tp paralysis, Ti inflammation and Th hereditary dislocation. The direction of instability is marked Ia as anterior, Ip as posterior or Ii as inferior. If instability is present in two directions the combination of two letters is used with the capital I, while Im marks the instability that is present in more than two directions. If the instability is confirmed under anaesthesia the letter marking the direction of instability should be underlined. The direction of dislocation needing reduction is marked with a capital letter (e.g., IA). Voluntarism is classified as V0 if absent, V1 if doubtful, and V2 if apparent. In addition the degree of instability can be classified into four categories (-, +, 2+, 3+). With the use of this system every type of instability can be classified, but it is too complex for everyday use.

Incidence of multidirectional shoulder instability

About 45% of all major joint dislocations are shoulder dislocations. The majority of dislocations are traumatic anterior dislocations. The incidence of traumatic posterior dislocation is estimated at 2%, but the exact figures are unknown because of the high number of cases not officially recorded. Although in 1956 Rowe showed that 96% of shoulder dislocations were traumatic and only 4% atraumatic, with our increasing understanding of the mechanism of shoulder instability, and with more precise clinical and radiological examinations, atraumatic MDI is much more commonly diagnosed now than earlier. The exact incidence of MDI has still to be defined.

Emery and Mullaji (1991) found signs of shoulder laxity in 57% of boys and 48% of girls in a study of 150 shoulders of 75 asymptomatic schoolchildren (aged 13–18 years). Most of the laxity signs were bilateral. Twenty-three percent of the children showed signs of multidirectional laxity. Generalized joint laxity was not a common feature among children with signs of shoulder laxity, in this series.

Most authors have found that MDI (symptomatic laxity) is equally common in boys and girls, and is often bilateral, with a high recurrence rate. The majority of patients treated in the reported series were aged 15–30 years.

Aetiology of multidirectional shoulder instability

The aetiology of MDI is multifactorial. There are four major aetiological factors that can lead to instability either on their own, or in combination (Mallon & Speer, 1995) (Table 7.2).

Bony and labral constraints

According to measurements, the hollow of the glenoid–labral socket is about 9 mm deep in its supero-inferior direction and 5 mm deep in its anteroposterior direction. Approximately 50% of this depth is produced by the fibrous labrum. Because of the saucer shape of the glenoid some lateral translation is needed to allow

Table 7.2 The aetiology of MDI.

Bony and labral constraint
Capsular and ligamentous restraints
Impaired muscular control
Collagen abnormalities

inferior, anterior or posterior subluxation of the humeral head. Therefore, compression forces play an important role in stabilizing the glenohumeral joint. The anteroposterior orientation of the glenoid is variable but averages 7° of retroversion. There is debate in the literature regarding the amount of supero-inferior tilt. Some investigations have suggested a few degrees superior tilt, while other studies have suggested the glenoid has a slightly inferior tilt (Morrey and An, 1990; Mallon and Speer, 1995). Obviously, a shallow glenoid–labral socket (due to a labral or a bony glenoid anomaly) and any significant changes in the anteroposterior or supero-inferior tilt of the glenoid may predispose the patient to shoulder instability, but the authors are impressed by the number of patients with bony glenoid abnormalities who have a stable shoulder.

Capsular and ligamentous constraints

The capsule of the glenohumeral joint is flexible and loose to allow a large range of movement. Some parts of the capsule are thickened and have specially orientated collagen fibres, which are important stabilizers of the shoulder. These are the superior, middle and inferior glenohumeral ligaments and the coracohumeral ligament. These ligaments tighten up, and provide stability, in different positions of the arm. With the arm at the side of the body the superior capsule, especially the superior glenohumeral ligament (SGHL), and also the rotator interval and the coracohumeral ligament (CHL), are the structures that prevent inferior translation. With 45° abduction the anterior and posterior portions of the inferior glenohumeral ligament complex (IGHLC) become the inferior stabilizers, while at 90° abduction the posterior band of the IGHLC is the prime stabilizer. Anterior translation is primarily prevented by the middle glenohumeral ligament (MGHL), the SGHL, and the subscapularis tendon with the arm at the side of the body. With increasing abduction the anterior band of the IGHLC is acting as the main anterior stabilizer but to achieve anterior dislocation, elongation of several structures is necessary, in addition to detachment of the anterior band of IGHLC from the glenoid (Bankart lesion). Posterior translation is prevented by the posterior band of the IGHLC, and by the anterosuperior capsule when the arm is abducted. (Matsen *et al.*, 1990; Morrey and An, 1990; Mallon and Speer, 1995).

In addition to their stabilizing function, the ligaments, the labrum, and the capsule contain proprioceptive mechanoreceptors that provide the sensation of joint motion (kinaesthesia) and joint position (joint position sense) (Lephart *et al.*, 1994). Any damage to the capsular, labral, or ligamentous system, therefore, not only weakens the mechanical support of the joint but also leads to disruption of the sensory afferent-feedback mechanism.

Impaired muscular control

Movement of the glenohumeral joint is controlled by the simultaneous action of the deltoid, rotator-cuff and biceps muscles. These muscles are active during the entire arc of movement, but to a different extent. The muscles about the shoulder have not only a motor function, but they contain spindle receptors that are thought to be part of the proprioceptive feedback mechanism in conjunction with the capsulolabral mechanoreceptors (Lephart *et al.*, 1994). The subscapularis, the infraspinatus, and the teres minor pull the humeral head downwards, and also towards the glenoid while the supraspinatus predominantly generates a compression force. The action of the cuff muscles is to provide a stable fulcrum for the action of the deltoid. As a consequence of these muscle actions the humeral head remains centred during movement. The compressive force provided by the cuff muscles is probably the main stabilizer in midrange movements, while at the extremes the ligaments are more important. The scapulothoracic muscles enhance glenohumeral stability, and without these muscles the lateral scapula, with the glenoid, would rotate downwards and encourage inferior translation of the humeral head. Different studies have shown that patients with MDI have poor coordination of their rotator-cuff muscles, and of the scapulothoracic muscles (Rowe *et al.*, 1973; Matsen *et al.*, 1990; Morrey and An, 1990; Kronberg *et al.*, 1991; Mallon and Speer, 1995).

Collagen abnormalities

The shoulder capsule contains predominantly Type-I collagen with some Type-III collagen. The amount of collagen is similar in loose and normal shoulders, but the number of cross-links is significantly reduced in loose shoulders (Tsutsui *et al.*, 1991). Patients with MDI have a significant increase in their rate of collagen formation. Thus collagen abnormalities, without the presence of a definite collagen disorder, may predispose an individual to shoulder instability.

Assessment of the patient with multidirectional shoulder instability

The diagnosis of MDI requires a careful history, a skilled physical examination, proper radiological investigation, and sometimes additional investigations such as neurological assessment, psychological assessment, electromyography (EMG) studies, and special laboratory tests.

History

The history of a patient with MDI shows a wide variation compared with that of a patient with traumatic shoulder instability. The primary complaint is often pain, and not instability. The pain is usually located around the shoulder area, but sometimes it can be referred into the arm. The pain is often aggravated by any use of the arm, but typically by carrying a bag or other object, and is probably the result of subluxation of the shoulder and stretching of the supporting structures. Girls sometimes describe that they have more trouble with the shoulder around the time of their periods.

Many patients complain about tingling or numbness of the fingers, or even the whole arm, with momentary paralysis of the whole area, aggravated by different positions or by the use of the extremity. This phenomenon was named by Rowe *et al.* (1973) as 'dead-arm syndrome' and can mimic a thoracic-outlet syndrome (TOS). The cause of these symptoms is not established, but is probably associated with the altered position of the scapula relative to the rib cage, and the neurovascular bundle of the upper extremity.

Some patients describe a clicking sensation, caused by subluxation of the shoulder in different positions, but most commonly, during forward elevation. Other patients describe full dislocation with spontaneous reduction. Occasionally, patients will present to the emergency room with a dislocated shoulder.

Patients, or their parents, often mention that they have been able to voluntarily dislocate their shoulder(s) as a 'party trick' since the age of 6–10 years without any problem, but as a teenager the shoulder has become painful, or feels unstable.

An association with an episode of minor trauma is not uncommon. Patients may describe an episode when the arm was pulled during an assault, or the shoulder was pushed in a crowd, or injured during sport, or the shoulder was injured at work while lifting a heavy object. These episodes were not in fact the cause of the shoulder dislocation, but simply converted a previously asymptomatic but lax shoulder into a symptomatically unstable shoulder. Compensation claims are not uncommon in this group of patients. Less commonly, patients can have a frank dislocation, caused by significant trauma, and in such cases the differentiation from traumatic unidirectional instability can be very difficult.

Patients also come to light, as referrals to the shoulder specialist, following failed previous surgical stabilization procedures (sometimes even a series of operations) on the shoulder, when either the previously diagnosed instability re-occurs, or when there is instability in the opposite direction. These are patients who have subtle forms of MDI that is superimposed on a more apparent unidirectional instability.

There are a further group of patients who, either at the first consultation, but most commonly after repeated consultations, are suspected of having a psychological problem that may aggravate their symptoms.

Physical examination

As for all shoulder conditions the first step of the examination of the MDI patient is inspection. Patients who have a permanently dislocated or subluxed shoulder usually have an altered posture that can be obvious even when the patient is dressed. The patients should always be examined undressed (for girls their bra is left on), and it is very important to observe the patient while he or she is getting undressed. The way the patients use, or do not use, the arm during dressing can provide valuable information on the degree, and main direction, of the instability. Voluntary dislocators often forget about their shoulder problem while they are getting undressed, and the previously dislocated shoulder looks stable, even at the extremes of movement. The shape of the shoulders can be different, either due to subluxation or dislocation of the humeral head, or due to rotation and pseudo-winging of the scapula. Different shoulder shapes can also be associated with severe spasm of the trapezius muscle. The patient may keep the arm in internal rotation at the side of the body. Sometimes, in patients with a permanent dislocation, there can be discolouration and swelling of the upper limb. Muscle wasting can occur due to inactivity, but it can also be associated with a congenital anomaly, with injury, and with previous operations. Any scars about the shoulder can provide information on previous operations. A very thick broadened scar may suggest a collagen disorder and is known to be associated with excessive joint laxity.

On palpation, tenderness along the medial aspect of the scapula, or trigger areas over the trapezius, rhomboid, and levator scapulae may be observed. Tenderness of the greater tuberosity can be present in cases of subacromial impingement secondary to instability. Clicking or crepitus around the shoulder during movement is not uncommon.

The next step is to assess the active and passive range of movement. The patient should be asked to carry out active forward elevation, lateral elevation, and internal and external rotation of both arms, while their shoulders are inspected from the back. In the case of predominantly posterior instability it is common to see the shoulder posteriorly dislocate, at about 40° of active elevation, with a spontaneous reduction with further elevation of the arm, and a similar dislocation as the arm is brought back down. This phenomenon is usually associated with a pathological scapulothoracic movement pattern that includes an abnormal internal rotational movement of the arm and scapula, and also winging of the scapula; we call this pseudo-winging, because it occurs without muscle weakness. A disrupted movement pattern can often be observed in most MDI cases, even without spontaneous dislocation or subluxation of the shoulder. The range of passive movement and the stability of the shoulder(s) during passive movement is the next step in the assessment. Patients with MDI commonly have excessive ranges of internal and external rotation. The range of external rotation with the arm at the side of the body is often 90°. Internal rotation, by reaching behind the back, is a combination of both glenohumeral and scapulothoracic rotation and is recorded by indicating the highest spinous process that can be reached by the thumb. Frequently, this is also grossly excessive and reaches the T5 or even T4 level.

Generalized joint laxity should always be considered in patients who may have MDI. Carter and Wilkinson (1964) used five clinical signs to assess generalized joint laxity. These were: (1) passive opposition of the thumb to the flexor aspect of the forearm, (2) passive hyperextension of the fingers so that they lie parallel with the extensor aspect of the forearm, (3) more than 10° of hyperextension of the

elbow, (4) more than 10° of hyperextension of the knees, and (5) excessive dorsiflexion of the ankle with eversion of the foot. They considered the patient to have generalized joint laxity if three of the five signs were positive. The Beighton scale (1973) is probably more popular and this is a scale of nine points (Table 7.3). The first four features of the Carter scale are used, but both sides of the body are examined giving a score out of eight; the ninth point comes if the patient can place the palms of both hands upon the ground on forward flexion, with the knees straight. Five or more points are required, in an adult, for a diagnosis of generalized joint laxity, and six points are required in a child.

Patients with MDI usually have weak rotator-cuff muscles and scapular stabilizers (serratus anterior, trapezius and the rhomboids). The rotator cuff is tested in a standard manner, as described in chapter one. Pectoralis major and latissimus dorsi can be tested by asking the patient to adduct their arm against resistance. The patient is asked to shrug their shoulders to test the trapezius. The power of the rhomboids can be tested by asking the patient to pull the shoulder blades together, whilst holding the arms at 90° of abduction with the elbows flexed to 90°, and with the examiner providing resistance, by pushing forwards on the elbows. Weakness of the serratus muscles leads to winging of the scapula that is more obvious when the patient is asked to do a wall pushup (Matsen *et al.*, 1990; Silliman and Hawkins, 1993).

The assessment for instability is the most crucial part of the examination. This requires a degree of experience, and sometimes repeated examinations of the patient. The patient must be relaxed and the asymptomatic arm should be examined first.

Table 7.3 The Beighton scale for ligamentous laxity.

Thumb to forearm	R = 1	L = 1	Total = 2
Hyperextension little finger	R = 1	L = 1	Total = 2
Elbow recurvatum	R = 1	L = 1	Total = 2
Knee recurvatum	R = 1	L = 1	Total = 2
Excess spinal flexion			Total = 1
			Combined total out of 9.

The anterior drawer test, anterior apprehension test, crank test, load and shift test (Table 7.4), relocation test and release test should be performed as described in chapter one. The release test has not been previously described. In this test the patient has just had the relocation test performed and the posterior load has given the patient more confidence, as the head is relocated. In the release-test the surgeon then releases the located head, and it springs forward again giving the patient a second bout of apprehension.

The sulcus sign is the most important sign and is the test for MDI. (Fig. 7.1).

Posterior stability is tested with the posterior jerk test (Fig. 7.2) and the posterior drawer and load and shift tests.

It is essential that the drawer test, the sulcus test, and the apprehension tests should reproduce the usual symptoms complained of by the patient for the tests to be diagnostic of instability. Again this comes down to the difference between laxity and instability. Excessive translation alone does not diagnose instability, it only demonstrates laxity. The majority of patients with MDI have multidirectional laxity with symptomatic instability most commonly in one direction alone.

Neurological assessment is essential in these patients, for they often complain of numbness and weakness of the arm (dead-arm syndrome). The differential diagnosis in these patients is TOS, a condition which also presents in the late teenage girl. Cervical root compression syndromes are very rare in such a young group of patients. A neurological opinion may be needed in young girls with such a differential diagnosis.

Radiological assessment

The true anteroposterio (AP) radiograph and axillary view will show the majority of bony Bankart lesions, Hill–Sachs and reversed Hill–Sachs lesions as well as

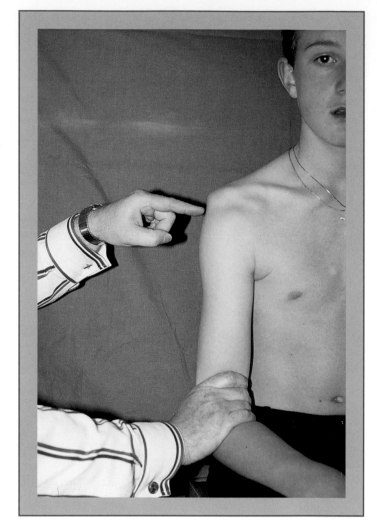

Figure 7.1 – *The positive sulcus sign (reproduced with permission from Shoulder Arthroscopy, Bunker and Wallace (eds), Dunitz).*

congenital anomalies such as humeral or glenoid dysplasia (Fig. 7.3) or increased glenoid retroversion.

Anterior and inferior translation can be visualized by using autotraction stress radiography. The use of an image intensifier in the operating theatre as part of the examination under anaesthetic can be helpful in these patients as well. Unlike the patient with traumatic dislocation, patients with MDI can be difficult to examine under anaesthetic because the shoulder is so sloppy that it is difficult to know when the joint is centred. The surgeon knows the shoulder has an excessive amount of translation, but, without knowing the centred position, he can not tell if the translation is anterior or posterior, this is where an image intensifier can be vital.

CT scanning can be used to assess glenoid retroversion. The retroversion of the glenoid surface in

Table 7.4 The load and shift test for laxity.	
Grade 0	Normal translation
Grade 1	Abnormal translation
Grade 2	Equator subluxes over glenoid rim
Grade 3	Full dislocation of the glenohumeral joint

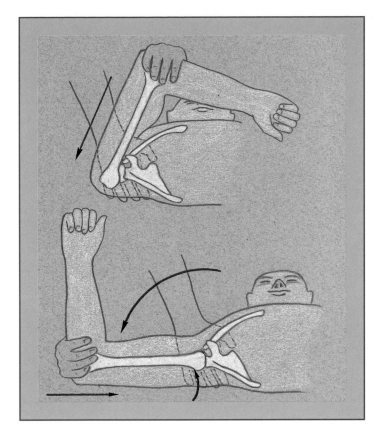

Figure 7.2 – *The posterior jerk test. The arm is flexed in internal rotation and slight adduction. The surgeon applies load to dislocate the joint and then reduces the joint with a 'thud'.*

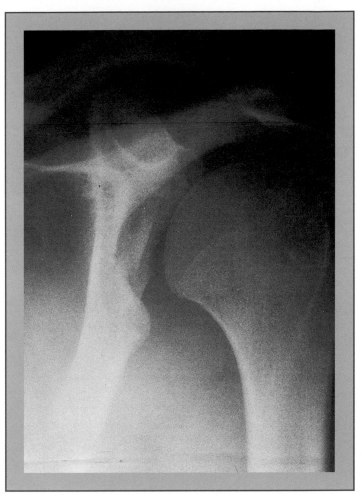

Figure 7.3 – *A radiograph of a patient with primary glenoid dysplasia.*

relation to the scapular blade is normally 4–12°. Double-contrast CT can be used to look for labral abnormalities.

Gadolinium-enhanced MRI can also be used to evaluate labral pathology. However, CT and MRI are expensive techniques and in the former deliver ionising radiation, which we want to avoid in teenage girls and young adults. These techniques are thus used only if the surgeon is considering surgical alteration of version (glenoid or humeral rotational osteotomy).

Static and dynamic Moire topography is capable of demonstrating minor asymmetry of scapulothoracic motion related predominantly to weakness of the trapezius and serratus anterior.

Examination under anaesthetic

Many patients with MDI experience pain or are just too apprehensive for a precise diagnosis to be made from clinical examination (Table 7.5). A full examination can only be made with an examination under anaesthetic (EUA). This procedure is used as a diagnostic test, so that a logical conservative treatment plan can be devised. It may also be used prior to surgical treatment. Both shoulders must be examined, even in the case of unilateral symptoms. The technique of laxity testing is similar to that described above. Because the patient is fully relaxed it is a lot easier to assess the laxity, but the examiner must recreate the forces of normal muscle action around the shoulder, by applying an axial load along the humerus, whilst carrying out these tests. This is the load and shift test. It must be kept in mind that most normal shoulders of anaesthetized patients allow some degree of translation, therefore the findings should be evaluated in conjunction with the clinical history and previous clinical examination. It can not be stressed too highly that under anaesthetic the surgeon can only test laxity, because by definition instability must be symptomatic and whilst anaesthetized the patient can not tell the surgeon whether their laxity is symptomatic.

Table 7.5 Investigation of the patient with MDI.		
Clinical	Sulcus sign	
	Anterior laxity	Apprehension test
		Relocation test
		Release test
		Anterior drawer
	Posterior laxity	Posterior drawer
		Posterior jerk test
	Glenohumeral and scapulothoracic movement pattern	
	Muscle strength	
Radiology	Primary dysplasia (Hill–Sachs) (Bony Bankart)	
	CT assessment of version	
EUA	Repeat clinical laxity testing	
	Load and shift test	
Arthroscopy	Capsular redundancy	
	Over-the-top Bankart lesion	
	'Drive thru' sign	
	'See-through' sign	
Neurology	EMG patterns	
Psychology		
Unusual	Skin biopsy for collagen disorders	
	Chromosomal analysis	

Always remember that even patients with TOS, or other mimics of MDI, can have shoulder laxity as well.

Arthroscopic assessment

In addition to EUA, arthroscopic evaluation may be necessary in some cases before deciding on treatment. The arthroscope can provide further information on the labrum, the capsule, the glenohumeral ligaments, the rotator cuff, the long head of the biceps tendon and its attachment, and the articular surfaces. Some fraying of the labrum at the site of the most dominant instability is a common finding. There is rarely a Bankart lesion, although a minor cleft or fraying is common enough. Dislocation or subluxation of the humeral head can often be demonstrated by stressing the shoulder. In MDI the joint is found to be very capacious. The positive 'drive thru' sign and positive 'see through sign' are often seen.

Neurophysiological testing

Electromyography examination of normal shoulders has revealed that muscle activity during shoulder motion occurs simultaneously in agonistic and antagonistic muscles. Patients with a disrupted scapulothoracic movement pattern may have voluntary, or involuntary, dysfunction of these muscles. Hyperactivity of some muscles, and reduced activity of other muscles, can be observed (Rowe *et al.*, 1973; Kronberg *et al.*, 1991). Differences in activity can often be detected within different portions of the same muscle such as between the anterior-, middle- and posterior-thirds of the deltoid, or the superior and inferior portions of the trapezius.

In patients with voluntary dislocation the muscles that pull the joint out of place can be felt to be inappropriately active as the shoulder dislocates, and can be felt to relax as the shoulder reduces. Pectoralis major and latissimus dorsi are the commonest offenders. Electromyography of these muscles may reveal high activity.

Psychological assessment

Occasionally at the first clinical consultation, but more commonly after repeated clinical examination, the orthopaedic surgeon or physiotherapist may suspect that the patient is psychologically disturbed.

Most voluntary dislocators have some degree of psychological problems. A psychologist must be sensitive to the emotional problems of adolescence in these young patients. A disrupted family life (divorced parents, child abuse) or school conflict are common causes of psychological disorders. Some young patients use their shoulder problem to 'control' their ambitious parents, who make them play musical instruments, do sports at a highly competitive level, or study in highly competitive independent schools.

Additional investigations

In some selected cases histological examination of the skin, connective tissue and muscle is necessary to diagnose a collagen disorder. Other patients may require special laboratory tests to confirm chromosomal anomalies or metabolic disease.

Treatment of multidirectional shoulder instability

Non-operative treatment

Most authors agree that the first line of treatment of MDI is non-operative (Rowe *et al.*, 1973; Neer and Foster, 1980; Matsen *et al.*, 1990; Burkhead and Rockwood, 1992; Wallace, 1993; Mallon and Speer, 1995). There have been several rehabilitation protocols published, but there is no evidence that any one is better than the other. The basic principle of every rehabilitation programme is to improve the muscle strength and coordination of the patient, whilst also encouraging a change in lifestyle or psychological treatment if this is felt necessary.

Rehabilitation programme

The rehabilitation of the patient with MDI should be carried out by an expert multidisciplinary team which should include a shoulder surgeon, a physiotherapist and an occupational therapist. The team leader is usually the orthopaedic surgeon who assesses the patient, makes the diagnosis, monitors the patient's progress, arranges additional investigations and makes decisions on methods of treatment. Additionally, a clinical psychologist and a psychiatrist may be involved in the treatment of these patients. Good communication between the team members is crucial.

Although, under ideal circumstances, the physician, the physiotherapist and the occupational therapist assess the patient together the physiotherapist must make his or her own assessment of the patient. The main elements of this evaluation are the posture of the patient, the shoulder position (scapulothoracic, glenohumeral), joint stability (hypermobility, instability), muscle length (contacture, looseness), muscle strength (isometric, concentric, eccentric), and proprioception (scapulothoracic, glenohumeral).

The programme is initiated with an explanation of the condition to the patient who must understand the importance of the rehabilitation and of his or her own active participation in treatment. The rehabilitation programme then concentrates on proprioceptive input, to improve joint-position sense, and the re-learning of the correct movement patterns, this is in addition to the development of strength and endurance

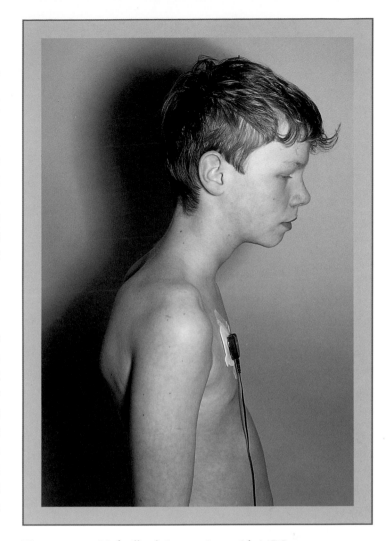

Figure 7.4 – *Biofeedback in a patient with MDI.*

in the scapulothoracic and glenohumeral muscles (Lephart *et al.*, 1994). Mirrors, closed-circuit television, proprioceptive neuromuscular facilitation (PNF, which includes methods of promoting or hastening the response of the neuromuscular mechanism through stimulation of the proprioceptors) and biofeedback (audible or visual stimuli which correspond to muscle activity, with relaxation and enhancement techniques to control this activity) (Fig. 7.4) can be used for the correction and retraining of scapulothoracic and glenohumeral movement patterns.

The stability of the glenohumeral joint, and of the scapula, will then be enhanced with an improvement of muscle balance due to strengthening exercises (Fig. 7.5), closed-chain exercises (wall pushups, knee pushups,

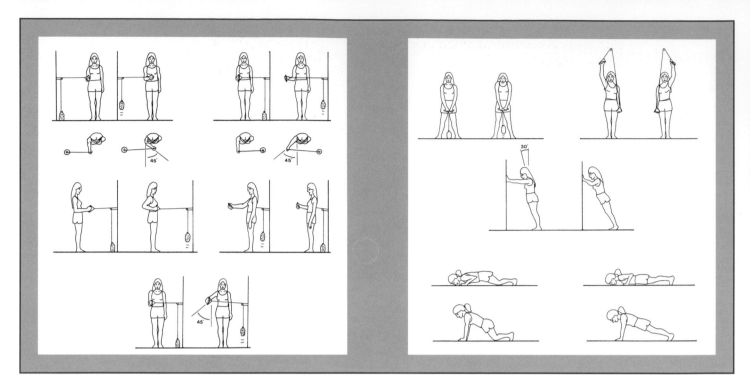

Figure 7.5 – *Short-arc exercises for strengthening the rotator cuff and deltoid using pulleys and weights (after Neer).*

Figure 7.6 – *Closed-chain exercises for strengthening scapular stabilizers (after Neer).*

regular pushups) (Fig. 7.6), and stamina training. Short-arc abduction exercises are recommended, throughout the strengthening process, to avoid instability during the arc of exercise.

The rotator cuff and deltoid are strengthened using TheraBand rubber bands, later to be replaced with a pulley with increasing weights. The strength of the scapula stabilizers is improved with shoulder shrugging and closed-chain exercises. The patients are instructed, on a number of occasions, regarding which exercises should be performed each day and the number of repitions to be done. The progress of the patient is monitored by the physiotherapist who instructs the patient to progress to the next stage when appropriate.

The final aim of rehabilitation is to improve the functional capacity of the patient with an increase in the complexity and intensity of the activities. Occupational therapy and a home-exercise programme, should promote and maintain the functional capacity of the shoulder.

Psychological treatment

Patients who have difficulty understanding their condition, patients who do not cooperate during their treatment and patients who might have a psychological element to the initiation of their instability (voluntary dislocation), or the persistence of their shoulder instability, should be assessed and treated by a clinical psychologist.

Many voluntary dislocators may have a psychological problem and need treatment for this, but children who use their shoulder instability as a 'party trick' can usually be stopped from dislocating their shoulder with appropriate explanation, and advice, and management by 'skillful neglect' may be very appropriate. Parents must also be aware of the condition, and of the importance of the rehabilitation programme, and the place of psychological support if needed.

Surgical treatment

Surgical treatment of antero-inferior instability

Patients who fail to respond to extended conservative management may be treated surgically, but generally no patient should be operated on if they are under the age of 16 years, or when the dislocation is voluntary. Following a careful clinical, radiological, and arthroscopic evaluation surgical management must address the underlying pathology. Usually, this means tightening up the antero-inferior laxity of the capsule. However, if other pathology is discovered at the time of surgery this must also be repaired.

The Neer inferior-capsular shift procedure. The inferior-capsular shift was first described by Neer and Foster (1980) and is the most commonly used surgical procedure for antero-inferior dislocation. The aim of the operation is to eliminate excessive capsular laxity, especially in the anterior capsule and inferior capsular recess.

It is important that a cosmetic axillary approach is used, because the patient is usually a teenage girl or young adult. The skin is mobilized widely upon the deep fascia so that the deltopectoral groove can be opened.

A standard deltopectoral approach is now used, preserving the cephalic vein but ligating and dividing the deltoid pedicle. For the inferior-capsular shift to be adequate the surgeon will need to make an adequate exposure of the inferior capsule. In order to do this safely the axillary nerve must be located and protected throughout the procedure. The suscapularis is tenotomized on stay-sutures, after ligation and division of the anterior circumflex humeral artery and its venae comitans. The whole of subscapularis must be divided in order to gain access to the inferior capsule. The capsule is now opened with a vertical capsulotomy on stay-sutures from the rotator interval down to the inferior glenoid recess, staying close to the humerus so as to avoid the previously seen axillary nerve. The humeral head is now externally rotated and the capsulotomy is taken around the neck of the humerus until the capsule is released from the postero-inferior humerus as well. The front of the capsule is then horizontally divided to form a T capsulotomy.

The inside of the joint is now inspected to see if there is an additional Bankart lesion. In the rare event of a Bankart lesion being present it is repaired with suture anchors.

The inferior flap is now pulled upwards and the apex is sutured to the humerus as high as it will go (usually at the level of the rotator interval). The humeral margin of this flap is now sutured to the stump of capsule left on the humerus. Once the lower flap has been advanced superiorly the laxity of the inferior capsular recess should have disappeared. The rotator interval is now closed, the sutures passing from the superior flap to the free anterior edge of the supraspinatus. This is a most important step. Finally the superior flap is pulled inferiorly, crossing the

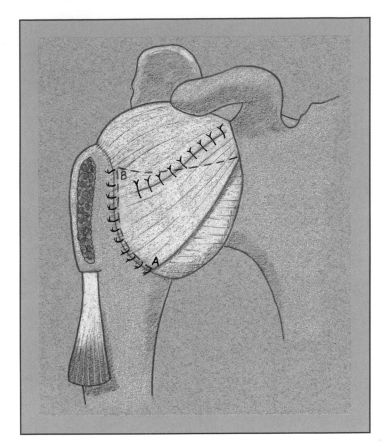

Figure 7.7 – *The Neer-capsular shift.*

inferior flap in a cruciate manner, and sutured both to the stump of capsule on the humerus and on top of the inferior flap, with a flap-to-flap suture (Fig. 7.7). Care must be taken to avoid over tightening of the capsule. If an anterio-inferior capsular shift is performed the inferior flap should be positioned while the arm is held in 45° elevation and 45° external rotation although Neer's original suggestion was in slight flexion and 10° of external rotation. Once the superior flap is positioned the arm is held at the side of the body, but still in 45° external rotation. After the operation the arm is immobilized in a broad arm sling and body bandage for 4 weeks.

Mobilization is carried out slowly, focusing more on isometric than strengthening exercises. Stretching of the capsule must be strictly avoided.

Neer and Foster (1980) reported only one recurrence out of 32 cases but with less than 2 years follow-up. Others have reported 9–11% recurrent instability after an average of 3–7 years (Cooper and Brems, 1992; Bigliani *et al.*, 1995). If other criteria, such as pain and limitation of activities, are also included in the evaluation then between 27 and 39% of the patients have only a fair or a poor result (Bigliani *et al.*, 1995; Mallon and Speer, 1995). It should be emphasized that this is a much higher proportion than after surgical treatment of traumatic anterior instability.

There is some early evidence that capsular tightening can be achieved by using lasers. The procedure, which is carried out arthroscopically, is relatively straightforward. Depending on the main direction of instability, different parts of the capsule are literally painted with the laser and the collagen is seen to shrink in the beam, much like bacon-rind crisping in the frying pan. The penetration of the laser is limited, therefore no extensive damage can be done. Although the patients probably do gradually loosen the capsule again, the early temporary stability obtained using this method can be extremely helpful in supporting the rehabilitation programme.

Some surgeons (Duncan & Savoie, 1993) have reported acceptable results with an arthroscopic inferior-capsular shift operation in a limited series of 10 patients. All of them had satisfactory results at a follow-up of 1–3 years. However, this should be looked upon as experimental surgery at this stage.

Surgery for postero-inferior dislocation

Recurrent posterior dislocation is a very rare condition. The results of treatment are poor, and the results of surgery worse. Few surgeons have published their results and those that have can rarely muster a series which goes into double figures. Authors of textbooks will glibly state that the Scott posterior-glenoid osteotomy is the procedure of choice for posterior dislocation, without telling the reader that Scott reported three cases, only two of which were his, and that of these cases only one was atraumatic, and one dislocated immediately postoperatively. Alternatively, they will state that the Neer-inferior shift from the posterior approach is the procedure of choice, without saying that Neer only described 15 cases, half had a follow-up of 2 years, with one dislocating in this time period.

Against this background Hawkins (1984) performed a careful retrospective study of all patients who had presented to his clinic with posterior dislocation. There were 35 patients of whom 26 underwent surgery, 13 (50%) of these re-dislocated following surgery. The average age at presentation was 16 years, and surprisingly there were twice as many boys as girls. This is in marked

contrast to antero-inferior MDI, which is far commoner in girls. Most had started as a voluntary dislocation, which became an unintentional instability. Eighty percent could demonstrate their dislocation to their surgeon. All the patients dislocated as the arm was elevated in slight adduction and internal rotation, and relocated with a clunk on full elevation. One-fifth of the shoulders could be dislocated by muscle action alone.

Seventeen patients had a posterior glenoid osteotomy, 7 (41%) re-dislocated and five had complications, which were severe in two, leading to arthritis of the joint. Six had a reverse Putti–Platt operation and 6 (83%) re-dislocated. Three had a Boyd and Sisk operation of whom one re-dislocated.

Tibone and Ting (1990) presented 20 patients who had undergone a posterior capsule repair with a staple. Nine had an unsatisfactory result, six having a recurrence and three continuing to experience moderate or severe pain. Five further patients suffered complications from surgery. Only one patient could throw as well after surgery as before.

Hawkins (1984) stresses that posterior dislocations should be classified into three types (Table 7.6).

Every surgeon is in agreement that habitual dislocators should not be considered for surgery. Voluntary dislocators, likewise, should not be considered for surgery. Only involuntary, or unintentional, dislocators should be considered for surgery, and then only if they have pain and functional disability and have failed to respond to the conservative treatment protocol shown above.

Postero-inferior capsular shift. The rationale behind this procedure is that the posterior capsule is lax and that the inferior capsule is too capacious in these patients. It appears logical therefore to reduce the dimension of the capsule with a Neer-capsular shift.

The operation is performed with the patient in the lateral decubitus position. A skin-crease incision is made

Table 7.6 Classification of posterior instability.		
(a)	Habitual	Psychiatrically disturbed; wilful
(b)	Voluntary	Intentional but not wilful
(c)	Involuntary	Unintentional

from the spine of the scapula aiming towards the axillary crease. Neer warns that the scar always stretches in these patients, and that patients should be warned of this pre-operatively. The deltoid is split in the direction of its fibres for a distance of 5 cm. The posterior deltoid has a thick deep fascia, which is split to reveal the infraspinatus and teres minor. Care must be taken not to damage the axillary nerve which is seen exiting the quadralateral space, along with the posterior circumflex humeral vessels.

The plane between the infraspinatus and teres minor must now be located, because this is the watershed between the axillary nerve and the suprascapular nerves and allows extensile exposure of the posterior capsule. Sometimes it is difficult to define this plane. One trick is to realize that the infraspinatus is a bipennate muscle. The central tendon is easily seen, so the surgeon can measure the distance of the spine of the scapular to the tendon; taking this distance again below the tendon will lead safely to the surgical plane.

The infraspinatus is retracted superiorly, and the teres minor inferiorly, to expose the capsule. The infraspinatus can be tenotomized on stay-sutures for a more extensile exposure. A 'T' capsulotomy is now performed in an identical fashion to the antero-inferior capsular shift. The joint is inspected and then the inferior flap is pulled up and sutured, so that the inferior recess is abolished. Then the top flap is brought down and sutured to overlap the inferior flap. If a postero-inferior capsular shift operation is performed the arm is held in slight extension and neutral rotation whilst the capsule is re-attached. The shoulder is then immobilized in a shoulder spica with the arm in 30° of abduction, 20° of flexion, and 10° of external rotation.

Neer (1980) reported on 15 patients undergoing a primary posterior repair. In five of these patients he found an anterior Bankart lesion and had to open the front of the joint as well as the back, performing an anterior Bankart procedure and a posterior shift. Only six cases were followed up for over 2 years. One patient had an axillary neurapraxia and one redislocated.

The problem with posterior soft-tissue procedures is that the posterior capsule is not as thick as the anterior capsule. In young adult males the posterior capsule may be strong enough to control instability when it has been double-breasted, but in many patients the capsule has the consistency of tissue paper. Any soft-tissue procedure will only convert single-ply tissue paper to two-ply tissue

paper, which lacks the strength to control a dislocating shoulder.

Scott posterior glenoid osteotomy. The rationale behind this procedure is that the glenoid is retroverted, allowing the humeral head to slip off the back of the glenoid. The osteotomy corrects this. As already stated Scott (1967) described the procedure in three cases.

The approach is the same as for the posterior shift. The joint is opened in order to fashion a vertical osteotomy of the glenoid, parallel to the joint surface. A bone graft is then taken from the posterior angle of the acromion and is tamped into the osteotomy to form an opening wedge. It is important to leave an intact anterior cortex, and to avoid coming inadvertently into the joint with the osteotomy.

Scott (1967) had one recurrence in three cases. Hawkins (1984) reported 7 recurrences in 17 cases. Wilkinson (1985) reported 4 recurrences in 23 cases. Rockwood (1993) reported a 69% recurrence rate in 23 patients.

Nobuhara has reported on his modification of the glenoid osteotomy using a purely inferior bone block. Postoperatively 26% of patients had pain on activity, 27% had a local discomfort and 32% had recurrent instability when lifting. Only 36% of patients returned to their pre-operative level of sports.

Gerber and Ganz (1984) commented that in a cadaver study of this procedure the humeral head is forced forward, on to the coracoid, causing coracoid impingement.

Internal rotation humeral osteotomy. The rationale of this procedure is that the shoulder only dislocates in internal rotation. If the humeral head is held in external rotation then the instability does not occur. It appears logical therefore to consider performing a humeral osteotomy, placing the humeral head in external rotation (internally rotating the humerus) and fixing the osteotomy with a plate (Fig. 7.8).

This procedure is performed through a cosmetic anterior-axillary approach. The humerus is approached through a standard deltopectoral approach. The osteotomy is performed at the level of the superior edge of the latissimus dorsi. The long head of the biceps is protected. Two 'K' wires are inserted and a 40° rotation is performed taking the head into external rotation and the shaft into internal rotation. The osteotomy is fixed with a third tubular plate, bent to form a condylar blade plate. The arm

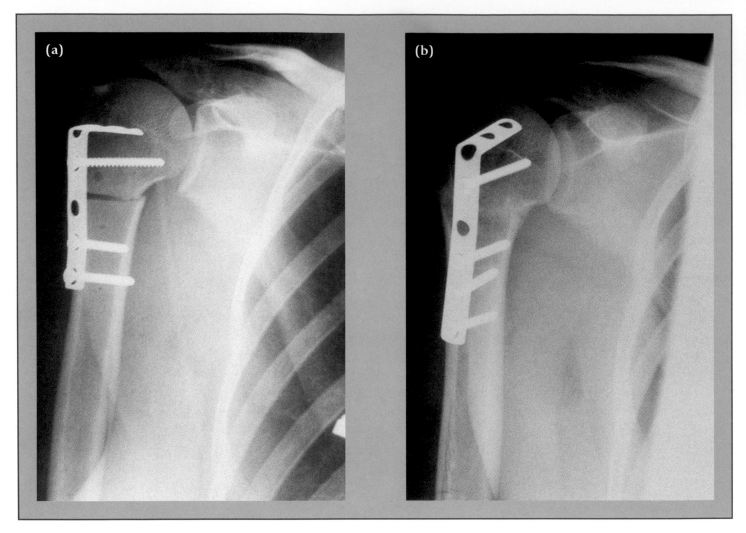

Figure 7.8 – *Internal rotational osteotomy of the humerus for posterior instability.*

is placed in a sling for 3 weeks postoperatively and then mobilized under physiotherapy control (Weber *et al.*, 1984).

There have only been two small series reported of humeral osteotomy for posterior dislocation. Surin (1990) evaluated 12 patients with one dislocation and one non-union. Welch from Toronto also reports a similar experience.

Posterior bone block. The rationale behind the posterior bone block is to provide an increased 'chock-block' effect which will prevent the humeral head from dislocating posteriorly.

The procedure is performed through the posterior approach as for a posterior shift. A bone block is harvested from the posterior iliac crest and is screwed to the posterior glenoid rim.

Mowery (1985) reported on five patients treated with a posterior bone block. Three of the five patients required a re-operation, one for anterior dislocation and two for scar revision of a very widened scar.

Warren (1989) treated 11 patients with a posterior capsulorrhaphy with or without a bone block and 10 of the 11 patients had a satisfactory outcome.

The Boyd and Sisk procedure. The rationale behind this procedure is to transfer the tendon of the long head of the biceps from its normal position, and to take it around the back of the humerus, and to staple it to the back of the glenoid. This has two effects, firstly it places a strong structure (the tendon) across the weakened area of posterior capsule, to physically prevent dislocation, and secondly the long head of the biceps tends to push the head back when the arm is internally rotated; by transferring the tendon this force is removed. Boyd (1972) reported his results in eight patients. Five of these patients had a traumatic dislocation, with a posterior Bankart tear in four. Only three patients were atraumatic. Boyd reports that the operation should not be performed with less than three assistants. The operation is complex because it requires a simultaneous anterior and posterior approach to the shoulder with the patient in the lateral decubitus position. However, the results were satisfactory, with no recurrences in this small series.

Arthroscopic posterior repair. Wolf has reported 15 patients, with traumatic posterior recurrent dislocation, who have undergone an arthroscopic reconstruction using suture hooks and anchors. Ten patients had an excellent result, 1 had a fair result and 1 had a poor result.

Botulinum injections and tenotomies. There can be occasional cases when the clinical and the EMG examination confirm overactivity of isolated muscles (pectoralis minor, pectoralis major, subscapularis). Botulinum toxin type A, which is a potent neurotoxin, prevents the release of acetylcholine from the presynaptic axon at motor end-plates. It can be used therapeutically to produce a reversible partial chemical denervation when injected directly into muscle. The method is mainly used in the treatment of neurological disorders, associated with severe muscle spasm, such as blepharospasm of the eyelids. It can be used in selected cases in the management of MDI patients, in addition to the rehabilitation programme, to allow retraining to occur. Its effects are currently being evaluated in our units in Nottingham and Exeter.

Tenotomies of overacting muscles have been used in the past. Their effect is usually short-lived and the instability often returns.

Summary

The diagnosis and treatment of patients with MDI is complex. Management depends upon having a multidisciplinary team, led by an orthopaedic surgeon. Each member of the team is responsible for certain aspects of the treatment of the teenager. If conservative management fails then the Neer inferior-capsular shift is a highly effective surgical solution for antero-inferior MDI.

The same can not be said for the surgical treatment of postero-inferior instability. Here there are a number of surgical options that sound attractive theoretically, but are poor in practice. Time will tell how we ought to manage this challenging condition.

CHAPTER 8

Frozen shoulder

T. Bunker

Introduction

Frozen shoulder is the most enigmatic of all the conditions that occur around the shoulder. Codman (1934), who coined the term frozen shoulder, stated 'It is difficult to define, difficult to treat and difficult to explain from the point of view of pathology'.

Recent research (Bunker & Anthony, 1995) has unravelled this enigma for we now know that the pathology of frozen shoulder is that of a fibrous contracture of the coracohumeral ligament and rotator interval of the capsule. Histologically, this tissue is composed of a dense matrix of mature Type-III collagen. The tissue is highly cellular, and the cells are fibroblasts and contractile myofibroblasts (Table 8.1). These findings are similar to Dupuytren's contracture and the two conditions share many other features. Frozen shoulder is a Dupuytren-like disease which affects the shoulder and leads to contracture of the capsule, which acts as a checkrein to external rotation, causing a global restriction of passive joint movement. This knowledge allows us, for the first time, to make rational decisions about how to treat the condition.

Table 8.1 Pathology of frozen shoulder.	
Fibrous contracture of	Coracohumeral ligament
	Rotator interval
	Capsule
Histology	Dense collagen matrix
	containing fibroblasts
	and myofibroblasts
Causing	Checkrein to movement

Definition

The general features of frozen shoulder are shared with many other forms of shoulder pathology, and its pathognomonic features are somewhat underplayed. Coming to a consensus on a definition for frozen shoulder has proved elusive.

Codman (1934) stated that patients with frozen shoulder shared certain common features. These features were slow onset, pain felt near the insertion of the deltoid, inability to sleep on the affected side, painful and restricted elevation and external rotation, with a normal radiological appearance. This description, like his description of the patient with a rotator-cuff tear, is difficult to better six decades later.

The problem is that this definition is still too general because it could be applied to a patient with a cuff tear, although the likelihood of an entirely normal radiograph is slim. This has led to confusion because any shoulder that is stiff and painful is described as frozen by general practitioners, and all too often even by orthopaedic surgeons. Wiley (1991) arthroscoped 150 patients referred with a given diagnosis of frozen shoulder and 113 turned out to have some other pathology, which illustrates the scale of the problem! Bayley (1994) arthroscoped a large series of patients with a presumed diagnosis of frozen shoulder and found that one half had some other pathology.

Lundberg (1969) tried to overcome this confusion by classifying the stiff, painful shoulder into two groups: (1) primary frozen shoulder occurs in those patients who fit Codman's criteria and in whom all other pathology is excluded; and (2) secondary frozen shoulder is an identical clinical syndrome caused by a clear cut, discernable condition, such as soft-tissue injury, fracture, arthritis, hemiplegia, or any other known cause. This classification of primary and secondary frozen shoulder is helpful because it allows us to focus on primary frozen shoulder, to which the rest of this chapter is dedicated.

Zuckerman (1994) attempted to get a consensus definition of frozen shoulder from his colleagues in the American Shoulder and Elbow Society (ASES). Ninety-eight percent agreed that frozen shoulder exists, 92% said that it was a condition with a global loss of both active and passive shoulder movement. Fifty-eight percent said that they would like a better or tighter definition.

We attempted to get a more comprehensive definition from colleagues in the British Elbow and Shoulder Society and the South West Orthopaedic Club, and our questionnaire was returned by 55 orthopaedic surgeons, 26 consultants and 29 trainees. Ninety-six percent stated that it was a condition characterized by loss of both active and passive motion. Eighty-seven percent stated that elevation should be less than 100°, 91% said that external rotation should be under 30°, and 96% said that internal rotation should be restricted to less than the L5 vertebral level. Ninety-one percent agreed that the onset of frozen shoulder is insidious. Ninety-eight percent stated that radiographs of the shoulder must be normal (Table 8.2). The pathognomonic sign in frozen shoulder is loss of passive external rotation. This feature only occurs in two other conditions — arthritis and locked posterior dislocation — both of which are excluded by a normal radiograph.

Frozen shoulder is also characterized by its course. Classically, it is said to have three phases, a painful phase, a stiffening phase and a phase of resolution (Fig. 8.1). Reeves (1975) in a prospective study of 41 patients with frozen shoulder, followed for five to ten years, found that the painful phase lasted 10–36 months, the stiffening phase 4–12 months and the recovery period 12–42 months. This shows frozen shoulder to be a most protracted disease, with the very shortest period to resolution being beyond 2 years, and the most protracted over 7 years.

Codman stated that 'even the most protracted cases recover with or without treatment in about 2 years'. Unfortunately, this has led to a somewhat nihilistic approach to the disease, and this statement needs to be reviewed in the light of the following 60 years of investigation into frozen shoulder. Although Codman stated that the condition 'clears up entirely', this he qualified in two ways; firstly he stated that 'recovery is by degrees, it is pretty hard even for the patients to say when they are well'; secondly what he meant by an entire recovery was that the joint was not left 'deformed or otherwise permanently damaged'. In other words the condition does not lead on to arthritis. The paper by Grey (1978) is often quoted by those who say that the condition always resolves. This is probably the shortest oft-quoted paper in orthopaedics for it is five paragraphs long! Contrast this with the statements of Simonds (1949): 'complete recovery... is not my experience', and of

Table 8.2 Definition of frozen shoulder.	
Symptoms	True shoulder pain
	Night pain of insidious onset
Signs	Painful restriction of active and passive motion
	Passive elevation less than 100°
	Passive external rotation less than 30°
	Passive internal rotation less than L5
	All other shoulder disease excluded
Investigations	Plain radiographs normal
	Arthrogram shows contracted joint
	Arthroscopy shows vascular granulation tissue at base of the long head of biceps (rotator interval)

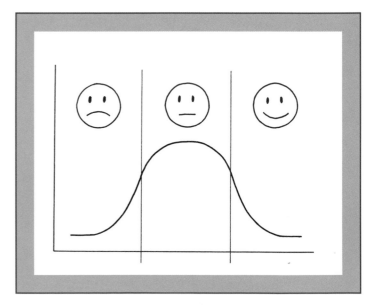

Figure 8.1 *The classic course of frozen shoulder. In reality the course may be more protracted and movement may not return to normal although functional impairment is small.*

DePalma (1952): 'It is erroneous to believe that in all instances restoration of function is attained'. Most papers show that 10% of patients have ongoing disability. Reeves' very detailed study, which had a 10 year follow-up, showed that of 41 patients 25 had a permanent loss of movement, although there was only a functional loss in 3 patients. The best paper on the natural history of frozen shoulder (Shaffer *et al.*, 1992) evaluated 62 patients both objectively and subjectively for an average follow-up of 7 years. They found that 50% still had either mild pain or stiffness of the shoulder, or both. Sixty percent still demonstrated some restriction of motion compared with study generated control values. Marked restriction of movement, when present, was most common in external rotation. The authors concluded that complete resolution was not universal and this brought them to question whether this is a self-limiting condition because half their patients remained symptomatic and more than half had a measureable loss of motion, although this caused little functional disability.

Terminology

Over a decade ago the author became intrigued by this conundrum and wrote an article entitled 'Time for a new name for frozen shoulder' (Bunker, 1985). I argued that the term frozen shoulder was being used as a dustbin diagnosis for any stiff and painful shoulder that was difficult to diagnose. This encouraged doctors to do as little as possible about this common, disabling, protracted and painful condition. Frozen shoulder has been plagued not only by a lack of consensus for a definition but also by the plethora of terms ascribed to it. Many of these give a false pathology to the condition. Periarthritis was the term used by Duplay in 1872, which is a confusing non sequitur. Many physicians and rheumatologists like to call frozen shoulder 'capsulitis', but this implies that it is an inflammatory condition. As we shall see, the condition is actually a fibrosing disease and although there is perivascular inflammation, and some inflammatory change in the synovium, inflammation is not the prime pathology. Neviaser (1945) called frozen shoulder 'adhesive capsulitis', which not only implies that it is inflammatory, but also suggests that there are adhesions within the joint (Neviaser said there were adhesions at the infraglenoid recess and that the capsule stuck to the head like adhesive); however, no one since has ever seen this intra-articular adhesions in this condition, and there are none in this condition. Quigley (1969) used the term 'checkrein shoulder', which, as we shall discover, was a very apt name indeed. However, frozen shoulder remains the most popular term for this condition and has the merit of implying no false pathology.

Incidence

Frozen shoulder is actually quite a rare condition. Of 1324 consecutive new patients attending my shoulder clinic 70 fitted the criteria of primary frozen shoulder, an incidence of just 5%. The diagnosis was confirmed by shoulder arthroscopy, unless specifically contraindicated.

Previous studies have probably over-reported the incidence, as other shoulder disease was not so rigorously excluded. Lundberg (1969) suggested an incidence of 2% of the population and Bridgeman (1972) suggested an incidence of 2.3%.

The condition occurs with equal frequency in the right shoulder as in the left shoulder. As far as dominance is concerned most people are right-handed, but this does not mean that frozen shoulder is commoner in the non-dominant hand! Frozen shoulder is not affected by dominance. Roughly 10% of cases will get the condition in the second shoulder within 5 years of the initial diagnosis. Bilateral frozen shoulder is commoner in diabetics.

Clinical presentation

The patient, who is in late middle age, (average 56 years) presents with an insidious onset of true shoulder pain. Men are affected as commonly as women and the left shoulder is affected as commonly as the right shoulder. Severe and unrelenting shoulder pain is the cardinal symptom and this pain is particularly severe at night. The shoulder subsequently stiffens, the stiffening being both abrupt and severe. Both stiffness and pain limit the patient in terms of their activities. Function is severely impaired, particularly those functions which require rotation (doing up the bra, hitching up the trousers [for internal rotation], dressing and combing the hair [for external rotation]).

The patient will usually have tried all conservative methods of treatment, without success, before attending the shoulder clinic. Most have had at least one steroid injection and prolonged physiotherapy.

On examination the patient may appear depressed due to relentless night pain. Examination of the shoulder is unremarkable. There is usually no wasting, and in particular no wasting of the infraspinatus. The deltoid may be slightly wasted due to disuse. There may be tenderness lateral to the coracoid process, but this is unpredictable. The acromioclavicular joint is normal. Movement is markedly restricted, both actively and more importantly passively. Most authors suggest that combined elevation is less than 100°. In our series combined elevation was 83.2°.

Most authors agree that passive external rotation should be less than 50% of the unaffected side. A reduction of external rotation is the pathognomonic sign of frozen shoulder. Patients with rotator-cuff disease will often have restriction of elevation, although the passive range is greater than the active range. However, most patients with cuff disorders maintain a good range of passive external rotation. In massive rotator-cuff tears there can be secondary shortening of the coracohumeral ligament, which acts as a checkrein to external rotation, but usually the other signs of cuff tear (sulcus, eminence, wasting of cuff, subacromial crepitus, upward subluxation of head, weakness of cuff) are quite obvious by this stage. Gross limitation of passive external rotation is only present in three other conditions — arthritis, locked posterior dislocation and frozen shoulder. In our series the average external rotation was 9.4°. Internal rotation is similarly restricted both actively and passively. Usually the patient can just reach to buttock level. The shoulder, being stiff, is clearly stable. Neurological examination is normal.

Associated conditions

Diabetes mellitus
The relationship between diabetes and frozen shoulder is well documented (Bridgeman, 1972; Lequesne *et al.*, 1977; Fisher *et al.*, 1986; Pal *et al.*, 1986). Diabetic patients have a 10–20% incidence of frozen shoulder, which rises to 36% in insulin-dependent diabetes. Of patients with bilateral frozen shoulder 42% are diabetic. Diabetic patients often fail to benefit from manipulation (Janda & Hawkins 1993), although this has been disputed by Sneppen (1997). Twenty-seven percent of our patients had diabetes mellitus (fasting blood sugar measured in all patients) (Table 8.3).

Table 8.3 Associated conditions.

Diabetes	10% NIDDM have frozen shoulder
Dupuytren's	18–25% of patients with frozen shoulder
Cardiac disease	Elevated serum lipids
Personality	No evidence
Minor trauma	
Neurosurgery	? Phenytoin and phenobarbitone

This association may give some clues as to the pathogenesis of frozen shoulder. Angiogenesis is common in diabetes, and from our studies of the pathology of frozen shoulder, and those of others, we have found that angiogenesis is common in frozen shoulders as well. Kay and Slater (1981) found fibroblasts and myofibroblasts in the capsule of a diabetic with frozen shoulder. They suggested that myofibroblast proliferation appears to be related to high levels of some growth factors, such as platelet derived growth factor (PDGF), and suggested that release of PDGF from abnormal diabetic vessels may be a stimulus to local myofibroblast proliferation. We have found abnormalities of growth factors and cytokines in frozen shoulders, such as fibroblast growth factor, interleukin and tumour necrosis factor, PDGF levels were only mildly raised above normal.

Dupuytren's contracture
Meulengracht and Schwarz (1952) found evidence of Dupuytren's contracture in 18% of their patients with frozen shoulder. Schaer (1936) found Dupuytren's contracture in 25% of their patients. The incidence was far higher in our series. I personally examined the hands of all 50 patients in my initial study, 29 of 50 patients had a pit, nodule or band of Dupuytren's disease in their hands. The associations of diabetes and of Dupuytren's contracture has been noted by Edelson *et al.* (1991), who comment that Peyronie's disease is also common in this group. Of course Dupuytren's disease is also associated with diabetes and so once again we find an uncanny series of interconnecting associations.

Cardiac disease

Frozen shoulder has been associated with cardiac disease (McLaughlin, 1951; Wright & Haq, 1976). Many patients with cardiac disease have raised serum lipids. We tested 43 of our patients for fasting serum-lipid levels and found a significant elevation of cholesterol and triglyceride in frozen shoulder (Bunker & Esler 1995). The patients were fasted for 10 hours prior to venepuncture. Age- and sex-matched controls were taken from consenting orthopaedic patients admitted to the hospital for arthroscopic surgery to the knee and for foot surgery. There were 23 men (average age 59 years) and 20 women (average age 56 years) with frozen shoulder. The mean serum-cholesterol concentration in patients with frozen shoulder was 5.92 + 1.17 mmol/l compared with 5.14 + 1.13 mmol/l in the control patients ($p < 0.0l$, Student's t-test). The mean serum triglyceride concentration in the frozen shoulder patients was 2.24 + 1.38 mmol/l and in the controls 1.62 + 0.64 mmol/l ($p < 0.01$). The exclusion of nine patients with diabetes from the frozen shoulder group did not alter the significance levels of frozen shoulder from the control series. Raised serum lipids are also found in patients with Dupuytren's contracture (Sanderson *et al.*, 1992), and in patients with diabetes (Havel, 1979). The astonishing connections continue to appear.

Personality

Coventry thought that patients with frozen shoulder had an abnormal emotional affect. Quigley (1969), on the other hand, stated that the abnormal emotional responses of patients with frozen shoulder could be 'as often the result of the painful shoulder as the cause'. No evidence has been found of personality disorders, in patients with frozen shoulder, on standard psychological testing (Wright & Haq, 1976).

Minor trauma

There may be an association between minor degrees of trauma and the onset of frozen shoulder. Frozen shoulder may, for instance, come on after a Colles fracture. Dupuytren's disease may also be initiated by minor trauma to the hand or, for instance, a Colles' fracture.

Neurosurgery

Frozen shoulder has been recorded in patients recovering from neurosurgery. It is highly likely that these patients were on anti-epileptic treatment, the commonest combination at the time being phenytoin and phenobarbitone. Phenytoin is associated with Dupuytren's disease and phenobarbitone with frozen shoulder. Phenobarbitone is also associated with raised serum-lipid levels. So the coincidences continue.

Investigations

Haematological and biochemical tests

Full blood count (FBC), erythrocyte sedimentation rate (ESR) and HLA B27 are all normal in frozen shoulder. Calcium, phosphate, serum globulins and bone alkaline phosphatase are all normal (Table 8.4).

Plain radiographs

By definition these must be normal although some disuse osteopenia is allowed.

Arthrography

Neviaser (1975) showed that there was a characteristic reduction in joint volume in frozen shoulder with a lack of filling of the axillary fold (Fig. 8.2) and the subscapular recess (the rotator interval). The bicipital sheath is well visualized. Arthrography after manipulation under anaesthetic showed that the capsule of the axillary recess tore away from the humeral neck, allowing extravasation of contrast material.

Table 8.4 Investigations in frozen shoulder.

FBC, WBC, ESR	Normal
HLA B27	Normal
Serum lipids	May be elevated
Calcium, phosphate, serum globulins and bone alkaline phosphatase	Normal
Radiographs	Normal
Arthrograms	Contracted joint
MRI	Thickened capsule
Arthroscopy	Matted granulation-tissue in rotator interval
	Contracted joint space
	Tight infraglenoid recess

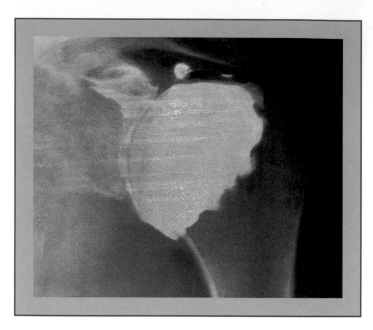

Figure 8.2 – *An arthrogram of frozen shoulder showing a contracted joint.*

Magnetic resonance imaging

Very few studies have been performed on magnetic resonance imaging (MRI) of frozen shoulder. Emig *et al.* (1995) examined nine patients with frozen shoulder and found that the capsule was thickened, being an average 5.2 mm thick in the frozen shoulder group versus 2.9 mm thick in the control group ($p < 0.01$). They could find no significant difference between coracohumeral thickness or the rotator interval on coronal oblique scans, but this is a difficult plane for examining such structures.

We took 14 patients with frozen shoulder and performed coronal oblique scans of the rotator interval and although there was clear thickening of the coracohumeral ligament on some of the scans this was not significant.

Arthroscopy

We performed a shoulder arthroscopy on 30 patients with primary frozen shoulder prior to manipulation. Twelve were re-arthroscoped following the manipulation. The major finding was a consistent abnormality arising out of the subscapularis bursa, at the base of the origin of the long head of the biceps (Fig. 8.3). Twenty-seven patients had an abnormal villous fronding of the synovium, which was clearly highly vascular, arising from the subscapularis bursa and spreading to a variable extent across the rotator interval area. In some patients there was

a nodular appearance of the synovium, with finger-like projections and in others a synovial fronding like seaweed. The final three patients also had an abnormality of the rotator interval, which was covered in a mature sheet of dense scar tissue, the average duration of symptoms for these three was greater than for the whole series (24 months compared to 14 months for the series), and there was no increase in vascularity in these patients. These changes are so consistent as to be pathognomonic for primary frozen shoulder.

The tendon of the long head of biceps was normal in 24 patients. The tendon had a top surface vasculitic change where it entered its tunnel in four patients, a common feature of impingement. In one patient there were petechial haemorrhages at the base of the long head of biceps, and in one patient the long head of biceps was entirely enclosed in scar tissue from the rotator interval area of the capsule. One patient had a mesentery, or vincula of the long head of biceps. The tendon of supraspinatus was normal in all patients but the scar from the rotator interval reached on to the tendon in one case.

There was minor cartilage fibrillation of the humeral head in three patients, two patients had a licheniform or geographical marginal erosion of the humeral head, the remaining 25 patients had a completely normal humerus. The glenoid had minor cartilage fibrillation in two patients, the remaining 28 patients were normal. The labrum was normal in all patients, there was a Buford complex in one patient and a Detrisac Type II sublabral hole in another patient. The middle glenohumeral ligament was normal in all cases (one was affected by the Buford complex), although the scar from the rotator interval merged with two. The subscapularis was normal in all cases, although the rotator interval changes reached on to the subscapularis in two cases. The inferior glenohumeral ligament was normal in all those cases where it could be seen, in six patients the joint was so contracted and of such small volume that it was not possible to see the ligament. There was only one patient with any evidence of adhesions and these were within the rotator interval area.

The infraglenoid recess was too tight to access in four patients (in two patients we were able to navigate into the infraglenoid recess, despite not being able to see the inferior glenohumeral ligament). The infraglenoid recess was of small capacity in all but two cases, and was more vascular than normal in seven patients.

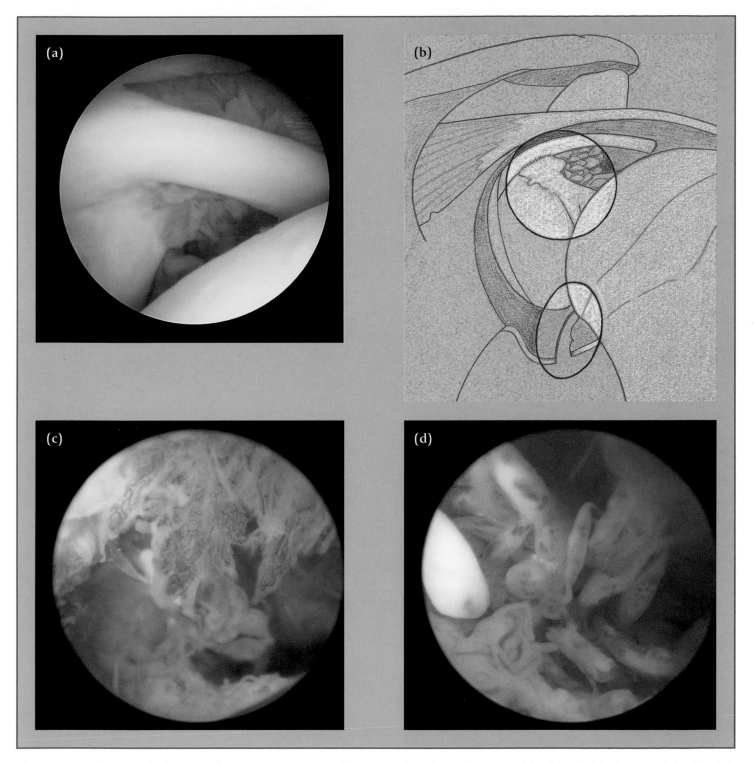

Figure 8.3 – *The main finding at arthroscopy is a synovitis obliterating the subscapular recess (a), (b) and (c) close-up of the fronded, vascular synovitis, (d) villonodular synovitis.*

This study shows that the pathognomonic change is within the rotator interval area of the capsule. The entrance to the subscapular recess (the foramen of Weitbrecht) is filled with highly vascular nodular or fronded tissue in the early stages, and dense scar tissue in the more protracted cases. The secondary change is a tight infraglenoid recess.

Twelve patients were re-arthroscoped after manipulation. In 11 cases there was an avulsion of the capsule in the infraglenoid recess from the humeral neck

(Fig. 8.4). In one patient this tear extended into the inferior glenohumeral ligament. In three patients there was petechial haemorrhage from the rotator interval area. These changes are similar to the arthrographic changes of Neviaser (1975), and are borne out by the arthroscopic changes reported by Uitvligt (1993).

What of the literature concerning arthroscopy in primary frozen shoulder? A review of the arthroscopic findings made in frozen shoulder is given in Table 8.5. The first report of arthroscopy for frozen shoulder was by Ha'eri and Maitland in 1981. They studied 24 patients with primary frozen shoulder, and found the joint capsule was contracted in 60%, but there were no intra-articular adhesions, the joint surfaces were normal, and they suggested that this study implicated an extra-synovial cause for frozen shoulder.

Ogilvie-Harris and Wiley (1986) reported on 439 cases of arthroscopic surgery of the shoulder. Of these, 40 cases had primary frozen shoulder. The patients appeared to have an extrasynovial contracture of the anterior capsule, which could be seen to tighten on external rotation, causing the loss of motion. These cases had a reduced joint capacity, mild synovitis and no adhesions. Wiley (1991) refined this study. Of 150 patients referred with frozen shoulder, 37 qualified for the diagnosis of primary frozen shoulder and were arthroscoped. The appearance was uniform; there was a patchy, vascular, matted area of granulation tissue around the origin of the long head of the biceps tendon, and the opening into the subscapularis recess. The scar tissue appeared as a small, red, nodular area of granulation tissue filling the subscapularis recess. The joint capacity was reduced, but there were no adhesions.

Our first report (Bunker *et al.*, 1993) on 10 patients with primary frozen shoulder showed a characteristic vascular papillary infolding of the synovium, obliterating the subscapularis recess. Uitvligt *et al.* (1993) reported on 20 patients with primary frozen shoulder. Entry to the joint was difficult. There was a synovitis between the biceps and subscapularis (the subscapular recess) in 19 of the 20 patients, in 12 patients this affected the subscapularis bursa. There were no adhesions. Duralde *et al.* (1993) performed an arthroscopy on 11 patients with primary frozen

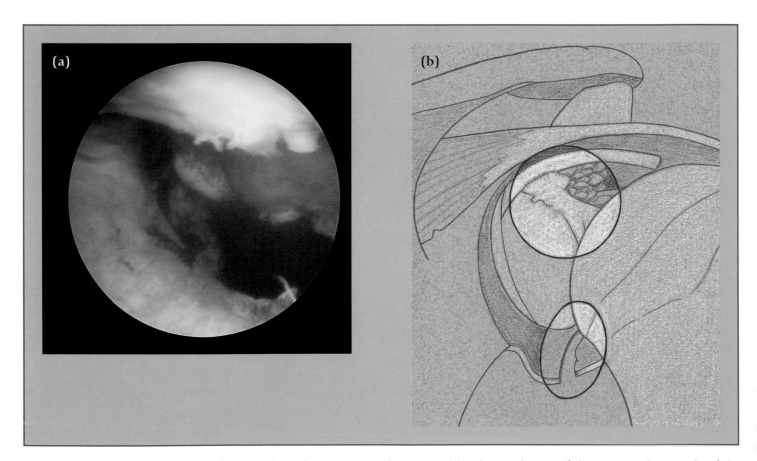

Figure 8.4 – *After manipulation the infraglenoid recess tears. The humeral head is at the top of the picture, the capsule of the infraglenoid recess at the bottom and the crescentic tear can be seen clearly.*

Table 8.5 Review of arthroscopic findings in frozen shoulder.

Ha'eri *et al.*	n = 24	1981	Contracted joint
			No adhesions
			Imply extra-articular cause
Ogilvie-Harris	n = 40	1986	Extrasynovial contracture
			Synovitis
			Reduced joint volume
			No adhesions
Wiley	n = 37	1991	Granulation tissue
			In subscapular recess
			No adhesions
Bunker *et al.*	n = 10	1993	Villous hyperplasia
			In rotator interval
			Tight infraglenoid recess
Uitvligt *et al.*	n = 20	1993	Entry difficult
			Synovitis subscapular recess
			No adhesions
Duralde *et al.*	n = 25	1993	Synovitis
			Subacromial adhesions
Hannafin *et al.*	n = 15	1994	Vascular synovitis
Esch	n = 50	1994	Scarred rotator interval
			Synovitis
			Subacromial bursitis
Midorikawa		1994	Contracted coracohumeral ligament
Segmuller	n = 24	1995	Proliferative synovitis
Bunker *et al.*	n = 35	1996	Scarred rotator interval
			Tight infraglenoid recess

shoulder, 14 with primary frozen shoulder who were diabetics; and 20 patients with secondary frozen shoulder. They found a synovitis in 42 shoulders and extra-articular subacromial 'adhesions' in 40 shoulders. Hannafin *et al.* (1994) arthroscoped 15 patients with primary frozen shoulder. They found a diffuse vascular synovitis in the 13 patients with Phase 1 or 2 disease and minimal synovitis in Phase 3. They took biopsies of the capsule and found that in Phase 1 there was an inflammatory synovitis with a normal capsule, in Phase 2 a vascular synovitis with fibroplasia of the capsule, and in Phase 3 minimal synovial hyperplasia, with capsular fibroplasia and scar formation. Esch (1994) arthroscoped 50 patients with primary frozen shoulder and found a thickened, scarred, rotator interval, a synovitis with adhesions around subscapularis, and a chronic subacromial bursitis. Midorikawa *et al.* (1994) found that the coracohumeral ligament was contracted and performed arthroscopic release to good effect. Segmuller *et al.* (1995) assessed 24 patients with primary frozen shoulder and invariably found a proliferative synovitis just beneath the biceps insertion, i.e. in the subscapular recess.

These 11 studies show a consistent pattern of arthroscopic findings in frozen shoulder. The major pathognomonic finding is an obliteration of the subscapularis recess with scar tissue covered by a highly vascular papillary infolding of the synovium. The axillary recess is tightened and the joint is of a reduced volume. There are no adhesions. Whatever pathology there is appears to be extrasynovial, or within the capsule and concentrated around the subscapularis bursa, this area of the capsule is a somewhat complicated area called the rotator interval.

Functional anatomy of the rotator interval

The rotator interval is the area of the capsule which lies between the front edge of the supraspinatus tendon, and the top edge of the subscapularis tendon (Fig. 8.5). This area is made more complicated by the subscapularis recess, which herniates under the coracoid process. The capsule is thin at this point, and if the joint is filled with fluid under pressure, for instance during arthroscopy, the rotator interval will bulge out at this point. However, normally there is negative pressure within the shoulder joint, so at open surgical exploration this area is felt as a sulcus, above the top edge the of subscapularis, dipping into the joint. The long head of the biceps passes obliquely across this area before entering into the pulley system of the intertubercular sulcus. The capsule of the rotator interval is strengthened by the coracohumeral ligament, which originates from the coracoid process and inserts into the intertubercular area of the humerus. With the arm in neutral rotation this ligament is lax, it only becomes noticeable during external rotation of the shoulder. It also lies at an inaccessible area of the shoulder, high up under the coraco-acromial ligament,

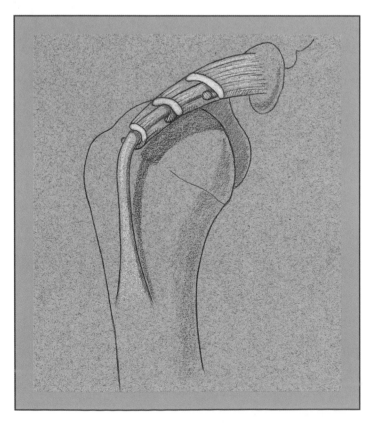

Figure 8.5 – *The rotator interval area of the capsule.*

and because of this it is a somewhat neglected ligament. Edelson (1991) suggested that in order to understand the coracohumeral ligament we ought to look at its counterpart in the hip. The analagous structure in the hip is the Y shaped iliofemoral ligament of Bigelow, which although not a true ligament, but rather a thickening of the joint capsule of the hip, is still regarded by some as the strongest ligament in the body. The iliofemoral ligament arises from the inferior iliac spine, which is the analogue of the coracoid process, and runs down to insert between the greater and lesser trochanters. The reflected head of the biceps femoris is the analogue of the long head of biceps and runs over the iliofemoral ligament; in this it differs from the long head of the biceps in the shoulder, which runs under the coracohumeral ligament. However, in evolutionary terms the long head of biceps was also extra-articular, indeed if you dissect a shoulder of lamb you will find it to be extra-articular. The long head of the biceps seems to have dropped down through the coracohumeral ligament as the coracoid enlarged.

The coracohumeral ligament, although neglected, is by virtue of its strength and strategic position a pivotal element in the control of shoulder movement. Nobuhara and Ikeda (1987) have reported good results in shoulder instability achieved merely by closing the rotator interval and reinforcing this repair with the coracohumeral ligament. Gagey *et al.* (1987) liken the action of the coracohumeral ligament and the inferior glenohumeral ligament to the cruciate ligaments in the knee in regard to the intricate and coordinated way in which they guide and stabilize movements of the joint.

Boardman *et al.* (1996) demonstrated that the coracohumeral ligament is a large and powerful structure. In cross section the ligament averaged 16 mm by 5 mm, compared to the superior glenohumeral ligament which measured 4 mm by 4 mm. The strength to failure of the coracohumeral ligament was 360 N compared to the superior glenohumeral ligament at 102 N.

Harryman *et al.* (1992) examined the role of the rotator interval in a carefully controlled laboratory study. They performed a cadaver test on the shoulder first dividing the rotator interval and then imbricating it (Fig. 8.6). They found that imbricating the interval limited shoulder-joint movement globally, but mostly restricted external rotation. Conversely dividing the rotator interval allowed an increase in global shoulder movement and particularly external rotation. They concluded that the

146

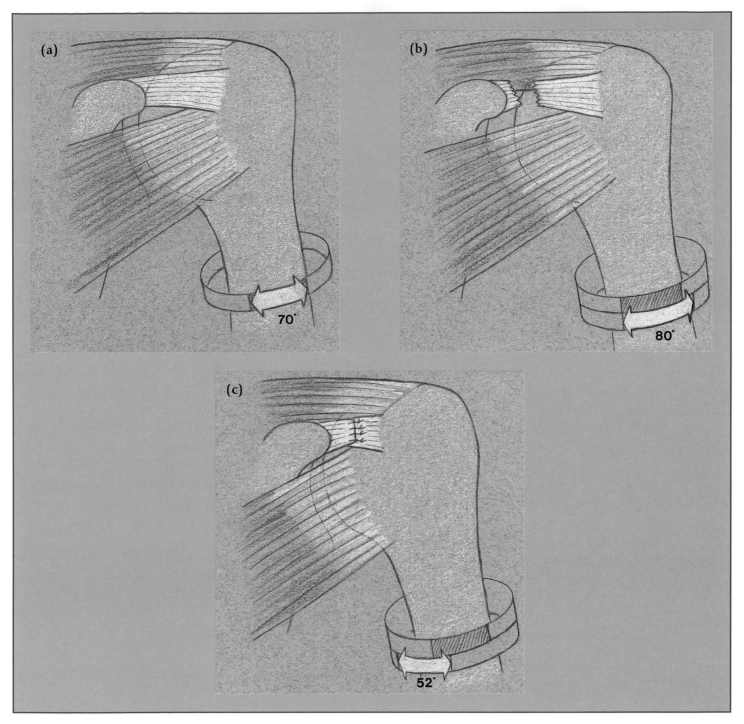

Figure 8.6 – *Harryman's experiment (1992). Release of the rotator interval allows an increase in external rotation (b). Imbrication of the rotator interval causes a contracture of external rotation (c).*

rotator-interval capsule plays an important part in glenohumeral motion and stability. They stated that release of this part of the capsule may improve the range of motion of shoulders that have limited flexion and external rotation.

Neer *et al.* (1992) found the coracohumeral ligament to be a well defined structure in 63 anatomical specimens. They found that the coracohumeral ligament originated from the coracoid and inserted variably into the rotator interval, supraspinatus or subscapularis. They found that division of the coracohumeral ligament alone allowed an increase in external rotation of 32°, and suggested that it may be contracted in frozen shoulder, old fractures and arthritis, and that it may need to be released in these conditions. Conversely, Cooper *et al.* (1993) stated that the coracohumeral ligament is not a real ligament, but merely a folded part of the capsule of the joint, which becomes prominent when the shoulder is externally rotated.

Ozaki *et al.* (1989) went further than Neer and stated that contracture of the coracohumeral ligament and rotator interval appears to be the main lesion in frozen shoulder, and, moreover, release of these structures relieved pain and restored movement to the shoulder.

Findings of surgical exploration

The early macroscopic descriptions of frozen shoulder, which the early pioneers left as their legacy, cannot be bettered. Neviaser (1945) reported that the thickened and contracted capsule peeled from the humeral head like adhesive plaster from the skin (Table 8.6). This he termed 'adhesive capsulitis'. No adhesions have been reported in numerous recent arthroscopic studies (Wiley, 1991; Uitvligt *et al.*, 1993; Bunker *et al.*, 1994).

Simmonds (1949) described the rotator cuff as 'looking like a vascular, leathery hood with no obvious demarcation between the tendons'. We now term the demarcation between the tendons the rotator interval. It is the rotator interval which is seen to be obliterated on arthrograms and at arthroscopy.

DePalma (1952) stated that the coracohumeral ligament is 'converted into a tough inelastic band of fibrous tissue spanning the interval between the coracoid process and the tuberosities of the humerus. It acts as a powerful checkrein...division of the coracohumeral ligament allows early restoration of scapulohumeral movement'.

Ozaki (1989) found that the major cause of restricted glenohumeral movement was a contracture of the coracohumeral ligament and rotator interval. The coracohumeral ligament was contracted and converted into a thick, fibrous cord. Release of this contracted ligament relieved pain and restored motion.

Neer *et al.* (1992) stated that he had found that the coracohumeral ligament may become shortened in frozen shoulder, and may have to be released at surgical reconstruction to restore external rotation.

Over the past 5 years I have explored 20 patients with frozen shoulder through an acromioplasty incision. The findings are consistent. The coraco-acromial ligament is always normal. When the coraco-acromial ligament is excised, an abnormal thickening can be seen in the rotator interval area. I say the rotator interval area because the anatomy is distorted by the scarring and contracture of the coracohumeral ligament, which obliterates the normal sulcus of the rotator interval. Indeed it is difficult to define exactly where the superior edge of the subscapularis tendon is, which is highly abnormal. It is also difficult to define where the anterior edge of the supraspinatus tendon is. If the arm is now externally rotated this scarred area tightens, and then can be seen to be acting as a checkrein to external rotation. Division of this scarred area allows immediate, and complete, external rotation in the vast majority of patients. The scarred area is highly vascular, and when divided bleeds forcefully. In two or three patients the contracture extended into the anterior and superior capsule and external rotation was regained with a manipulation at this point.

With the rotator interval now opened, I excised the whole of the rotator interval area to reveal a normal long head of biceps tendon, a normal humeral head, a normal glenoid and no adhesions.

Table 8.6 Surgical findings.

Neviaser	n = 10	1945	Thick contracted capsule
Simmonds	n = 3	1949	Vascular leathery hood
DePalma	n = 35	1952	Coracohumeral ligament becomes thick fibrous cord
Neer	Many	1992	Coracohumeral ligament may be shortened
Bunker	n = 20	1996	Coracohumeral ligament thick and scarred

Pathology

The cause of frozen shoulder has been uncertain since it was first described by Codman in 1934. Postulated causes include an autoimmune connective tissue disorder, recurrent haemarthrosis, reactive arthropathy, infection, trauma, algodystrophy, suprascapular nerve entrapment, and rotator-cuff degeneration. All these factors have been examined and disproven (Hazelman, 1991). Let us examine the macroscopic and histological evidence collected by those few surgeons who have performed open surgical release of frozen shoulders.

The few studies of tissue from patients with frozen shoulder have suggested either an inflammatory process (Neviaser, 1945; Simmonds, 1949; DePalma, 1952) or a fibromatosis (Lundberg, 1969; Kay & Slater, 1981; Ozaki et al., 1989; Hannafin et al., 1994; Bunker & Anthony, 1995).

Neviaser's (1945) study of 10 cases is often cited. He found thickening and contracture of the capsule, and increased vascularity, with considerable or extensive fibrosis, in six cases, but interpreted the increased cellularity as due to inflammatory changes. Simmonds (1949) reported four cases that showed dense collagen fibres, increased vascularity and the presence of 'histiocytes' (which we now term fibroblasts); however, he also concluded that frozen shoulder was an inflammatory condition.

De Palma (1952) explored 32 cases of patients with frozen shoulder. He described the histological findings in some, but not all, of his cases. He found degeneration of collagen fibres, round cell infiltration, increased vascularity, thickening of the synovial membrane and evidence of increased fibrosis. He also concluded that the cause was a low-grade inflammation. It should be noted that all these studies were performed between 1945 and 1952 when small round cell infiltration was nearly always inflammatory; although Simmonds recognized that some of these cells were fibroblasts, such techniques as immunocytochemistry, which are available to us now to differentiate small round cells into fibroblasts and inflammatory cells, were not available then.

Lundberg (1969) noted that the capsule was dense or compact, with an increased cell population, most of which were fibroblasts. His pathologist, Norden, suggested that, histologically, this tissue was identical to Dupuytren's tissue. In 1981 Kay and Slater described the histology of the capsule in a diabetic with frozen shoulder and stated that it was similar to Dupuytren's tissue. They stated that the cells were purely fibroblasts and myofibroblasts, and that there were none of the inflammatory changes as reported by Neviaser. Ozaki et al. (1989) examined 17 cases of patients with frozen shoulder, and reported that histologically the capsule showed fibrosis, but they did not examine cell type. Hannafin et al. (1994) took arthroscopic biopsies in 15 patients which showed diffuse capsular fibroplasia, thickening and contracture.

Open surgical release gave us the opportunity to subject the excised tissue from 12 patients with primary frozen shoulder to histological and immuno-cytochemical examination. The excised tissue from patients' shoulders measured from 1.0 × 1.0 cm to 5.0 × 3.0 cm (average 2.4 × 1.5 cm) (Fig. 8.7). Van Gieson and MSB stains showed that this tissue was made of nodules and laminae of dense collagen (Fig. 8.8) which was of the 'mature' Type-III category. This was also confirmed by strong birefringence under polarized light. Nodules consisted of a collagen matrix amongst which there is a proliferation of fibroblasts arranged alongside layers or bundles of dense collagen. The cell population was moderate to high (Fig. 8.9). A striking feature was increased vascularity in seven cases (Fig. 8.10).

The histological appearance of tissue excised from Dupuytren's contractures of the hand were similar in all respects, with a tendency to strings of nodules and a slightly greater cellularity and vascularity.

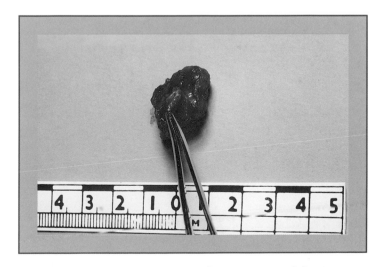

Figure 8.7 – *Macroscopic view of tissue removed from rotator interval. Note that it is enlarged vascular and nodular tissue. The forceps are holding the normal coracoacromial ligament, abnormal tissue below.*

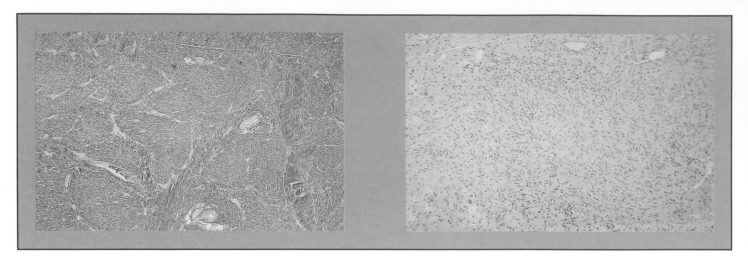

Figure 8.8 – *Histology shows this tissue to be composed of a dense collagen matrix (reproduced with permission from Bunker T., Journal of Bone Joint Surgery, 1995).*

Figure 8.9 – *Histology shows the tissue to be highly cellular (reproduced with permission from Bunker T., Journal of Bone Joint Surgery, 1995).*

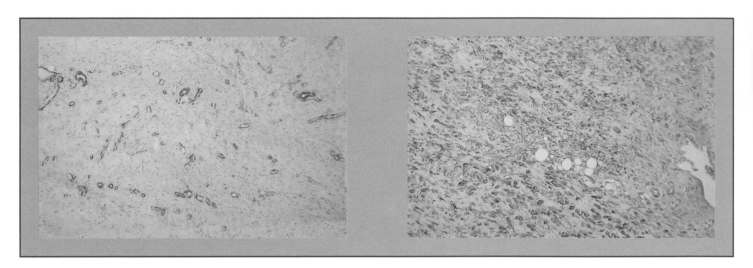

Figure 8.10 – *Histology shows the tissue to be very vascular (reproduced with permission from Bunker T., Journal of Bone Joint Surgery, 1995).*

Figure 8.11 – *Immunocytochemistry shows the cells to be fibroblasts and myofibroblasts (reproduced with permission from Bunker T., Journal of Bone Joint Surgery, 1995).*

With regard to the results of immunocytochemistry, vimentin was strongly expressed by the cells in the collagen matrix, which confirms that the cells are fibroblasts. Some of these fibroblasts also expressed alpha smooth muscle action, thus displaying a differentiation or a change to a myofibroblastic phenotype (Fig. 8.11). The myofibroblast, or contractile fibroblast, is the pathognomonic cell of contractile scar tissue such as found in Dupuytren's and the other fibromatoses. Leucocytes and macrophages were scanty and were never seen in the nodules or laminae, only on the periphery and usually around small vessels.

Synovium was present in seven cases and was either entirely normal, or showed minimal papillary infoldings without hyperplasia (Fig. 8.12). Tissues from Dupuytren's contractures produced the same range of results. These findings show that primary frozen shoulder is a fibrosing condition rather than an inflammatory condition and that it is, in its general histology and immunocytochemistry, indistinguishable from Dupuytren's contracture. It appears therefore that frozen shoulder is a disease characterized by fibrosis of the shoulder joint capsule, histologically similar to Dupuytren's contracture, leading to a contracture of the

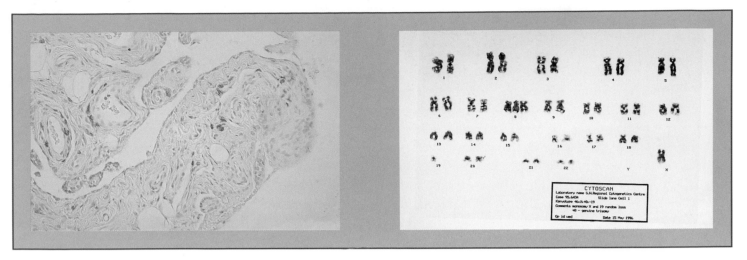

Figure 8.12 – *Inflammatory cells are only seen in the periphery and the synovium (reproduced with permission from Bunker T., Journal of Bone Joint Surgery, 1995).*

Figure 8.13 – *Chromosome analysis of patients with frozen shoulder showing trisomy 8. Trisomy 7 is actually more common.*

coracohumeral ligament, which acts as a checkrein to passive glenohumeral movement, and external rotation in particular.

If frozen shoulder is a similar disease to Duypuytren's contracture then it would fall into the group of diseases that are termed the fibromatoses. The fibromatoses are tumorous proliferations intermediate in their biological behaviour between benign fibrous lesions, such as nodular fasciitis, and malignant lesions such as malignant fibrous histiocytoma. The superficial fibromatoses are Dupuytren's contracture of the palm, Garrod's knuckle pads, plantar fibromatosis of Ledderhose, and Peyronie's penile fibromatosis. Clonal chromosomal abnormalities have been found in many of these conditions, clonality being defined as the observation of two or more cells with the same structural abberrations or supernumary chromosomes.

In Dupuytren's contracture, clones of cells trisomic for chromosome 8 have been noted (Sergovich *et al.*, 1983; Wurster Hill *et al.*, 1988; Bonnici *et al.*, 1992) and trisomy 8 has also been found in Peyronie's disease. We cultured tissue from the capsule of the shoulder in seven patients with frozen shoulder and examined them for chromosomal abnormalities. We found trisomy 7 and trisomy 8 in these patients (Fig. 8.13). This lends further weight to the hypothesis that frozen shoulder is a fibrosing disease.

Abnormal growth factor and cytokine expression has been shown in Dupuytren's tissue using reverse transcription, polymerase chain reaction techniques (Baird *et al.*, 1993). Dupuytren's tissue has been shown to have an increased prevalence of interleukin-1α, interleukin-1β, transforming growth factor β, and basic growth factor. The significance of this is that the cytokines interleukin-1, basic fibroblast growth factor and transforming growth factor β stimulate the growth of fibroblasts, whilst transforming growth factor β enhances the production of collagen. We decided that since frozen shoulder and Dupuytren's contracture shared so many other features in common, that we should test the hypothesis again, by examining the cytokine expression in tissue from frozen shoulder.

The excised rotator interval tissue from eight patients with frozen shoulder was quick-frozen and then processed using the reverse transcriptase polymerase chain reaction technique. The cytokine expression was compared with the Dupuytren's results and controls from the same laboratory as the original work on Dupuytren's contracture. Every frozen shoulder specimen strongly expressed interleukin-1α, and tumour necrosis factor β. These levels are not only significantly raised over controls but are higher than the levels found in Dupuytren's contracture. The levels of interleukin-1β, transforming growth factor β and basic fibroblast growth factor are raised above controls but are not as high as the levels found in Dupuytren's tissue. Thus we have shown that frozen shoulder also shares abnormal cytokine expression with Dupuytren's disease and moreover it is the same cytokines which are elevated, the cytokines which cause fibroblast proliferation.

This leaves two outstanding questions. If frozen shoulder is a Dupuytren's-like condition which is not painful and does not heal, why should it be so painful?; and why should it get better? In the formative phase Dupuytren's contracture can be painful but patients rarely present until the final stage of contracture. The pain of frozen shoulder, however, is severe and it is unlikely that it is caused by the forming contracture itself. The same is true of plantar fibromatosis, it is rarely painful except when the nodule is large enough to feel like a pebble upon which the patient is walking. However, if the pain of frozen shoulder was due to the nodule pressing on the coraco-acromial ligament it should remain painful and not ease, as it does. Arthroscopically a vascular synovitis is noted and it is possible that the synovitis is responsible for the pain. Some of the abnormal cytokines that we have found in

frozen shoulder lead to a synovitis and increased prostaglandin production, both of which may cause pain. The answer probably lies not in the disease itself but in the situation in which it occurs. We have already mentioned Harryman's (1992) study in which imbrication of the rotator interval was shown to lead to obligatory anterosuperior translation of the humeral head, which in turn leads to impingement (Fig. 8.14).

When the condition passes into the second and third phases the tissue stops forming and then the capsule can be stretched out, or torn by manipulation, or divided by surgical release which allows the humerus to centre again on the glenoid. This in turn allows the impingement pain to settle.

Regarding the reason for frozen shoulder getting better in contrast to Dupuytren's contracture which does not, all is not as it seems. Schaffer (1992) showed that

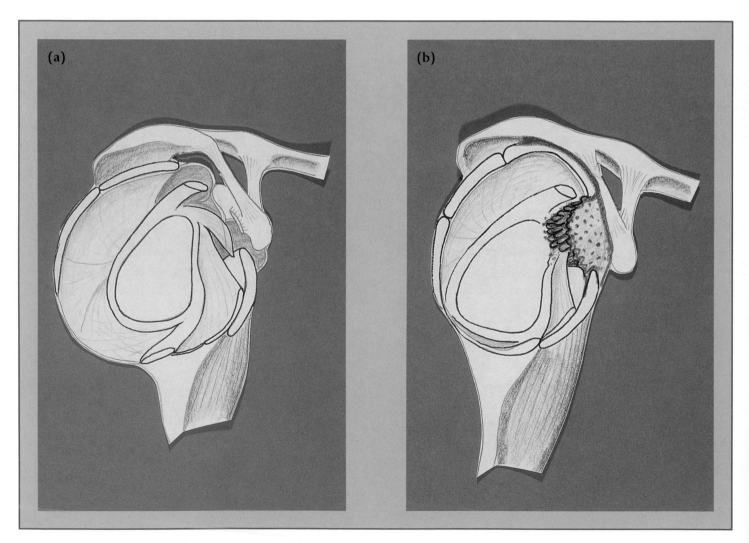

Figure 8.14 – *Contracture of the rotator interval causes obligatory superior translation leading to impingement. (a) normal, (b) contracture drags the head upward causing impingement pain.*

Table 8.7 Natural history of frozen shoulder.		
Codman	1934	Nil by 2 years
Simmonds	1949	70% disabled at 3 years
DePalma	1952	10% disabled at 4 years
Meulengracht	1952	30% disabled at 3 years
Charnley	1959	7% disabled at 3 years
Lloyd-Roberts	1959	30% disabled at 4 years
Lundberg	1969	Stiffness persisted
Reeves	1975	61% disabled at 10 years
Grey	1978	All better
Shaffer	1992	50% disabled at 7 years

the natural history of frozen shoulder is actually one of continuing disability, just as one would expect in a Dupuytren's-like condition, the difference being that although there is continuing mild discomfort in 50% of cases and measureable limitation of movement in 60% of cases, there is little functional disability (Table 8.7). There may be several reasons why the literature is biased towards optimism in terms of the natural history of this condition. Many of the original studies had no consensus on diagnostic criteria, poor methodology with no controls and poor follow-up. However, the most likely reason for such optimism is that ultimately the residual functional disability is neither frequent nor substantial, and that most people adapt to their restriction. Neer (1990) stated that elevation of 150°, external rotation to 50° and internal rotation to T8 is sufficient for normal function. Older patients with less functional demands can tolerate even more restriction in one plane. Finally, since restriction is mainly in external rotation and most functional demands of the shoulder depend upon elevation, it may be easier for the patient to compensate for this loss.

Treatment

Conservative treatment

'The most successful physician is one who amuses his patient sufficiently whilst nature affects a cure' (Voltaire). Many conservative cures have been tried — from mud packs to radiotherapy — and their limited success may well have been due to the fact that they amused the patient whilst nature took its course!

For the first time we are now beginning to understand the cause of frozen shoulder which gives this generation an immense advantage over our forebears. The cause of frozen shoulder is fibrosis of the rotator interval tissues, leading to a checkrein effect restricting glenohumeral movement. Treatment must be aimed at stretching, softening, breaking or excising rotator interval tissue. In effect this means physiotherapy manipulation, steroid injection and manipulation under anaesthetic.

Physiotherapy

Physiotherapy and home stretching means performing passive stretching and range of motion exercises. This starts with warming of the tissues and is followed by pendulum exercises, pulley exercises, wallbars, pushing, in order to force external rotation, with a stick, and forcing internal rotation by towelling the back.

During the formative phase these exercises may be painful and, theoretically, could cause microtearing of the forming contracture, and stimulate further fibrosis. However, these exercises are very helpful in the late stages of the disease, acting in one of two ways. If the fibrosing checkrein is small and thin then at this stage it may be stretched out. If the fibrosing checkrein is too thick to stretch, then the other areas of the capsule that are not affected to such a degree, such as the infraglenoid recess, can be stretched up. This leads to gains in elevation, and therefore function is greatly improved, although external rotation may remain restricted, much as in Shaffer's long-term study of the natural history of the disease. Such physiotherapy stretching exercises are essential after manipulation under anaesthetic or surgical excision in order to keep up the benefit attained during manipulation.

Steroid injection

Steroid injections have been given empirically in frozen shoulder. There are some studies that show a beneficial effect from intra-articular steroid therapy.

Fazzi (1995) injected steroid subcutaneously around the nodules of patients with Dupuytren's contracture prior to excision. Those injected 24 hours prior to excision showed no changes within the tissue although the lumens of the vessels on the periphery of the nodules, which were normally occluded, were opening. When he examined the tissue, which had been injected 4–6 days preoperatively, there were striking changes histologically. There were numerous ghost-cells among the fibroblasts. The absence of an inflammatory reaction in association with this cell death suggests that a process of planned cell death, or apoptosis, was occurring rather than necrosis. The normally present pro-inflammatory cytokines were all absent. These changes only affected nodules that were active and did not cause changes in the collagen of mature cords.

Whilst the histology of frozen shoulder and Dupuytren's contracture is similar, we should not extrapolate too far, but these findings certainly give food for thought concerning steroid injection in frozen shoulder.

Manipulation under anaesthetic

Manipulation under anaesthetic has had an extraordinarily chequered career in the management of frozen shoulder.

Codman (1934) stated that 'breaking up of adhesions even under ether was always an unpleasant business, that sometimes great force was required, and as the adhesions yielded there was often a loud snapping sound which vibrates down the humerus and gives the sensation to the operator that the bone has been broken or the ligaments at the elbow torn'. On one occasion Codman had opened the subacromial bursa surgically and placed his finger inside to break up the adhesions but the joint still would not yield, he therefore forced external rotation whilst his finger was still in the bursa and distinctly felt some of the fibres of subscapularis give way. This was probably the contracted rotator interval and scarred subscapularis recess giving around the top edge of the subscapularis.

Codman, in 30 years' experience, found that manipulating shoulders yielded few miracles, and that most cases had many uncomfortable, restless nights and slow recoveries, but recovery was always sure. He concluded that a good vacation under pleasant healthful circumstances seemed to be more desirable to the patient than any form of treatment!

Concern that manipulation could cause tearing of the rotator cuff, dislocation or humeral fractures meant that manipulation under anaesthetic went out of vogue through the middle part of this century.

Professor Sir John Charnley was intrigued by frozen shoulder as well as by joint replacement. In 1959 he published a paper on his personal results of manipulation in this condition. Prior to this investigation he set out to determine what the prevailing orthodox attitude to manipulation was. He sent out a questionnaire to Fellows of the British Orthopaedic Association and 70% of those replying stated that they would never manipulate a frozen shoulder, as all would eventually get better, and some could be harmed by it. Always the iconoclast he set out to prove that he new better. Charnley (1959) manipulated 35 patients with frozen shoulder and showed that none came to any harm, that early manipulation did not prolong treatment, that pain relief was the most important result of manipulation and that the duration of symptoms postmanipulation was fairly constant, averaging 10 weeks, irrespective of how long the symptoms had been present before manipulation. Charnley insisted on one matter of technique — that external rotation should be released before abduction was attempted, because otherwise dislocation could occur.

Manipulation has attained the status of the most predictable form of treatment for frozen shoulder in the last half of this century. Sneppen (1997), in a very carefully controlled study, showed that 75% of cases obtained a near normal range of motion, and 79% of cases were relieved of their pain. Seventy-five percent returned to work within 9 weeks of manipulation.

There is one group of patients, however, who have a poor response to manipulation — that is diabetic patients. Janda and Hawkins (1993) showed that any improvement in movement and diminution in pain disappeared by 4 weeks postmanipulation and suggested that manipulation should not be attempted in diabetics.

Surgery

Surgical release

Surgical release for frozen shoulder has been undertaken in very limited numbers, and with limited evaluation in the past (Neviaser, 1945; Simmonds, 1949; DePalma, 1952; Lundberg, 1969; Neer, 1992). In 1989, Ozaki *et al.* described their method of open surgical release for frozen shoulder in 17 patients and recommended this form of release in patients who failed to respond to non-operative treatment. Despite this, open surgical release remains a poorly recognized and little performed procedure.

We have performed an open surgical release in 20 patients who failed to respond to conservative methods and manipulation. The release is performed through a deltoid muscle-splitting incision centred over the medial third of the coraco-acromial ligament (Fig. 8.15). The fibres of the deltoid lie in a plane perpendicular to Langer's lines at this point, and so a gridiron incision has to be made, the skin being incised along Langer's line, and undermined so that the gridiron split can be made in the deltoid. The whole of the coraco-acromial ligament is then cleaned with a pledget before being completely excised (Fig. 8.16). The scarred nodular area of the coracohumeral ligament now comes into view and is better appreciated with the arm in external rotation, when the ligament can be seen and felt as a checkrein from the coracoid to the intertubercular sulcus. Because the rotator interval is obliterated by scar, it is difficult to judge where rotator interval ends and subscapularis or supraspinatus start. The checkrein is divided, being careful not to incise the long head of biceps which runs just below the checkrein. The edges of the rotator interval can be seen and felt more easily from inside the joint, and all the tissues that make up the rotator interval are now excised so that there is a gaping hole between the top edge of the subscapularis and the leading edge of the supraspinatus (Fig. 8.17). Finally, an arthroscopic duckbill punch is taken and the scarred area is excised down to and below the coracoid process. At the time that the checkrein is incised and divided the shoulder contracture is felt to release and external rotation is regained; occasionally a final manipulation is required to regain a full 80° of external rotation. The shoulder is then flexed to split the infraglenoid recess. Bupivacaine with adrenaline 1:200 000 is instilled. No attempt is made to close the rotator interval, the split in the deltoid is allowed to close and the skin closed with a subcuticular suture. Postoperatively the patient is placed in a roller-towel support overnight. No sling is allowed and physiotherapy is instituted to maintain the gained range of motion.

Arthroscopic surgical release

If an open surgical release can be performed then it is only a matter of time before an arthroscopic technique will supersede it.

There have been several series of arthroscopic surgical release conducted for resistant frozen shoulder, but most

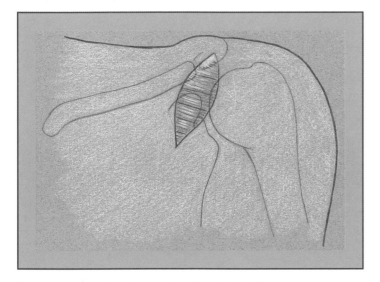

Figure 8.15 – *The skin incision for the Ozaki release.*

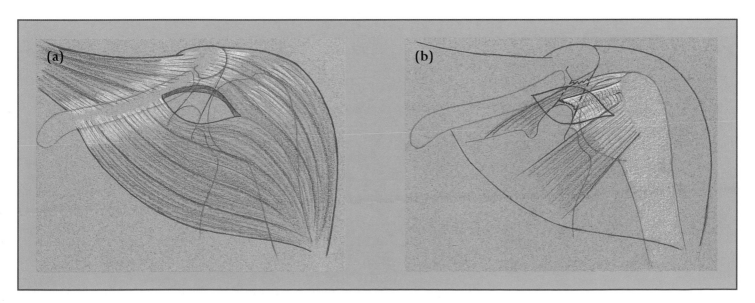

Figure 8.16 – *The deltoid is split to reveal the coraco-acromial ligament.*

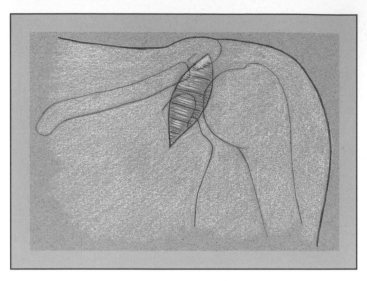

Figure 8.17 – *The coraco-acromial ligament is excised and the underlying scarred rotator interval is totally excised to release the joint and reveal the long head of biceps.*

of them have been blunderbuss treatments aimed at everything and nothing in particular, with a bit of manipulation thrown in at the end for good luck.

Esch (1994) performed an arthroscopic debridement of the joint following manipulation in 40 patients. In a further 10 patients he was more selective, performing an arthroscopic release of the rotator interval in some, and in others undertaking subacromial bursectomy, an arthroscopic acromioplasty, or excision of the coraco-acromial ligament and the coracohumeral ligament.

Segmuller *et al.* (1995) performed an arthroscopic release of the infraglenoid recess followed by a gentle manipulation in 26 shoulders.

Midorikawa *et al.* (1994) sectioned the coracohumeral ligament with electrocautery and then performed a subacromial bursectomy, and finally a manipulation in 14 cases with satisfactory results in all patients. This was a resistant group of patients, all of whom had failed to improve with manipulation.

Arthroscopic excision of the rotator interval and coracohumeral ligament shows promise, both theoretically and practically, in selected patients with primary frozen shoulder who have failed to respond to conservative measures or manipulation under anaesthetic.

Summary

Primary frozen shoulder is a disease characterized by insidious onset of true shoulder pain with a global restriction of both active and passive shoulder movement, especially external rotation.

Primary frozen shoulder is caused by a fibrous contracture of the rotator interval and coracohumeral ligament of the shoulder joint. Histologically, this tissue is composed of a dense collagen matrix, consisting mainly of mature Type-III collagen. The tissue is highly cellular and the cells are fibroblasts and contractile myofibroblasts. These findings are similar to Dupuytren's contracture and the two conditions share similar abnormalities of growth factor and cytokine expression, clonal chromosomal abnormalities and serum-lipid elevation. Both conditions are common in diabetes mellitus and can occur after minor trauma.

Elucidating the pathology of frozen shoulder allows us to comprehend the clinical features and natural history of the condition, and to formulate a logical plan of treatment. Clinically, the contracted tissue acts as a checkrein to external rotation, and causes a global loss of active and passive movement. The contracture causes obligate superior translation of the head, leading to impingement and pain. In mild cases, once the contracture has matured either it, or more likely the unaffected part of the capsule, can be stretched out such that the head centres again on the humerus, and the pain fades. Although a measureable amount of restriction remains, the patient compensates well, the disability is small, and the patient stops visiting his physician. In the more contracted cases, if treatment is to be effective it must be aimed at stretching, breaking, or surgically dividing the abnormal tissue and preventing it from recurring. Surgical release, and in particular arthroscopic surgical release, show promise in the management of this common, disabling, protracted and painful condition.

CHAPTER 9

Stepping stones towards the ideal shoulder replacement

T. Bunker

Introduction

The ideal joint replacement should have three goals: firstly it must abolish the patient's pain, secondly it should restore a functional, and ideally a normal range of motion, and thirdly the implant should integrate securely and indefinitely with its host, and wear so little as to outlast the host. Hip replacements can now predictably achieve the first two, and often the third of these criteria, but shoulder replacements continue to fall far short of all of these objectives (Table 9.1).

The majority of patients, following shoulder replacement, are forever grateful to their surgeons for the relief of pain, which although often incomplete, makes such a dramatic change to their lives. Ensuring a lifelong bond between prosthesis and bone as well as wear characteristics so low as to outlast the patient is a challenge facing all joint replacements. This is not peculiar to the shoulder, but still just as difficult to achieve.

Patients undergoing shoulder replacement expect a shoulder that is less stiff and allows more movement in order to improve their ability to undertake everyday tasks.

The shoulder with a full range of movement is the aim of all shoulder surgeons, but remains elusive. This is the challenge that makes shoulder surgery so rewarding both practically and intellectually.

The surgeon faces three major challenges which are peculiar to the shoulder. These are: (1) to ensure that the soft tissues around the shoulder (muscles and capsule) are allowed to function in the best and strongest fashion; (2) to restore the bony anatomy and prosthetic geometry to as near perfect as possible; and (3) to ensure that the frictional resistance of the joint is as close to normal cartilage-on-cartilage as possible.

Factors under the surgeon's control, as far as the soft tissues are concerned (Table 9.2), are a surgical approach

Table 9.1 Goals of shoulder replacement.	
● Pain relief	Glenohumeral joint
	Rotator cuff
	Acromioclavicular joint
● Restore movement	Functional
	Normal
● Outlast host	Osseo-integration
	Low wear

Table 9.2 Soft tissue procedures related to a good outcome.	
Extensile surgical approach	
Intact deltoid	Origin
	Insertion
Soft tissue releases	Rotator interval
	Coracohumeral ligament
	Anterior capsule
	Inferior capsule
	Posterior capsule
Restoring resting length to muscle	
Repair of cuff defects	
Relief of impingement	
Acromioclavicular joint excision	
Secure closure	Early rehabilitation
	Restores function

Table 9.3 Geometric variables.
Diameter of head
Retroversion angle
Facing angle
Distance above tuberosity
Medial offset
Posterior offset
Neck length
Joint line
Diameter of glenoid
Glenoid thickness
Surface shape (mismatch)
Glenoid facing angle
Glenoid retroversion angle

which causes the least damage to the deltoid muscle and the rotator cuff; soft-tissue release of contractures of the capsule and rotator interval; restoration of normal resting length to all muscles around the shoulder (rotator cuff and deltoid); repair of any cuff defects; relief of impingement and arthroplasty of the acromioclavicular joint if required; and a surgical closure that allows early rehabilitation and restoration of function.

In returning the anatomy of the shoulder to as near perfect as possible there are a number of variables that are under the surgeon's control, and each must be corrected (Table 9.3).

Factors under the surgeon's control that affect frictional torque are head size, joint conformity, glenoid size and the material surface properties of the prosthesis.

Obviously many of these factors are interdependent, but it can be seen that the surgeon's task is daunting and far more complex than is required of hip replacement or knee replacement.

Pathology

Joint replacement surgeons will recognize that the technical problems of the protrusio hip are quite different from those of superolateral arthritis of the hip, just as the valgus knee presents a different set of challenges to the varus knee. So it is in shoulder replacement, but amplified 10-fold. Why should this be? The first reason is that the shoulder is far more complex

than the knee or the hip in terms of geometric considerations, ligament balance and rotator-cuff reconstruction. The second reason is the extraordinary variety of disease processes that present with an arthritic shoulder. Some of the forms of secondary arthritis that present, not uncommonly, in the shoulder are quite exotic, such as acromegalic arthropathy and syringomyelia. Surgical reconstruction for traumatic arthritis is common following three- and four-part fracture dislocations. The problems of rheumatoid reconstruction are far more involved around the shoulder and the shoulder presents with unique problems, such as cuff arthropathy, which are not seen in any other joint.

Each of these diseases present specific clinical challenges in terms of pathology, indications for surgery, technical problems of reconstruction and complications.

Primary osteoarthritis

The patient with primary osteoarthritis is a delight to the shoulder surgeon because these patients present the least challenge in every way.

Rotator-cuff tears are uncommon in primary osteoarthritis (about 5%), and the quality of the muscles and tendons are usually good. The shoulder capsule is rarely contracted, indeed it is often quite distended by joint fluid. External rotation deficits are due to locking of the posterior rim osteophytes rather than by capsular contracture. If there has been long-standing posterior erosion of the glenoid, leading to an internal rotation contracture, then the anterior capsule may be tight, but this is unusual. The humeral head has an encircling osteophyte rim. Although on radiographs this is recognized as the characteristic inferior osteophyte (Fig. 9.1), the anterior and posterior osteophytes are usually just as florid. Superior osteophytes are minimal. There is central loss of cartilage and sclerosis. The glenoid is flattened, eroded on the posterior rim, and although there are peripheral osteophytes these are much smaller and lie within the capsule origin. The surface of the glenoid is usually sclerotic with tiny buds of regenerating cartilage.

The indication for shoulder replacement in osteoarthritis is pain that can not be controlled by conservative methods. Gain in motion and function are secondary benefits.

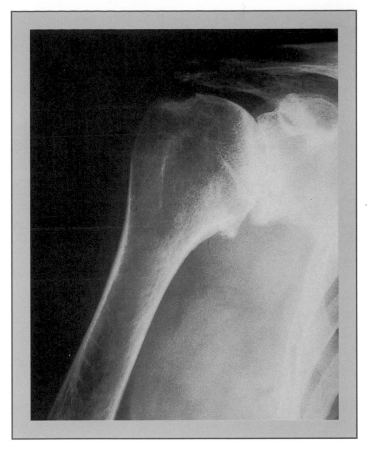

Figure 9.1 – *Primary osteoarthritis on plain radiography.*

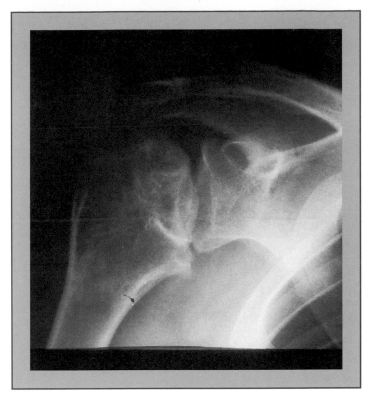

Figure 9.2 – *Avascular necrosis of the head of the humerus. Note how the head is very flattened compared to the glenoid. This is stage-V disease.*

Surgery is straightforward. The approach is standard. The osteophytes can jam on the posterior rim of the glenoid, but since the joint is relatively capacious it is just a matter of recognizing this possibility and using a lever to distract the joint and then externally rotating it to dislocate the head. Complications are uncommon.

Secondary osteoarthritis

Avascular necrosis

There are many causes for avascular necrosis of the head of the humerus. These include steroid therapy, sickle cell disease, decompression in divers and tunnel builders, alcohol abuse, gaucher's disease, lymphoma and systemic lupus erythematosus (SLE). The humeral head shows changes in the subchondral bone, including small fractures (the crescent sign) leading on to subchondral collapse and arthritis, whereas the glenoid remains relatively normal (Fig. 9.2). As in the hip, the early stages of avascular necrosis are difficult to recognize. The patient should be removed from further harm, for instance if steroid treatment can be stopped it should be.

The indications for surgery include pain associated with progressive collapse of the humeral head (Stage-IV disease). These patients are often younger than average. At surgery if the glenoid is well preserved then a hemiarthroplasty is the treatment of choice. In these patients the rotator cuff is usually intact and of good quality, reflecting their young age. Results of shoulder replacement are very satisfactory. If the glenoid is involved (Stage-V disease), then a total shoulder replacement should be performed rather than a hemiarthroplasty.

Acromegalic arthropathy

Acromegalic arthritis often affects the shoulders (Fig. 9.3) and hips. It has the distinction of being the only form of arthritis where the joint space can actually widen instead of narrow. The patient will have the usual features of the disease, growth of the tongue, jaw, hands and feet. Radiographs of the sella turcica will show enlargement. There may be visual field abnormalities due to the pituitary tumour encroaching upon the optic chiasm. The patient may have an element of gigantism

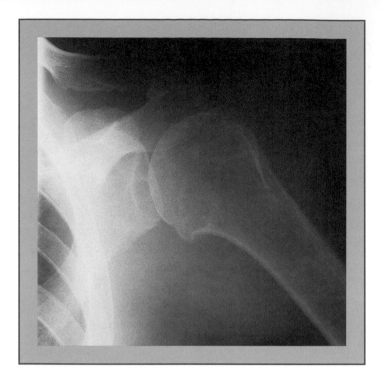

Figure 9.3 – *Acromegalic arthropathy of the shoulder.*

and the shoulder joint itself can be massive, the largest humeral head and glenoid available may be needed. The problem here is that all manufacturers make large heads of 50 mm diameter and 25 mm neck length, but oversized glenoids are not available. Consideration should be given to a custom implant in these patients.

Ablation of the pituitary tumour takes precedence over shoulder disease. Once the neurosurgeons have ablated the pituitary the patient will need to undergo hormone replacement and this will mean that they will require steroid cover during the stress of surgery. One-quarter of patients develop diabetes, which again complicates anaesthesia and postoperative recovery of the patient. These medical problems predominate over the surgical problems.

Ankylosing spondylitis

Shoulders and hips are commonly affected in ankylosing spondylitis. The features of the disease lead to joint stiffening and decreased pulmonary reserve. Ectopic bone formation is common and the patient should be given indomethacin prophylaxis for a period of 3 weeks during and after the surgery.

Psoriatic arthropathy

Psoriatic arthropathy presents little in the way of either medical or surgical challenges during shoulder replacement. Psoriatic plaques on the elbow may act as a portal for ingress of infection.

Haemophiliac arthropathy

Haemophiliacs should be treated on a haemophiliac unit. The two main problems are management of the bleeding diathesis, during and after surgery, which must be controlled by a haematologist and not by the surgeon. The second problem is that these patients have been exposed to concentrated blood products which originated from pooled sources and, between 1980 and 1985, in many countries included the human immunodeficiency virus (HIV) and hepatitis B and C. Many HIV-positive haemophiliacs have now died. This makes hepatitis B and C the most dangerous element to surgical and nursing staff. Special precautions must still be taken to screen for HIV and hepatitis in these patients and to protect surgical and nursing staff from exposure to body fluids. Once again these medical problems predominate over surgical problems.

Pigmented villonodular synovitis

This unusual form of secondary arthritis presents as an erosive arthritis of the shoulder. Surgery is as for primary osteoarthritis, but the surgeon should remove as much of the synovium as possible. The synovium often strips away from the capsule quite easily.

Synovial chondromatosis

The patient may present early in the disease with locking and loose bodies apparent on the radiograph (Fig. 9.4). Early disease can be treated by arthroscopic removal of

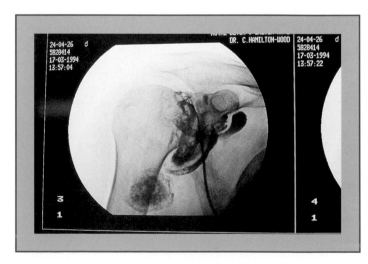

Figure 9.4 – *Synovial chondromatosis of the shoulder. Multiple loose bodies can be seen in this arthrogram.*

the loose bodies and synovectomy. Shoulder replacement is indicated in late disease when there is severe secondary osteo-arthritis and intrusive pain. The loose bodies may hide in the recesses of the joint, and in particular the subscapularis recess. As complete a synovectomy as possible should be undertaken, including these recesses.

Septic arthritis

Septic arthritis used to be a contraindication to shoulder replacement. However as experience has been gained of single-stage and two-stage exchange for infected hip and knee replacements some surgeons are now performing shoulder replacements, on selected patients, who have had sepsis in the past, and in whom the sepsis has cleared clinically and radiologically, and in whom the serum markers for infection C-reactive protein (CRP) and erythrocyte sedimentation rate (ESR) are within normal limits (Fig. 9.5). Biopsy should be performed at the time of surgery. Prophylactic antibiotics should be given, not on induction, but immediately after the biopsies have been taken. Resection of the synovium should be aggressive and the operation should only go ahead if the surgeon is confident that there is no active infection once the joint is open.

Consideration should be given to performing a surface replacement rather than a stemmed replacement, in these patients, as this leaves the possibility of prosthesis removal and fusion should the worst happen and the infection return. Antibiotic-loaded cement should be used, basing the choice of antibiotic upon the sensitivities of the organism, if it was recorded during the original septic episode. Antibiotics should be given postoperatively for 48 hours.

Arthritis of dislocation

This may occur due to the first or multiple episodes of dislocation causing severe damage to the head and the glenoid, but is usually caused by overtightening of the repair or scoring of the joint surface by screws or staples. Hovelius *et al.* (1996) showed a 20% incidence of radiographic arthritis, 10 years after initial dislocation (Fig. 9.6).

Shoulder replacement is a challenge in this group of patients because previous surgery has been undertaken and the surgical planes are difficult to define. The patient should be warned that in this situation there is a higher risk of nerve injury than during primary surgery. The two nerves most at risk are the musculocutaneous and axillary nerves. Taking down Bristow procedures for arthritis of dislocation is particularly taxing because the anatomy is so distorted and the musculocutaneous nerve is particularly vulnerable.

Neuropathic arthropathy

Neuropathic arthropathy remains a contraindication to shoulder replacement unless it is very mild, the muscles

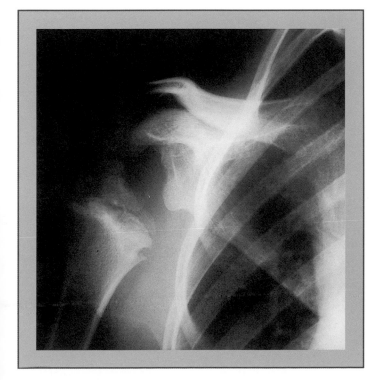

Figure 9.5 – *Old septic arthritis of the shoulder. The epiphysis was damaged by the infection.*

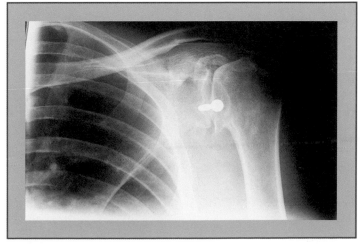

Figure 9.6 – *Arthritis of dislocation. The screw from the Bristow procedure can be seen.*

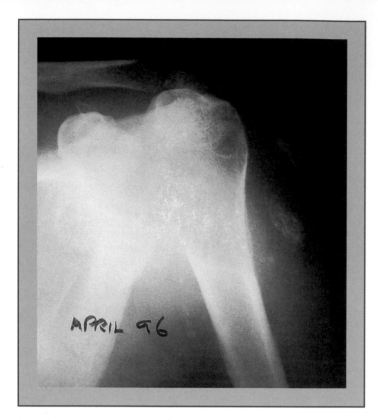

Figure 9.7 – *Neuropathic joint consequent upon syringomyelia.*

are well balanced, there is no rotator-cuff tear and there is minimal joint destruction. The usual cause of neuropathic arthritis in the shoulder is syringomyelia. Less common causes are diabetic neuropathy and syphilis. If there is severe bone destruction, or unbalanced muscle action, then shoulder replacement should not be undertaken (Fig. 9.7). The alternative is shoulder fusion. Even fusion is difficult to attain in neuropathic joints, although using a double-plating technique with bone grafting will lead to a higher success rate. Following shoulder fusion the patient should achieve one-third of the normal joint movement.

Rheumatoid arthritis

Rheumatoid arthritis is a systemic disease. The patients will often have lower-limb problems, which will make mobilization difficult, particularly if they have previously relied on crutches to walk. The arm will usually show typical rheumatoid deformities in the hand, wrist stiffness, elbow stiffness, and rheumatoid nodules as well as shoulder disease.

Remember that the shoulder girdle is a complex of joints, all of which may be affected by rheumatoid arthritis.

Do not make the mistake of thinking that because the patient has rheumatoid arthritis and complains of shoulder pain that they automatically need a shoulder replacement. The acromioclavicular joint may be affected and so may the 'subacromial joint'. Local anaesthetic injection studies may be needed to differentiate the pain source. The subacromial bursa is often involved by rheumatoid and may lead to gross swelling of the shoulder. The bursa is filled with solid tissue identical to a rheumatoid nodule, and it therefore can not be aspirated. This alone may lead to an impingement-like pain, which may be abolished by excision of the bursa and performing an anterior acromioplasty. The bursa may be so enlarged and inflamed that it can extend right down to the axillary nerve as it passes around on the deep surface of the deltoid muscle. The nerve is thus in danger during removal of such a bursa, particularly as the whole area is inflamed and the tissue planes are hard to dissect cleanly.

The Larsen classification is used for the evaluation of rheumatoid shoulder disease. This is based upon radiographic findings ranging from zero — a normal looking shoulder — to Grade V — severe bony destruction. An extra-articular cause for the pain should be sought in patients below Larsen Grade IV, but in patients with Larsen Grade IV and V the pain source is usually the glenohumeral joint, and shoulder replacement should be considered in these patients if their symptoms warrant it.

Neer has described two forms of rheumatoid disease, the 'dry' type and the 'wet' type (Fig. 9.8). It is very important to understand this distinction because the

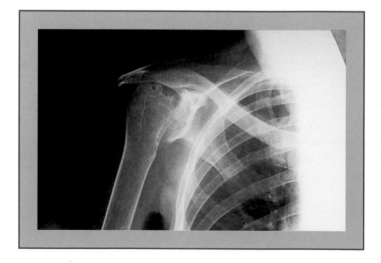

Figure 9.8 – *Wet or erosive arthritis of the rheumatoid shoulder. Note the periarticular erosions.*

patterns of disease are markedly different. The dry type looks more like osteo-arthritis, a stiff, sclerotic joint in a rheumatoid-positive patient; it also behaves more like osteo-arthritis, it progresses slowly and the bone quality remains good, with minimal erosion. The 'wet' type acts entirely differently. Here the synovium is highly aggressive, vascular, wet and thick. The radiographs show periarticular erosions which can be very large. The bone quality is poor and bone resorption can occur. Progression can be extremely rapid in these patients. Consequently, they need to be kept under close review and their shoulder replacement carried out earlier rather than later.

The usual deltopectoral approach is required in the rheumatoid patient. If there is gross medialization (Fig. 9.9) then a predrilled coracoid osteotomy may be required. Beware the bone may be very soft and it is not unknown for the screw to pull out of the coracoid postoperatively due to the bone being so soft. The screw should be backed-up by sutures from the pectoralis minor tendon to the conjoined tendon. The brachial plexus is surprisingly close to these medialized shoulders and again great care should be taken.

The rotator cuff is often of poor quality secondary to disuse and neglect, but is rarely torn. The literature states that a quarter of patients with rheumatoid disease have a full-thickness rotator-cuff tear, but this is an overestimate. The cuff often appears to be dysfunctional, but this is due to bone resorption, leading to medialization, and due to disuse.

The capsule is often contracted because the patient has been neglected. These contractures will need to be released. The rotator interval needs to be opened, the coracohumeral ligament released, the anterior capsule released from the glenoid, the inferior capsule released from the humerus and the posterior and superior capsule incised.

Bone grafting may be required to the glenoid, but fortunately this is extremely rare. The resected humeral head may be used, either as a block, or as cancellous morcels packed into the defect. However, the glenoid is osteopenic and does not hold screws well. If there is gross medialization, such that only a thin sliver of glenoid is left, it may be better to accept a limited-goals approach and insert a hemiarthroplasty.

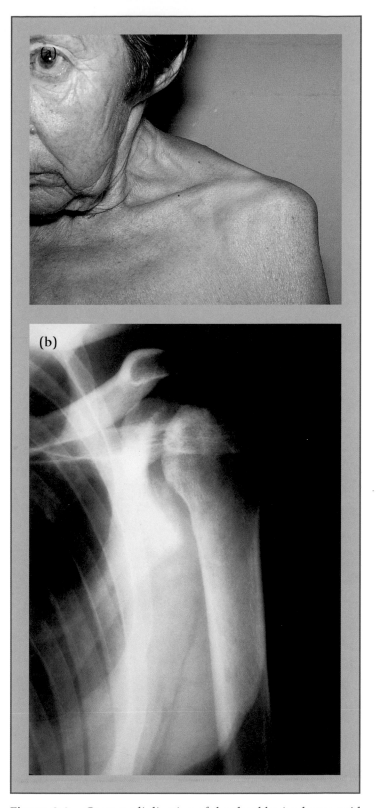

Figure 9.9 – *Gross medialization of the shoulder in rheumatoid disease due to glenoid bone loss, (a) clinical appearance, (b) radiographic appearance.*

Fracture dislocations

The use of hemiarthroplasty in acute fracture dislocations is dealt with in the chapter on three- and four-part fracture dislocations. However, patients may present at a late stage, following fracture, with a painful arthritic joint. These patients may have malunion of any or all of the four segments, the head to shaft, the lesser and the greater tuberosities. If there is a malunion of the shaft-to-head segment, then the malunion may have to be taken down, as an osteotomy before the prosthetic stem is inserted (Fig. 9.10). If not then the head will not be in its anatomical position in relation to the shaft; in other words the normal posterior and medial offsets will be wildly out, and the shoulder will function poorly. Commonly, a varus angulation is present between head and shaft and if this is not corrected the greater tuberosity may impinge.

If the greater tuberosity is malunited it is usually situated more posterior and superior than normal. Again, if an osteotomy is not performed, then the greater tuberosity will remain proud, in other words the distance above the tuberosity will be too small, and the tuberosity will impinge. If the greater tuberosity is left posteriorly and superiorly misplaced then the rotator cuff is dysfunctional. Additionally, in the fracture situation, the axillary nerve is often at risk from the callus formed at the site of union of head to shaft. The author has even found the axillary nerve travelling through a tunnel within this area of fracture union. The shaft is often medialized which brings it into closer proximity to the brachial plexus, and once again this means that even more care is required than in the normal situation.

If there has been a fracture dislocation the capsule or rotator cuff may have been torn leading to a higher risk of postoperative dislocation.

Shoulder replacement, in the late situation following fracture dislocation, is a very high risk-setting for surgery. The anatomy is highly distorted, the cuff defunctioned, the nerves are in jeopardy, osteotomies are complex and harder to perform in reality than their planning suggests, and complications are common. Pain is reduced, but the patient is always somewhat disappointed because the range of movement achieved after surgery is never as good as prior to their fracture and the function of their shoulder is always limited.

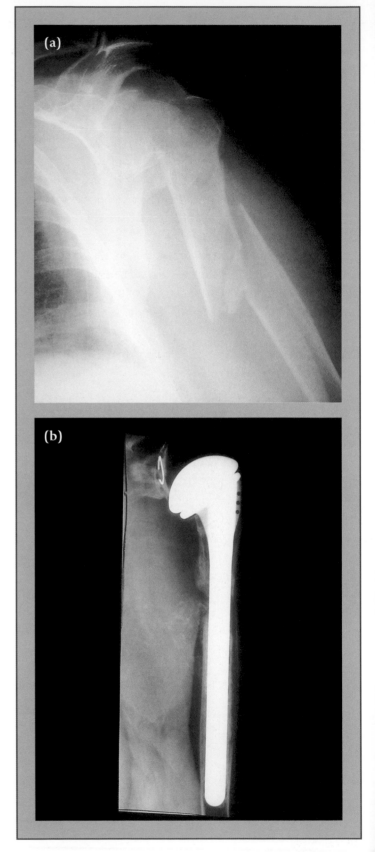

Figure 9.10 – *Severe fracture of the shoulder (a) treated with a long-stem shoulder replacement (b).*

Cuff arthropathy

The worst results of shoulder replacement occur in patients with cuff arthropathy. Any joint requires both a fulcrum and motors to power it. Unless these motor units (the rotator cuff) can be repaired then function will remain poor, the prosthesis will sublux, and the patient may even suffer from impingement pain (Fig. 9.11).

Reconstruction of the shoulder with cuff arthropathy remains one of the outstanding unresolved problems of shoulder surgery. Every shoulder surgeon will espouse their own favourite methods ranging from hemiarthroplasty to bipolar hemiarthroplasty, massive head hemiarthroplasty to constrained total replacement to shoulder fusion.

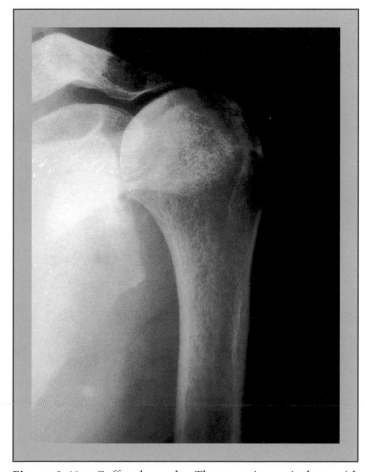

Figure 9.11 – *Cuff arthropathy. The acromion articulates with the head and there is gross destruction of the head, the glenoid, and the acromion.*

Reconstructing the soft tissues

The surgical approach

A prerequisite of any approach to shoulder replacement is to gain an excellent exposure of the humeral head and the glenoid cavity. The approach must be extensile, must not damage the deltoid muscle, must minimally interfere with the rotator cuff, must allow capsular release and rebalancing, and must protect the axillary nerve, the musculocutaneous nerve, the brachial plexus and the major vessels.

The patient is intubated and the anaesthetist and anaesthetic machine are positioned at the foot-end of the operating table, leaving the head end free for the surgical team. Prophylactic antibiotic (cefuroxime) is given. The patient is positioned supine, with the shoulder over the edge of the table. The humerus will be extended down by the side of the table to dislocate the humeral head. The head of the patient is placed on a head ring and a nurse's hat is used to hold the hair in place and away from the surgical site. A sandbag is placed between the table and the scapula to push the shoulder forward. Some surgeons place the head on a neurosurgical support, but this is not necessary and adds to the complexity of the procedure and set-up time.

The key to the surgical approach is the coracoid process. An 18 cm incision is made in a straight line from the clavicle, over the coracoid, and in line with the deltopectoral groove (Fig. 9.12). This line is infiltrated with bupivacaine hydrochloride and 1:200 000 adrenaline, in order to limit skin edge bleeding. The patient is then prepared with chlorhexidine or iodine skin preparation, from the nipples to the ear and from the operating table to the midline. A surgical glove covers the hand and an arm stocking is rolled up the free draped arm. Adhesive U-drapes are used to seal off the surgical site superiorly and inferiorly and then drapes are used to expose the surgical site. The clavicle, coracoid and surgical-incision line are marked with a skin marker pen and finally a face is drawn on the drapes over the patient's face to prevent assistants from inadvertently leaning on the patient! Lastly an opsite seal is applied. A straight 18 cm incision is made. The deltopectoral groove is defined and opened in its entirety. Three structures cross the groove; all must be ligated and divided. The first is the cephalic vein, the second is the deltoid artery and its venae comitantes, and the third is the acromial

165

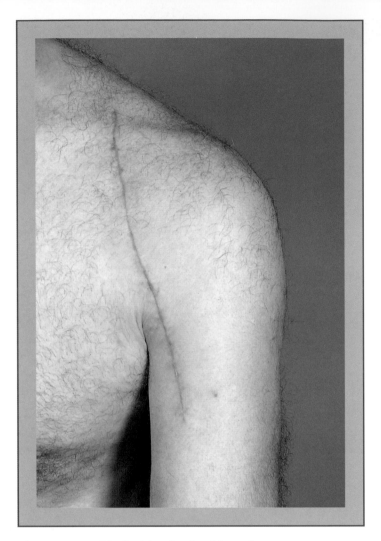

Figure 9.12 – *The incision for shoulder replacement.*

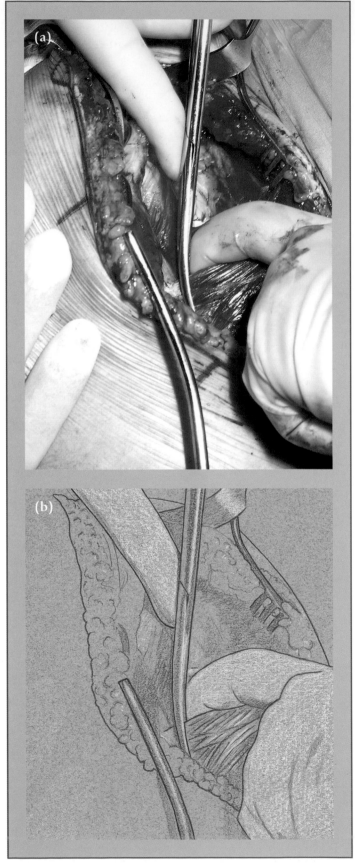

Figure 9.13 – *In the Perthes' approach to the shoulder a complete pectoralis major tenotomy is performed.*

artery. The deltoid and acromial arteries are branches of the thoraco-acromial artery. It is essential that the deltoid itself is not released from its origin on the clavicle because the anterior deltoid is vital to postoperative shoulder rehabilitation.

Three steps are now required for adequate exposure. The first is a complete tenotomy of the tendon of the pectoralis major leaving an 8 mm strip on the humerus for re-attachment (Fig. 9.13). Some surgeons will say this is unnecessary and that an incomplete tenotomy is adequate. Adequate is not good enough in shoulder replacement. A complete tenotomy makes a great difference to the exposure of the head and glenoid, and is safe, easy to repair, heals strongly and is cosmetically imperceptible. The second step is to abduct the arm 90° and free the undersurface of the deltoid muscle from the subacromial bursa and the rotator cuff. The third step is to insert a self-retaining shoulder retractor. The quadralateral space is now dissected to expose the axillary nerve, which must be protected. The anterior circumflex humeral artery is ligated and divided. The upper border of the tendon of the latissimus dorsi is tenotomized at its insertion, exposing the humeral neck, and improving access to the inferior capsule and the quadralateral space. The space is then dissected using a pledget on a Kocher clip to demonstrate the posterior circumflex artery and vein, behind which lies the axillary nerve.

Inspection of the subacromial space

The coraco-acromial ligament is incised, and if the surgeon feels that it is impingeing upon the cuff it is excised. The acromion is inspected and, if necessary, an anterior acromioplasty is performed, excising the inferior acromioclavicular joint osteophytes. The need for either of these procedures is exceedingly rare. It is essential that the deltoid insertion to the acromion remains undisturbed and strong during debridement of the subacromial space. The cuff is inspected and the bursa is released. It is very unusual to have to perform an excision of the acromioclavicular joint.

Release of the capsule and cuff

A Trethowan spike is then passed into the rotator interval to define the upper border of the subscapularis muscle. After placing stay-sutures (from top to bottom) in the subscapularis a vertical arthrotomy is made through the tendon and continued through the inferior capsule where it inserts into the humeral neck, keeping well clear of the axillary nerve. If there is a pre-operative internal rotation contracture, the subscapularis muscle must be Z-lengthened so that on closure 30° of external rotation is achieved (Fig. 9.14). The rotator interval is released and incised down to the rim of the glenoid the at 2 o'clock position. Finally the inferior capsule is further released from the neck of the humerus, whilst the humerus is externally rotated until the head of the humerus dislocates into the wound. The osteophytes which encircle the head are now excised to expose the normal shape and size of the head. Usually, a coracoid osteotomy is not required. In severe rheumatoid arthritis, however, where the glenoid has been markedly eroded, or in a posttraumatic case where the brachial plexus has to be exposed, a predrilled coracoid osteotomy should be undertaken.

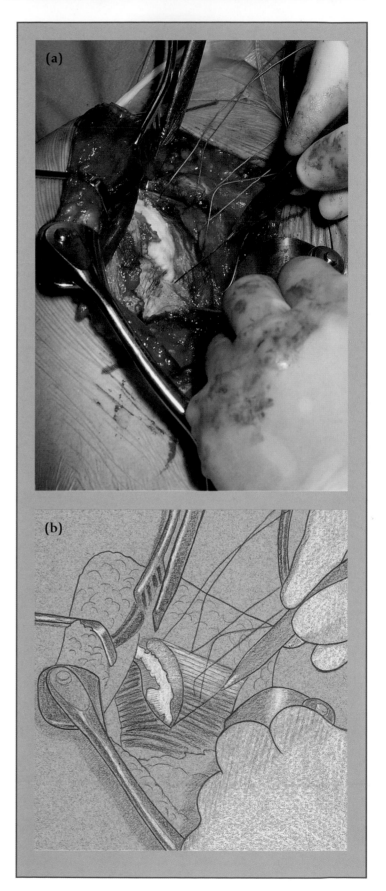

Figure 9.14 – *A vertical arthrotomy is made in the subscapularis.*

Geometric restoration of the joint

The humeral head

Diameter of the head. Boilleau and Walch (1992) used an industrial computerized measuring device to investigate humeral head size in 160 cadaveric humeri. They found that the head was a section of a sphere (Fig. 9.15) and that the diameter varied from 37 mm to 57 mm, the average being 46 mm; Ianotti *et al.* (1992) in a similar study of 140 shoulders found that the average diameter was 48 mm, with a range from 38 mm to 56 mm. In this study half the measurements came from cadaver humeri and half from magnetic resonance imaging (MRI) scans, but 60% of the cadavers and 67% of the MRI films were from men. Why is this important? the answer lies in the population who require shoulder replacements. Looking at my last 200 shoulder replacements, 76% were female, and would therefore have smaller head sizes. The Neer prosthesis was designed to replace the large humeral head of young men with fractures of the proximal humerus, and thus was manufactured with a 50 mm head diameter. The shoulder is an anatomical replacement like the knee, but unlike the hip. In the knee no self-respecting surgeon would contemplate putting an extra large femoral component into a lady with a small size knee because it would overstuff the joint, lead to an overtight flexion gap, and a terribly stiff joint. The case is the same with the shoulder. For this reason many manufacturers now make modular prostheses, where the head size can be templated preoperatively, and made to match as close as possible. On the other hand, if an undersized component is inserted there is a theoretical danger of postoperative instability.

Retroversion angle. The retroversion angle is determined by the saw cut that sections the head. This is determined by the surgeon. The retroversion angle is highly variable, varying even between the two sides of a single patient. Neer (1955) stated that the retroversion angle was 21°. This has been confirmed using modern industrial coordinate measurement machines by Roberts *et al.* (1991), who studied 29 humeri and measured the angle at 21.4°. Boilleau and Walch (1992) found the angle to be somewhat less at 17.9° but found great variability from minus 6.7° to plus 47.5° (Fig. 9.16). So, the question is 'why do surgeons tend to use a retroversion angle of 30° during shoulder replacement when they should be aiming at between 18° and 21°?' The answer

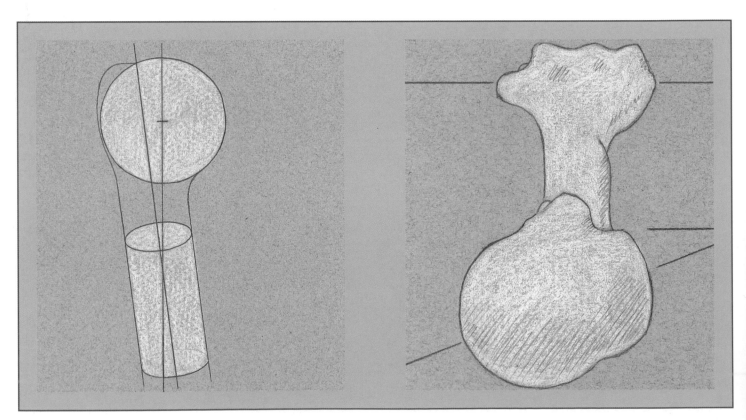

Figure 9.15 – *The proximal humerus is an epiphyseal sphere sitting upon, but not in line with, a cylindrical metaphysis.*

Figure 9.16 – *The retroversion angle varies, but averages 18° to 21°.*

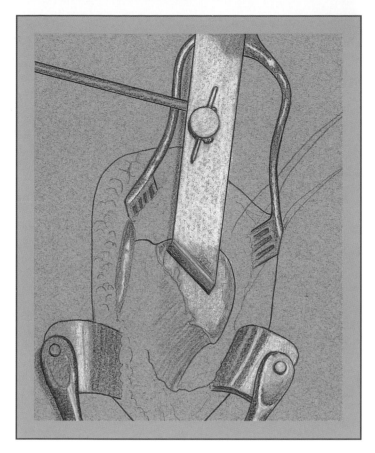

Figure 9.17 – *The facing angle is sectioned on the jig.*

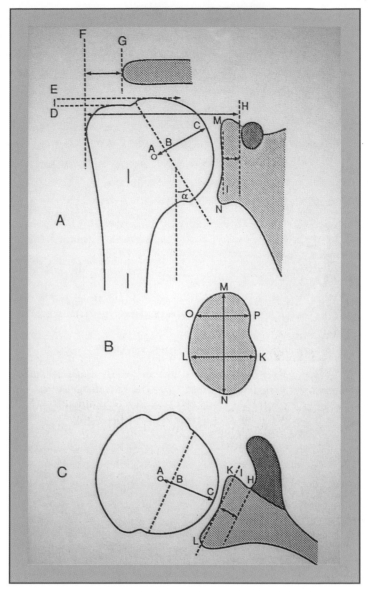

Figure 9.18 – *The distance above the tuberosity should be 8 mm (from Ianotti et al., reproduced with permission from Journal of Bone and Joint Surgery).*

lies in two factors. Firstly, increasing the retroversion angle to 30° decreases the risk of postoperative anterior dislocation. The second reason is slightly more difficult to grasp, and is that increasing the retroversion angle decreases the posterior offset of the head. We will discuss this in more detail later.

As improved prostheses become available to the surgeon allowing variability of posterior offset, retroversion angle can be planned, such that it is maintained at around 20°. Postoperative instability does occur following shoulder replacement but, again with growing confidence, the modern shoulder surgeon can tailor the soft tissue releases and balance to prevent this complication. The degree of retroversion is determined by the surgeon, and can be dialled into the cutting jig in many modern instrumentation systems. If the surgeon requires 20° of retroversion then that is how he sets the jig prior to sectioning the humeral head.

Facing angle. The facing angle is the neck shaft angle of the humerus. This determines the varus/valgus angle of the neck. The neck shaft angle is highly variable but averages 130°. Most prostheses are designed with a neck

shaft angle of 135°, and the jigs are designed to make the cut at this angle (Fig. 9.17) so that the prosthesis fits snugly on the cut surface of the bone. If the angle is cut incorrectly then, with a cemented stem, the surgeon can correct for the poor cut by placing a downsized stem in varus or valgus. However, if an uncemented press-fit stem is used there will be a gap between the collar of the prosthesis and the sectioned end of the humerus.

Distance above tuberosity. When the prosthesis is inserted it should protrude 8 mm above the tip of the greater tuberosity (Fig. 9.18). If the head protrudes less the tuberosity will be too prominent and will lead to impingement. However, if the head protrudes too far it may damage the rotator cuff, and must, by definition, be too big, causing overstuffing of the joint and decreased movement.

Achieving the correct distance above the tuberosity requires cutting the head at the correct level. In order to do this the surgeon must have a 'key point' reference against which the make the cut. The key point is the sulcus at the reflection of the head and the greater tuberosity, 6 mm behind the bicipital sulcus; the surgeon must place the cutting block of the cutting jig to ensure that the cut exits at this point (Fig. 9.19).

Therefore the surgeon must think of three variables when sectioning the humeral head: (1) the retroversion angle, (2) the facing angle, and (3) the key point. Getting these and the head size right is half the battle towards getting the head geometry correct.

Medial offset. The proximal humerus is a metaphyseal cylinder mated to an epiphyseal sphere. The problem is that the axis of the cylinder and the centre of the sphere do not lie in the same plane. The centre of the head is medial to the axis of the humeral shaft by some 7 mm (Fig. 9.20). Unfortunately, some designs of humeral head do not take this offset into account and thus may lead the head to abut against the rotator cuff and

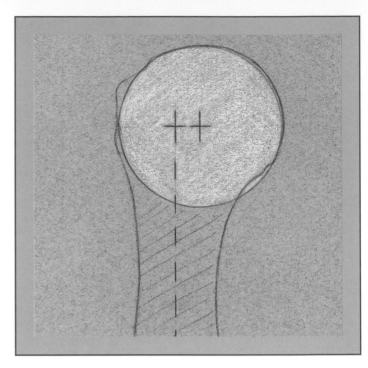

Figure 9.20 – *The medial offset. The centre of the head lies medial to the axis of the shaft of the humerus.*

damage it. Once again, if the offset is too great it will decrease the distance above the tuberosity and may lead to impingement of the greater tuberosity against the acromion.

Neck length. The neck length and the medial offset are related. The average neck length is 15 mm, with a range of 12–18 mm. Most modular prostheses have a variety of humeral heads of the same diameter, but of varying depth; the greater the depth, the longer the neck length. The choice of neck length may vary from 11.25 mm to 25 mm for each head size. Surgeons use this ability to increase the neck length in two ways. Firstly, if the surgeon is faced with a joint that has glenoid erosion he can use a prosthesis with an increased neck length to make up for the bone loss and to re-tension the rotator cuff. Without the ability to increase the neck length the shoulder would remain medialized, the rotator cuff would be lax and dysfunctional, and the shoulder would not work and would remain unstable.

Alternatively, if the surgeon is faced with a contracted joint in a small lady he may be faced with a situation where, despite capsular releases, the cuff itself is so contracted that he can not get a prosthesis with a normal neck length in, and the only prosthesis that will fit is one with a smaller neck length.

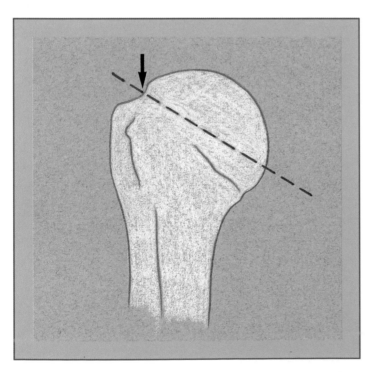

Figure 9.19 – *The key point is the synovial reflection of the superior articular surface.*

Tiny changes in neck length can lead to radical changes in shoulder function. Harryman and Matsen (1995) took two shoulder replacements (Fig. 9.21). One had a normal neck length and the other had a neck length that was increased by just 5 mm. They then applied the same torque force to each shoulder and found that the prosthesis with the increased neck length moved just half as far as the anatomical one. This leads to a stiff shoulder.

Joint line. When faced with a medialized shoulder with glenoid erosion, the surgeon would ideally bring the joint line back to normal by fitting a deeper glenoid. Since these are not available the neck length of the humeral component has to be increased; this may make the shoulder stiff.

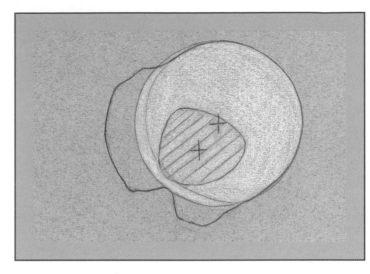

Figure 9.22 – *The posterior offset. The centre of the epiphyseal sphere lies behind the axis of the shaft of the humerus.*

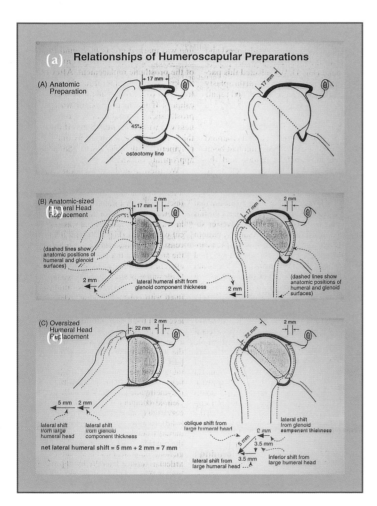

Figure 9.21 – *Matsen showed that a small increase in neck length radically altered the force required to achieve the same degree of elevation (from Matsen et al., reproduced with permission from the Journal Bone and Joint Surgery).*

Posterior offset. Finally, in discussing the geometry of the head we have to consider posterior offset. We have already said that the proximal humerus is like a metaphyseal cylinder surmounted by an epiphyseal sphere, and that the centre of the sphere is medial to the line of the axis of the cylinder. However, the centre of the sphere also lies behind the axis of the sphere (Fig. 9.22), and this is termed the posterior offset. The posterior offset is variable and measures from 3 mm to 5 mm. The problem is that most prostheses are made with no posterior offset and this can lead to the head being too far forward, causing interference with joint kinematics and leading to coracoid impingement. By a quirk of geometry increasing the retroversion angle decreases the posterior offset. Increasing the retroversion angle to 30° reduces the posterior offset to insignificant levels.

The glenoid

The glenoid is technically the most difficult part of shoulder replacement, perhaps the most technically difficult part of any joint replacement. The glenoid offers a tiny surface for osseo integration of a prosthesis. The surface of the glenoid is only 35 × 25 mm and the depth of the glenoid is only some 30 mm. Although most textbooks describe the glenoid as offering a cone of cancellous bone to the surgeon for fixation, the shape is actually quite complex (Fig. 9.23). The glenoid is indented, both on its superior and its posterior aspects, by the suprascapular artery

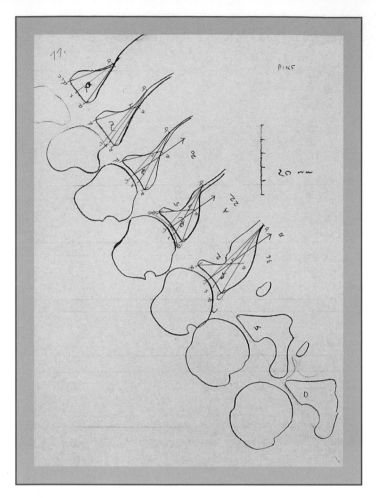

Figure 9.23 – *The glenoid is not a pyramid but is actually quite a complex shape.*

and nerve. As if this was not bad enough, the glenoid is often eroded. In osteoarthritis the posterior rim is eroded, leading to increased retroversion of the surface. In cuff deficient shoulders the superior aspect is eroded. In rheumatoid disease there may be superior erosion or gross medialization, such that only a thin sliver of bone presents itself to the surgeon, in which case the glenoid can not be replaced and a hemiarthroplasty must be performed. Despite the frequency of glenoid erosion most surgeons prefer to avoid bone grafting if possible. Neer and Morrison (1988) used an internally fixed bone graft in just 20 out of 463 total shoulder replacements, and smaller non-fixed grafts in a further 45 patients.

Added to these difficulties the exposure of the glenoid is difficult and because the glenoid is at the very depths of the surgical exposure any blood will tend to pool on the surgical field.

Biomechanically the resultant force at the glenoid starts at the inferior glenoid on initiation of elevation, moves to the superior glenoid at 30° elevation and then back to the central glenoid at 60° elevation. This produces the so-called rocking horse effect which may lead to glenoid component loosening. Any rotator-cuff dysfunction or tear accelerates this effect. There is also obligate anteroposterior translation of the humeral head on the glenoid during flexion (Harryman *et al.*, 1990; Collins *et al.*, 1992), causing an anteroposterior rocking horse effect. Rotational torque forces are also applied to the glenoid during elevation and we have recently reported rotational dissociation of modular glenoid prostheses from these forces (Bunker & Feldman, 1997).

The forces on the shoulder can be great. The compressive load across the joint is 0.89 times body weight at 90° abduction. This force is increased by 60% for each kilogram held in the outstretched hand. Recently, it has been calculated that five times the body's own weight is born by the shoulder whilst doing a press-up.

It is no wonder that many of the complications of shoulder replacement are related to the glenoid. Brems (1993) performed a meta-analysis of nearly 1400 shoulder replacements which showed that 38% had lucent lines around the glenoid (Fig. 9.24). The incidence of lucent lines around the glenoid was as high as 89% in some cases. The importance of meticulous cementation techniques was shown by Brems when he noted that 69% of lucent lines were visible on recovery-room radiographs, and that the presence or absence of lucent lines was statistically correlated with specific surgeons. Despite such high lucency rates, the 15-year survivorship of shoulder replacement is 85% and the revision rate for the glenoid just 3%. The problem with survivorship analysis is that such a low revision rate may mean that lucent lines are not important around the glenoid, or it may mean that glenoid revision is such a daunting operation that most surgeons persuade their patients to accept the situation!

Problems with the glenoid have led some surgeons to adopt a nihilistic approach to the glenoid, and they just insert hemiarthroplasties instead of total shoulders. However, this approach should be countered by the study of Gshwend (1991) who compared the degree of improvement in patients with hemiarthoplasty with degree of improvement following total shoulder replacement. He showed that in patients with osteo-arthritis, 83% were greatly improved following total

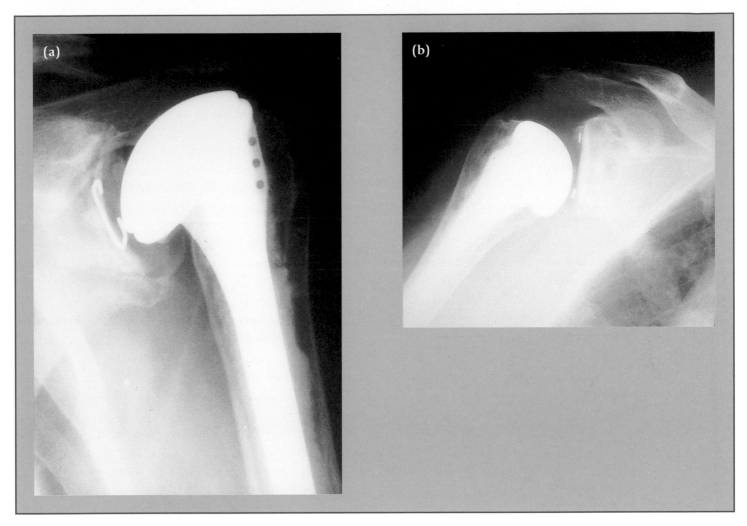

Figure 9.24 – *Lucent lines in the glenoid, (a) nil and (b) partial.*

shoulder replacement, whereas only 33% were greatly improved by hemiarthroplasty. These figures were confirmed in rheumatoid patients, where 70% were greatly improved following total shoulder replacement, and only 38% by hemiarthroplasty. So, despite the difficulties, the glenoid should be replaced if possible. These results have been confirmed by others (Norris & Iannotti, 1996).

Geometric considerations in relation to the glenoid should include the diameter of the glenoid, the surface shape, the thickness of the glenoid, the facing angle of the glenoid, and the retroversion angle of the glenoid.

Diameter of the glenoid

The diameter of the glenoid component should equal the size of the glenoid it replaces. However, attempts have been made to implant oversized glenoids in order to obtain greater stability, particularly in the cuff-

deficient shoulder. Neer made components that were oversized by 200 and 600%. However, these increased-size components made cuff repair more difficult, increased friction and led to an increased failure rate. Undersized components are also made for small rheumatoid ladies, but suffer from having a smaller surface for fixation to the bone.

Surface shape

There is great controversy over the best surface shape for the glenoid. On the one hand there is Neer's school, who believe that the humeral head and glenoid should match perfectly, i.e. have the same radius of curvature. The opposite school (Rockwood & Matsen, 1996) state that if a radiograph of a shoulder, or dried bones of a shoulder are examined, the glenoid is seen to be shallower than the humeral head; in other words there is a mismatch in the radii of curvature. This school has also shown that there is obligatory anteroposterior translation during flexion and that this can only occur with sliding of the surfaces one on the other; in turn this can only occur if there is a shallower glenoid than humerus.

Neer's school counters this by saying that although radiographs and dried bones appear mismatched, in real life, there is a cartilage cover to these bones. The cartilage of the glenoid is thicker at the periphery of the glenoid than centrally (Fig. 9.25). Arthroscopically we can see this thin central area and it is called the 'grey spot'. Neer's school has used ultrasound to measure this change in cartilage thickness across the glenoid and has proven that the cartilage surfaces of the glenoid and head are perfectly matched. Moreover, they state that the obligate translation is very small and only occurs at the extremes of motion, which are hardly ever reached following shoulder replacement. Since Neer's school has a perfectly matched prosthesis and Rockwood and Matsen's school a perfectly mismatched prosthesis the controversy surrounding this issue is set to continue.

The shape of the back of the glenoid prosthesis is almost as important as the articular surface because this is the surface which bonds to the bone. Because of the rocking horse motion it has been shown that a perfect match between prosthesis is vital in preventing deformation, warp or loosening. Mating two curved surfaces is difficult, even if shaped reamers are used, and for this reason some prostheses are flat in order to match a sawn flat section of the glenoid.

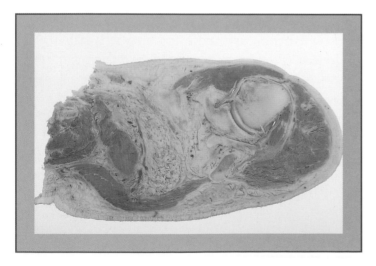

Figure 9.25 – *Anatomical section through the shoulder showing the perfect match of the cartilage and labrum, and the bony mismatch.*

Glenoid thickness

Most glenoids are 3 mm thick. Fortunately, the glenoid is protected from high peak loads due to the shock absorbing mechanism of the scapula and its supporting muscles, for such a thin layer of polyethylene would prove a disaster in a joint such as the knee or the hip.

Finite element analysis of glenoid loading led surgeons to believe that metal backing would distribute the loads from the glenoid in a more favourable manner. Such prostheses necessarily have to be far thicker (up to 10 mm), but turned out clinically to be a retrograde step, and most surgeons have returned to an all-polyethylene glenoid component.

Glenoid facing angle

The normal glenoid points upwards 5° compared to the medial scapular border. However, an upward facing glenoid appears to be detrimental in shoulder replacement and there may actually be some benefit in attempting to build in an element of downward facing to the glenoid.

Retroversion angle

Clearly the glenoid version angle must mate with the axis of the head in order to ensure maximal rotation and stability. The problem here is the degree of erosion caused by the arthritic process. Most glenoids have an element of posterior erosion. This should not be made up by methyl methacrylate. If the erosion is severe then a bone graft should be used.

Factors affecting frictional torque

The search for low frictional torque is the tribologists eternal quest because low frictional torque will lead to greater joint movement along with lower wear and loosening rates. Factors affecting frictional torque include size of the humeral head, glenoid size and material surface properties.

Head size

As we have already seen unconstrained shoulder prostheses depend upon copying nature, and thus the size of the humeral head should reproduce that found in the individual in question. Certainly head size, or increased neck length should not be used if at all possible, because we have seen how just a 5 mm increase in neck length forces the patient to double the muscle forces across the shoulder to achieve the same degree of elevation. Likewise head size can not be reduced as this would lead to tuberosity impingement and instability.

Some surgeons have elected to use a bipolar head to reduce friction. The problem is that a bipolar prosthesis uses a 22 mm internal head which is housed in a prosthesis with a 45 mm neck length. Since the normal neck length is 15 mm, if a 45 mm neck length prosthesis is inserted the cuff can not be closed unless there is 30 mm of glenoid erosion, or a cuff deficient shoulder.

Joint conformity

Rockwood and Matsen's school of thought, in which, as discussed earlier, a mismatched humeral head and glenoid is considered desirable, will result in point loading, which in turn leads to a low friction situation. The down side of point loading on a polyethylene component which is only 3 mm thick is that there may be increased polyethylene wear, but only time will tell.

Glenoid size

Reducing glenoid size will decrease frictional forces. The trade-off here is in terms of stability, the smaller the glenoid the less stable the joint becomes. Additionally, the glenoid is so small already that fixation to bone is one of the greatest problems of shoulder replacement. Why tempt fate by making the greatest problem of shoulder replacement even worse? Certainly making the glenoid bigger will increase the frictional resistance. The Neer prosthesis was designed with an extra large glenoid for cuff-deficient shoulders, but this proved a failure and was withdrawn from the market due to problems with loosening.

Material surface properties

Most shoulder replacements are metal (usually chrome cobalt, but some are made from titanium nitride) on polyethylene. This combination has been shown to work well in the hip and knee. Just as low friction materials have been used in the lower limb so surgeons have looked at varying materials in the shoulder. Ceramic humeral heads are available and various other combinations are under investigation.

Assuring longevity

Bone preparation

The head is sectioned to gain the correct retroversion angle, facing angle and to enable correct posterior and medial offset. This cut is made in relation to the 'key point' using the appropriate cutting jig (Fig. 9.26). Most cutting jigs rely on an intramedullary rod which aligns the jig in terms of varus/valgus and flexion/extension, and in most cases the rod is also the humeral canal reamer. The reamed canal is now washed and a cement plug is positioned correctly, followed by a gauze roll soaked in diluted hydrogen peroxide which will act as a tampon and prevent blood from the canal from interfering with glenoid preparation or cementation. Some shoulder systems have a temporary prosthesis, which protects the soft bone of the humeral head from the glenoid retractors and this is inserted at this point.

Now that the humeral head has been dealt with, definitive capsular releases and balancing can be performed. Firstly the anterior capsule is taken off the anterior glenoid down to the 6 o'clock position. This allows assessment and removal of the anterior osteophytes. It also allows the surgeon to slide a finger down the front of the glenoid to orientate the position of

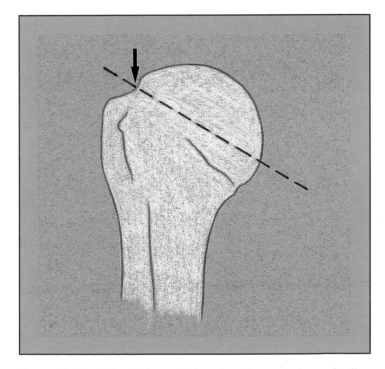

Figure 9.26 – *The jig is applied so that the cut exits at the 'key point', the highest point of the synovial reflection, in the valley between the head and the greater tuberosity.*

the glenoid keel this is necessary because often the glenoid has such severe posterior erosion that judging glenoid orientation off the face of the glenoid can lead to errors. The posterior capsule is now assessed. If the capsule is too tight then a scalpel is used to make an inside out capsulotomy close to and parallel to the posterior glenoid rim. Care is taken not to damage the long head of biceps tendon. The labrum is finally excised.

Attention is now turned to the glenoid, the most difficult part of shoulder replacement. As we have already mentioned there is considerable debate as to whether the glenoid should be replaced, because the incidence of lucent lines at the cement bone interface reaches 89%. In Sweden a register is kept of all shoulder replacements performed; in 1986, 112 hemiarthroplasties and 85 total arthroplasties were performed, compared with 110 hemiarthroplasties and only 6 total arthroplasties in 1989, reflecting this change in philosophy. Others (Brems, 1993) argue that the high incidence of glenoid lucent lines reflects poor technique, inadequate exposure and poor bone preparation (lavage and pressure). Brems believes that if adequate bone stock is present, then a total shoulder replacement is better than a hemiarthroplasty, both in terms of pain relief and function. In this respect, the shoulder is no different from any other major joint in the body. This point of view is backed up both by the study of Gschwend (1991) and by a recent multicentre study of 217 arthroplasties from the USA (Norris & Iannotti, 1996) which showed that total shoulder replacement was significantly better than hemiarthroplasty in terms of pain relief, sleep, overall shoulder function and movement in all directions. These findings were echoed by Jonsson *et al.* (1996) in a smaller prospective randomized study.

The glenoid is exposed by posterior displacement of the sectioned humeral head with a Fukuda retractor, or a humeral-head retractor (Fig. 9.27). A slot is then burred in the glenoid to accommodate the keel of the prosthesis. Care must be taken not to penetrate the back of the glenoid where the suprascapular artery and nerve lie in a groove, nor the anterior wall. Any breaches should be grafted with cancellous bone from the humeral head, to allow cement pressurization. The trial prosthesis is inserted and checked.

Cementation technique

Modern cementation technique is as essential in the shoulder as in the hip or knee. The bone should be cleaned with high-pressure lavage and cement

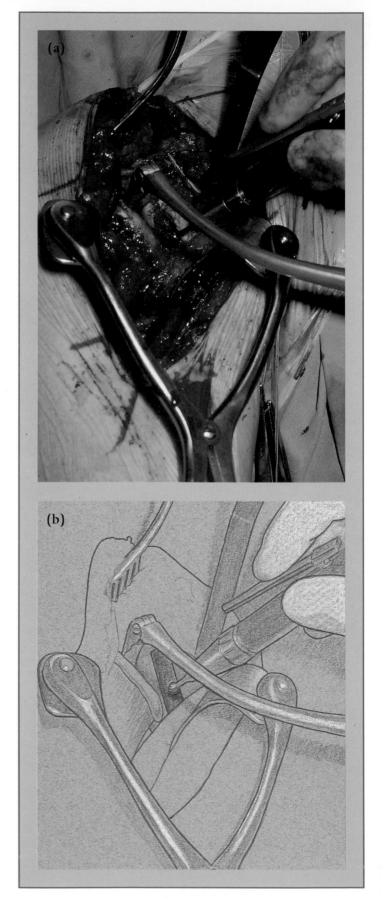

Figure 9.27 – *Glenoid exposure.*

pressurized into the glenoid, following which the glenoid component is inserted and pressurized until the cement has set. Undeniably the cementation technique is far more difficult in the shoulder than the hip or knee. The reasons for this are difficulties in exposure, and the fact that the glenoid lies down at the bottom of a sump where blood pools. Even the best surgeon cannot guarantee consistent excellence with cement under these conditions. This has led to many surgeons considering the use of uncemented glenoid components which use a combination of screws, studs and expanding bolts for initial fixation to the bone.

Attention is now turned back to the humerus. The protector and tampon are removed and the trial prosthesis inserted. A trial head is placed and trial reduction performed. The shoulder is now checked for cuff tension, range of movement, ligament balance and stability. The canal is now lavaged and antibiotic cement pressure-injected using a cement gun with a revision (narrow) nozzle and a cement restrictor to seal off the sectioned surface (usually a reversed femoral seal works well) (Fig. 9.28). The definitive stem is introduced and the retroversion angle is checked while this is being done. After the cement has cured, the definitive head is impacted and the prosthesis reduced.

Reconstructing the soft tissues

The two elements requiring reconstruction are: the ligaments which are often contracted and the rotator-cuff muscles which are shortened and need to be re-tensioned.

The arthritic shoulder is always stiffened and contracted. In particular, the coracohumeral ligament is contracted and requires release. The coracohumeral ligament makes up the roof of the rotator interval; it is important that both are released, the rotator interval along its length from the humerus to the base of the coracoid, and the coracohumeral ligament from the base of the coracoid. The anterior and inferior capsule are released when the arthrotomy is made, but the posterior capsule may be tethered and require release and balancing.

The muscles of the rotator cuff will be tensioned correctly if attention has been paid to regaining the lateral offset of the humeral head during insertion of the prosthetic components. However, the cuff muscles may have to be released both internally (taking care not to damage the suprascapular nerve) and externally from the bursa. The arthrotomy in subscapularis should be closed,

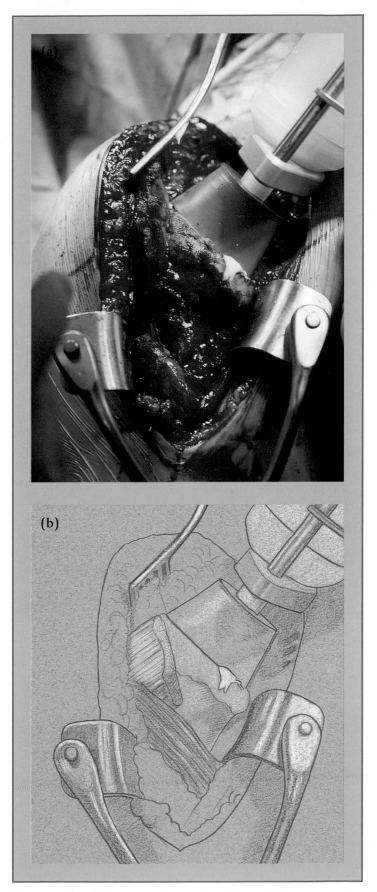

Figure 9.28 – *The cement is pressurized into the humerus using a cement gun and a seal.*

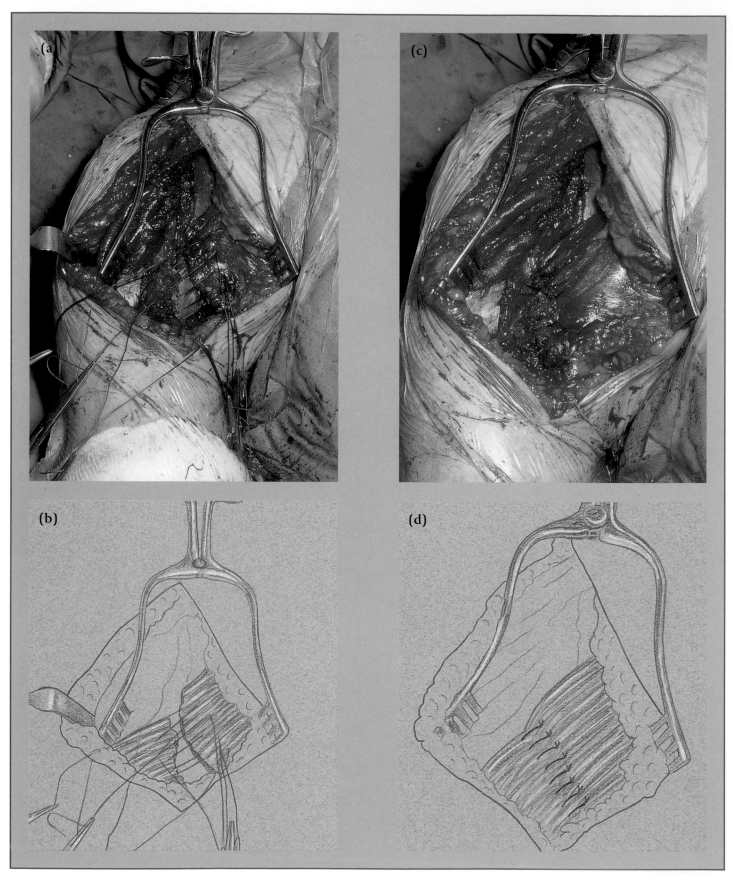

Figure 9.29 – *Pectoralis major is repaired with multiple mattress sutures. (a & b) The sutures are all placed prior to tying. (c & d) Secure repair of pectoralis major.*

allowing 30° of external rotation on the table. The rotator interval should be closed loosely or not closed at all, it should not be closed tightly because this will contract the shoulder.

The pectoralis major muscle should be carefully reconstructed (Fig. 9.29), and multiple mattress sutures passed through the thick sheet of the tendon on its deep surface. The skin is closed with a subcuticular suture.

Routine prophylactic antibiotics are given intravenously following surgery. The arm is placed in a sling for the first day and the sling is then worn, by night only, for the first 3 weeks following surgery.

Rehabilitation

Aggressive rehabilitation is as vital to outcome as the surgery itself. The patient must be motivated to comply with the physiotherapist. We tell the patient that 'The physiotherapist will visit to start the recovery exercise programme which is vital to your outcome. Remember that how quickly and fully you recover after shoulder replacement is, to a large extent, up to you. Your shoulder needs special exercises both whilst in hospital and when you return home in order to return the shoulder to full use'. This is further enforced in the written protocol which is given to each patient, a further copy being sent to the physiotherapist and family practitioner.

The rehabilitation protocol has a protective phase and then a strengthening phase (Fig. 9.30).

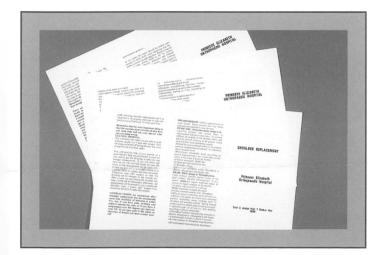

Figure 9.30 – *Postoperative protocols for shoulder replacement.*

Protective phase (weeks 1–4)

Goals: to protect the suture lines in the subscapularis and pectoralis major; to prevent stiffness developing in the shoulder, elbow and hand; to prevent wasting in all muscles that have not been sectioned during surgery.

Method: no active internal rotation; no passive external rotation beyond neutral; no elevation above shoulder level.

(i) *Pendulums.* The patient stands with the arm hanging down leaning the body forwards from the waist as far as possible. Slowly and gently the arm is swung backwards and forwards like the pendulum of a grandfather clock. It is then swung slowly in a circle clockwise five times, and then anticlockwise five times (stirring the porridge). This is called a set of pendulums. Each day the frequency and number of sets of exercises are increased. Gradually build, according to patient response, from one set, three times daily on day one, to four sets every 2 hours by 4 weeks.

(ii) *Elbow extensions.* The patient is instructed to stand up and remove the arm from the sling. The forearm is allowed to hang down so that the elbow is straight. This is repeated 10 times. Build sets.

(iii) *Hand and fist/wrist/twist sets.* The hand always gets a bit puffy following shoulder replacement and it is important to do gripping exercises to keep the hand pumping fluid away. These exercises should be performed 10 times each hour.

(iv) *Shoulder shrugs.* Submaximal isometrics using TheraBand to deltoid, infraspinatus and biceps only.

Range and strengthening phase

Entry criteria: pain-free passive range of one half normal. Healed subscapularis and pectoralis major.

Goals: to regain maximal range of motion; to regain strength in all muscles.

Use phase one exercises as warm up.

(i) Pulley exercises to regain elevation.

(ii) Active external rotation with TheraBand

(iii) Physiopassive stretching and mobilizations

(iv) Patient lies supine on couch with controlled passive stretching, using walking stick in elevation and external rotation. Sitting, internal rotation passive stretch, using a towel across the back.

Five repetitions per set of (i) to (iv). Sets building according to physiotherapist's instructions.

(v) TheraBand isotonic strengthening exercises to the deltoid, infraspinatus, subscapularis and biceps muscles.

(vi) Submaximal isotonic exercise to the deltoid, infraspinatus, subscapularis and biceps muscle.

(v) Corner pushups to strengthen scapular power.

(vi) Proprioceptive neuromuscular facilitation.

The patient leaves hospital only when safe to cope at home, usually 4 or 5 days after surgery. Three days postoperatively the sling can be left off during the day, but must be worn at night for the first 3 weeks following surgery. The patient will need the help of a partner, or a good friend, to help get dressed, to cook, and to get the shopping in until they can manage independently. The patient should not drive for 8 weeks following surgery.

Complications

There have been very few medium-term studies of shoulder replacement giving results and complication rates. Wirth and Rockwood (1996) in a meta-analysis of the world literature could only find five studies (391 shoulders) with a 5-year follow-up. Wallace *et al.* (1996), in the most honest appraisal of the complications of shoulder replacement, studied over 500 shoulder replacements performed by him or under his care and found that over 20% required re-operation. This is a far higher rate than would be expected after hip or knee replacement. He classified re-operations into four groups (Table 9.4).

(1) Revision operations in which a new humeral or glenoid component is inserted, this was the outcome of 10% of the original operations.

(2) Relining operations where a humeral head or glenoid insert was replaced (3%).

(3) Rotator-cuff operations in which the cuff is repaired, plicated or decompressed (3%).

(4) Supplementary operations, such as arthrolysis, acromioclavicular joint resection or stabilization, clavicular fractures or surgery to the deltoid (5%).

Loosening of the components is the single most common cause for re-operation. The major problem is glenoid fixation. Cofield (1995) reported that at 12 years radiolucent lines had developed at the bone–cement interface of 84% of their shoulders and definite loosening in 44%. There was a definite association between radiographic loosening and pain. The same group of shoulders were studied at 6 years follow-up and at 12 years; the rate of glenoid loosening quadrupled during the second half of the study (Fig. 9.31).

Instability is the second commonest cause of complication in shoulder replacement. Anterior instability may occur if the humeral head is too anteverted, or if the repair to subscapularis fails. Superior migration may occur with rotator-cuff dysfunction. Posterior instability can occur if the prosthesis is too retroverted.

Rotator-cuff tears are the third most common complication encountered after shoulder replacement. It occurs in about 2% of operations.

Table 9.4 Revision operations for shoulder replacement.

● Revision	New humeral component
	New glenoid component
● Relining	New humeral head
	New glenoid insert
● Rotator cuff operations	Cuff repair
	Cuff plication
	Cuff decompression
● Supplementary operation	Arthrolysis
	AC joint resection
	Periprosthetic fracture
	Surgery to the deltoid

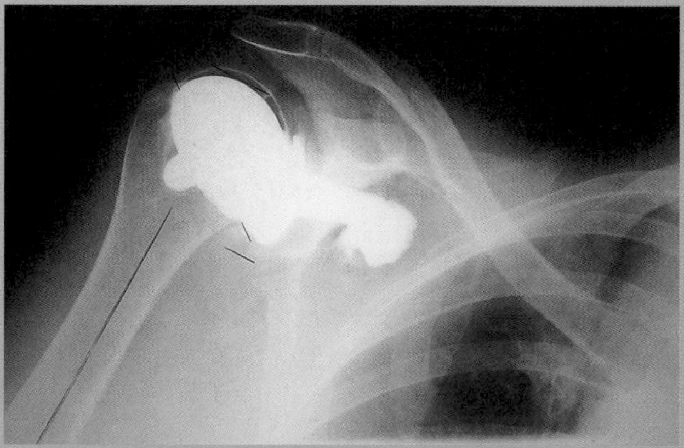

Figure 9.31 – *Loosening of the glenoid component. An arthrogram showing contrast material flowing around the keel of the prosthesis and escaping where the prosthesis has penetrated the scapula.*

Periprosthetic fractures are usually caused by failure in surgical technique (Fig. 9.32). Vigorous rotation of the humerus during dislocation, or excessive reaming of the canal, or heavy handed impaction of the components may lead to fractures.

Postoperative fractures will occur just as in every other joint replacement.

Infection is a rare, but potentially disastrous, complication of shoulder replacement. If an early infection is considered then an aggressive policy of urgent re-exploration and radical debridement of the operation site, with vigorous lavage using a high pressure system, followed by parenteral antibiotics, used according to sensitivities, should be undertaken until the CRP and ESR return to normal.

For late infection radical debridement should be undertaken and all prosthetic material, including cement, excised. An antibiotic spacer should be inserted and 6 weeks of antibiotic therapy should be administered. After 6 weeks, if the site is quiescent, and the ESR and CRP have returned to normal, and if cultures are negative, reimplantation can be considered. However, reimplantation through such a scarred field is a major and hazardous undertaking.

Nerve injury is rare following shoulder replacement, but has been reported in connection with the axillary and musculocutaneous nerves, and even to the other terminal branches of the brachial plexus.

Dissociation of modular components has been recorded on both the glenoid and the humeral side (Fig. 9.33).

Dysfunction of the deltoid muscle occurs after surgical approaches that damage the origin of this muscle and in which surgical repair is poor.

Survivorship analysis is presently enjoying a vogue in orthopaedic circles. The problem with survivorship analysis is what do you take as your criterion of failure? If re-operation is the criterion used a less experienced surgeon will undoubtedly have better survivorship figures than the highly experienced and more aggressive surgeon. The former will persuade his patients not to have a revision operation even in severe circumstances, but the latter will re-operate even if only to relieve some residual pain in the acromioclavicular joint. Thus survivorship, according to re-operation rate, varies from 97% at 5 years with less experienced surgeons to under 80% at 5 years with experienced surgeons.

If the criterion for survivorship is broadened to include re-operation or patient dissatisfaction, due to ongoing pain, then the figures drop to 70% at 10 years.

Summary

Shoulder replacement has come of age, it is no longer an experimental procedure. Attention to the details of

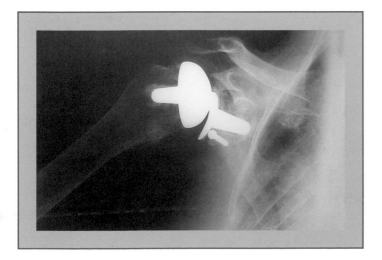

Figure 9.32 – *A glenoid fracture occurred during impaction of this uncemented glenoid component into the glenoid. It was primarily internally fixed with a lag screw and the patient had an excellent result.*

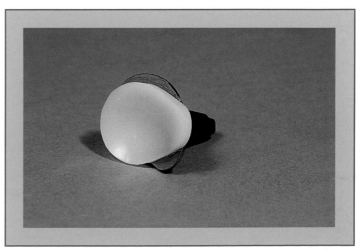

Figure 9.33 – *This metal-backed glenoid component has dissociated from the plastic liner.*

the operation has transformed the surgical results. The correction of geometric variables, in particular head size, posterior and medial offset of the head on the shaft, and retensioning of the rotator cuff muscles, has changed an operation from a method of painfree arthrodesis to a painfree, functioning and remarkably free moving joint.

Fixation of the glenoid component remains a challenge to the shoulder surgeon. However better exposure, instrumentation and prosthetic design has lead to significant improvement. Cementation of the glenoid has always been difficult because of its situation and the small area of fixation to the bone. Cementless fixation shows promise in giving long-term secure fixation.

CHAPTER 10

The acromioclavicular joint

C. Warren-Smith

Introduction

The acromioclavicular joint is a small, but vulnerable, and frequently injured joint. It is an unusual joint in that the articular cartilage is fibrocartilage rather than hyaline; this makes it particularly prone to early degenerative change. It has a pivotal position in that it lies just over the prime site of initiation of rotator-cuff tears, and forms the keystone of the coraco-acromial arch.

Because of the obliquity of the joint, and its position on the point of the shoulder, dislocations are very common. The management of dislocation of this joint is highly controversial. The arguments over operative and conservative treatment roll on and on. For those in favour of operative treatment, either immediate or delayed, the choice of operations is positively mouthwatering. This chapter aims to lead you through the good and bad points of the pathology and management of problems of the acromioclavicular joint, so that your patients can get the optimum treatment.

Functional anatomy

The acromioclavicular joint is diarthrodial (possessing two joint cavities, separated by a disc), and is located between the articular facet of the distal clavicle and the medial side of the acromion. The joint is orientated obliquely, with the clavicular surface facing outwards and downwards. The distal clavicle is usually thicker than the acromion, such that while the inferior surface of the distal clavicle lies at the same level as that of the acromion, the superior surface of the clavicle lies slightly superior to that of the acromion. There is frequently an articular disc, which is sometimes incomplete. There is a relatively weak capsule surrounding the joint, the main ligamentous thickening of the capsule being the superior acromioclavicular ligament. The strongest and most

important ligaments are extra-articular, they are the conoid and trapezoid ligaments; these are collectively called the coracoclavicular ligaments.

Fukuda et al. (1986) have indicated that the superior acromioclavicular ligament is the primary constraint to posterior displacement of the clavicle. It contributes to constraint in smaller amounts of displacement, whilst the conoid ligament limits larger amounts of displacement. The trapezoid ligament plays its major role when displacement and stress occur as the acromion is moved in compression towards the clavicle.

The joint is subcutaneous and is easily visible and palpable. The most prominent part is usually the distal end of the clavicle. The joint is abnormally prominent in some people (articulatio acromioclavicularis prominens) and the opposite side should always be examined in comparison, to avoid embarrassment, especially following trauma.

The deltoid takes origin from the lateral third of the clavicle and from the whole of the spine of the scapula, including the acromion. The trapezius attaches to the clavicle anteriorly, the medial acromion and the spine of the scapula posteriorly. The fibres of the trapezius and deltoid are, to all extents, contiguous. This continuous sheet of muscle and fascia is used in surgical exposure of the shoulder, as it can be split and the flaps raised; it can then be securely repaired, leading to early rehabilitation.

Immediately below the joint lies the anterior part of the musculotendinous junction of the supraspinatus muscle. The relevance of this in the aetiology of rotator-cuff tears is described in chapter four. Osteophytes on the inferior surface of the joint can cause impingement on the cuff and lead to cuff tearing.

The subacromial bursa does not usually lie beneath the joint, but is further anterior and lateral. Again the relevance of this is that arthroscopy of the subacromial bursa does not allow examination of the acromioclavicular joint unless the bursal wall is removed with a full radius resector during acromioplasty.

The scapula and the upper limb are effectively suspended from the end of the clavicle, which in turn is suspended from the neck by the trapezius muscle. The clavicle also acts as a spacer to hold the shoulder-complex away from the body axis, while the sternoclavicular joint acts as a pivot, and the scapula helps to stabilize the complex against the chest wall.

Clinical presentation

Pain is the predominant symptom of acromioclavicular pathology. When the patient is asked where their pain is they will point directly to the acromioclavicular joint with the index finger of the opposite hand (Fig. 10.1). The pain may be referred along the clavicle, or along the spine of the scapula, or rarely into the axilla. It should not be forgotten that the distal clavicle is broad from anterior to posterior, and symptoms may arise predominantly from the front or the back of the joint. This pain is classically accentuated by adducting the arm across the front of the patient, but adducting the arm across the back of the patient is a more specific test. In elevation, the pathological acromioclavicular joint will usually produce increasing pain towards the limit of movement. Classically, the last 30–40° of full abduction are painful, and the patient cannot 'get above the pain' as may be possible with a 'painful arc' due to supraspinatus impingement under the coraco-acromial ligament.

Disruption of the acromioclavicular joint may cause a significant mechanical disadvantage to the shoulder, with marked elevation of the distal end of the clavicle, and inferior and medial displacement of the shoulder from its normal position. Pain at the joint, clicking and catching, general aching, and weakness may result, particularly during work at or above shoulder level. There may be a tendency for the shoulder to tire rapidly during physical activity.

Radiography

The acromioclavicular joint is poorly seen on true anteroposterior (AP) radiographs of the shoulder. This is partly due to its subcutaneous position, which can cause relative over-exposure of the film, and partly due to the fact that on a standard view of the shoulder the joint overlaps the spine of the scapula and the acromion. For the acromioclavicular joint itself the X-ray beam should be angled upwards, by approximately 25°, centred on the acromioclavicular joint and coned down. This leaves the joint open to view without overlapping the spine of the scapula, and a clearer view of the acromion is also obtained (Fig. 10.2).

Radiology of the joint has traditionally been associated with weight-bearing views. However, the latter can be very misleading in that some dislocations may actually reduce with weight-bearing. There is no substitute for clinical examination if the history suggests instability of the joint (see below). If a picture is required, as a record of the instability, then this should

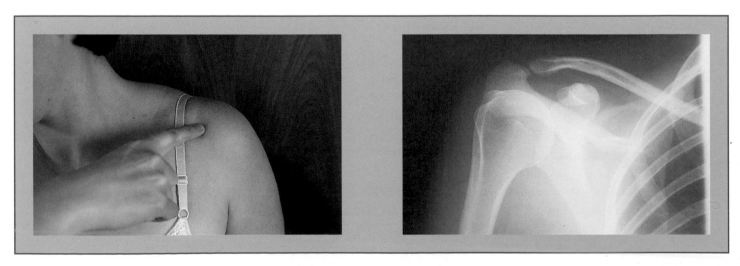

Figure 10.1 – *The patient can usually accurately localize pain at the acromioclavicular joint.*

Figure 10.2 – *Angling the X-ray beam upwards throws the acromioclavicular joint and acromion into prominence.*

be taken with forced adduction to sublux or dislocate the joint; the beam will need to be appropriately centred and angled, usually laterally, to display the joint properly.

Subluxation and dislocation of the acromioclavicular joint

Trauma to the acromioclavicular complex may take the form of some degree of injury to the joint alone, or may be associated with disruption of the coracoclavicular ligaments. There may be an associated fracture of the clavicle. Rarely, there may be a simultaneous disruption of the sternoclavicular joint. Extremely rarely, there may be an associated fracture of the coracoid.

Most commonly the disruption is associated with a direct fall on to, or a direct blow to, the point of the shoulder. Injury to the acromioclavicular joint is commonest if the shoulder is hunched forwards as the stress falls upon it.

Classification

The most commonly used classification is that of Allman (1967) (Table 10.1). Allman divided injuries into three grades:

- Grade 1. 'Sprain' of the acromioclavicular ligament without disruption. No X-ray abnormality.
- Grade 2. Disruption of the joint without disruption of the coracoclavicular ligaments. There is slight elevation of the distal clavicle on X-ray compared with the acromion, but the undersurface of the clavicle remains below the level of the superior surface of the acromion.
- Grade 3. The coracoclavicular ligaments are disrupted, and the whole distal end of the clavicle is above the level of the acromion on X-ray.

Tossy *et al.* (1963) divided injuries into similar grades, but with A and B subdivisions, where B indicated the presence of a fracture also. In his paper, Tossy had described Grade-3 injuries as separation at the acromioclavicular joint 'greater than one half its normal depth'. Allman's description is more commonly used.

It is important to note that Tossy radiographic Grade-3 injuries are not, in fact, always associated with complete rupture of the coracoclavicular ligaments. Lizaur *et al.* (1984) specifically noted that 13% of their series had intact coracoclavicular ligaments, but using the Grade-3 criterion of displacement > 75% width of articular surface of the acromion. This is a source of error in the comparison of different papers.

It should be appreciated that there are no absolute or clear-cut distinctions between the different grades of injury. There is a continuous spectrum of injury.

Rowe (1988) includes further grades of injury as detailed in Table 10.2.

Certainly it is the case that fractures of the tip of the clavicle, associated with disruption of the coracoclavicular ligaments, should be recognised for what they are; effectively they are equivalent to an acromioclavicular disruption, in terms of mechanical separation of the scapula from the clavicle, but leave the actual acromioclavicular joint intact. These fractures are commonly associated with posterior displacement of the clavicle, and symptomatic non-union is common.

Diagnosis

The diagnosis of a Grade-1 injury is a clinical one, supported by normal X-rays. There is tenderness at the joint, with no elevation of the clavicle. Grade-2 injuries show clinical evidence of a raised distal end of the clavicle at the joint. If the arm is held at the elbow by the examiner it may be possible to ballotte the end of the clavicle with a finger on its distal end. This should be compared with the opposite clavicle.

Table 10.1 Allman classification of injury.

Grade 1	Sprain	Coracoclavicular ligaments intact
Grade 2	Subluxation	Coracoclavicular ligaments intact
Grade 3	Dislocation	Coracoclavicular ligaments torn

Table 10.2 Rowe's additional classification.

Grade 4	Severe superior dislocation, tenting of skin
Grade 5	Posterior dislocation
Grade 6	Inferior dislocation
Grade 7	Bipolar dislocation

The diagnosis of Grade-3 acromioclavicular instability is a clinical one. In many Grade-3 injuries the displacement is obvious, but in some cases the clavicle may lie in a reduced position. Direct pressure downwards on the tip of the clavicle with the upper arm held steadied may demonstrate reduction of the subluxation, as with Grade-2 injuries. Hunching the shoulder forwards is a particularly useful test (Fig. 10.3), and will generally demonstrate instability immediately, as the tip of the clavicle dislocates. Protraction and retraction of the shoulder may be useful where there is posterior displacement. In the late case, where symptoms suggest instability, and no obvious upward displacement is apparent, it is particularly important to look for anteroposterior instability. Simply grasping the distal clavicle and moving it in an anteroposterior plane may demonstrate abnormal movement.

Treatment

Grade 1

Treatment of the sprain or Grade-1 injury is by simple rest and supportive measures, as required.

Grade 2

Treatment of the Grade-2 injury in the acute stage is the same as for the Grade-1 injury. A sling is more likely to be required, and the possibility of requiring subsequent surgical excision of the tip of the clavicle is worth mentioning to the patient. A number of methods of

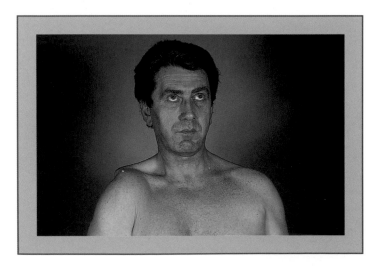

Figure 10.3 – *Hunching the shoulder forwards will usually readily demonstrate a dislocation.*

trying to hold the clavicle reduced have been advocated, but none have been shown to be better than a simple supportive sling. Indeed, many may cause complications including stiffness and skin problems. Urist (1946) gives a useful review of conservative methods that have been tried. Although traditionally these are said to be benign injuries, there is a significant incidence of troublesome long-term pain. Where symptoms do persist, or re-appear later, in relation to degenerate changes, it is usually the case that simple excision of the joint will alleviate the problem.

Treatment of acromioclavicular dislocation

Treatment of the acute dislocation, or Grade-3 injury, is controversial. There are proponents for early surgical stabilization of the joint, and there are those who favour conservative management, with repair of only those that remain symptomatic for an unacceptable time. It should be borne in mind that with early repair there is a reasonable chance of satisfactory healing of the coracoclavicular ligaments, and greater strength of repair may be achieved than with late repair, should this be necessary.

Conservative management

Several authors have concluded that a high proportion of patients will obtain a satisfactory result without surgery. Urist (1946), in a wide review of the literature, reported only 10–20% failure in those cases managed conservatively. Glick *et al.* (1977) reported no significant functional disability in 35 patients followed up at 3 years.

Dias *et al.* (1987) reviewed 44 patients at a mean of 5 years and found that none had changed their occupation and that only two had moderate discomfort. Ten patients however had difficulty carrying heavy loads, and six patients had a gross deformity, but did not complain about the appearance. Only four patients had a normal distal clavicle as seen on radiographs, 30 patients had expansion of the end of the clavicle, and 10 had atrophy. Thirty-six patients had an obvious deformity, and six of these had gross deformity.

Rawes and Dias (1996) reviewed 35 patients (out of the original 44 who presented in 1987) more than 10 years following injury and found that all, except one, had a good outcome. According to the assessment method of Imatani (1975), there were 14 excellent results, 15 good results and one fair result. Fifteen patients reported mild symptoms, and one reported moderate symptoms. Deformity was noticeable in 24 patients, but obvious in only 8, and in 14 patients the joint was ballottable. Neither deformity nor ballottability correlated with symptoms. None of the patients had changed their job or given up sport because of their shoulder.

Surgery

There is no doubt that despite the evidence suggesting that the majority of acromioclavicular disruptions may do well with conservative management, there is a steady flow of those who do not and who present to a shoulder surgeon.

Dawe (1980) reviewed 17 patients and reported that 13 had pain on exercise, 5 had changed to lighter jobs, 5 had stopped sport and 3 were concerned by cosmetic deformity.

In our series of 29 patients presenting late, with unacceptable symptoms, the majority had either gross subcutaneous dislocation, a fracture of the distal clavicle associated with disruption of the coracoclavicular ligaments, or jobs involving overhead work (Warren-Smith *et al.*, 1994).

Where surgical intervention is favoured there are a number of proposed lines of treatment, ranging from the most simple anatomical repositioning of the joint and internal fixation across the joint, to anatomical repositioning with stabilization to the coracoid by various means, to soft-tissue repair and resection of the distal clavicle.

Phemister (1942) described the simple use of percutaneous threaded pins to transfix the acromioclavicular joint from lateral position, with the wires being removed at 2 months. However this does not address the damage to the coracoclavicular ligaments (Fig. 10.4).

Paavolainen (1983) described the use of a malleolar screw to transfix the acromioclavicular joint, with repair of the coracoclavicular and acromioclavicular ligaments, and subsequent removal of the screw. Thirty-nine patients were treated, with 36 patients reviewed after 4 years. The positioning of the screw from the lateral position allowed rotation of the clavicle at the acromioclavicular joint even in the early stages. However, technical difficulties were numerous, occurring in 19 out of 39 patients, with only 80% of the joints accurately reduced. Despite this, long-term follow-up was reported as good in 92% of cases.

Bosworth (1941) described fixation of the clavicle to the coracoid by means of a single vitallium screw. The clavicle was overdrilled to allow some movement of the clavicle, while still preventing it from displacing upwards, and the procedure was carried out under local anaesthetic. A specially designed screw was advocated. The screw was to be left in indefinitely unless complications required its removal. However, this operation is not as easy as the line drawings seen in text-books would suggest. Screw misplacement is common, as are secondary operations for screw pull-out, misplacement or irritation.

Neviaser (1968) described the method of coraco-acromial ligament transfer, in which the coracoid end of the ligament is transferred to the superior surface of the distal clavicle. One-hundred and twelve patients were followed up, with 92% showing excellent results. Although coraco-acromial ligament transfer strengthens the acromioclavicular ligament, it does not address the problem of the more important rupture of the coracoclavicular ligaments.

Lizaur *et al.* (1984) reported a prospective study of 46 patients with acute complete dislocation of the acromioclavicular joint treated only by suture of the deltoid and trapezius and temporary fixation with two wires for 4–5 weeks. They reported that the coracoclavicular ligaments were intact in 13% of cases. Re-displacement, at a mean of 5.8 years, occurred in 10.9% of cases.

There has been recent interest in the use of non-absorbable ligament substitutes for reconstruction of the acromioclavicular joint. However, Takagishi *et al.* (1996) have shown that there is potential danger in this. Fifteen patients with complete acromioclavicular separation were re-examined at an average of 6 years. There was a satisfactory outcome in all patients, except for one with a traumatic brachial plexus lesion, but various changes were noted in the clavicle or coracoid, with erosion by the artificial implant; in a few cases, this was enough to suggest a significant possibility of breakage in the event of trauma.

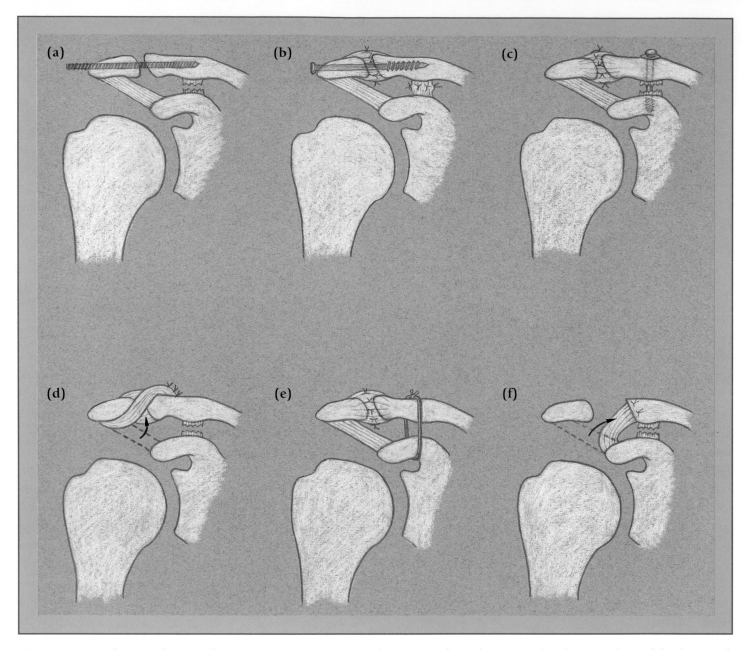

Figure 10.4 – *There are historically many ways to reconstruct the acromioclavicular joint. This diagram shows (a) Phemister's technique; (b) Paavolainen's technique; (c) Bosworth's method; (d) Neviaser's technique; (e) Takagishi's technique and (f) Weaver and Dunn's technique.*

Weaver and Dunn (1972) proposed that the ideal surgical treatment of the dislocated acromioclavicular joint should involve a single procedure, with no secondary operative site; no second procedure should be performed to remove metalwork; and there should be minimal risk of late degenerative change. They proposed that the joint be stabilized by resection of the distal clavicle to leave the cut surface facing obliquely downwards, with transfer of the acromial end of the coraco-acromial ligament into the medullary canal of the cut end of the clavicle, and repair

of the trapeziodeltoid raphe. This also avoids the late complication of acromioclavicular arthritis (Fig. 10.5).

In the original paper by Weaver and Dunn, 15 patients were followed up at an average of 35 months, with 11 good results, 3 fair results (due to objective cosmetic deformity only) and 1 poor result due to recurrence following inappropriate early return to physical activity.

We reviewed a series of 29 patients treated by this technique (Warren-Smith and Ward, 1987), and found

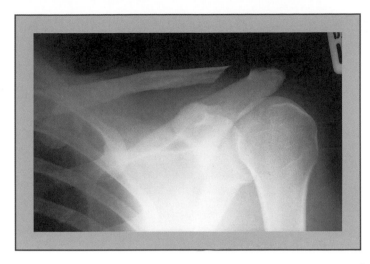

Figure 10.5 – *X-ray appearance following the procedure of Weaver and Dunn.*

17 excellent results, 11 good results, and 1 poor result (following the criteria of Imatani *et al.* [1975]). We also noted that suture of the deltoid to trapezius in closing was an important part of the repair.

Prospective trials

Bannister *et al.* (1989) compared conservative management and coracoid screw fixation, and found that conservatively treated patients regained movement more quickly and fully and had fewer unsatisfactory results than those treated surgically, but concluded that in those with acromioclavicular separation of 2 cm or more, early surgery produced better results.

Larsen *et al.* (1986) compared the outcomes of conservative management in 43 patients with a modified Phemister procedure in 41 patients. They concluded that the rehabilitation period was significantly shorter with non-operative treatment and, after 13 months, that there was no difference in the clinical results. About half of the operated group had problems with the metallic device, including migrations, breakages, and infections. They also concluded that operation should be considered in those who do heavy work, or whose daily work requires them to hold their shoulder in 90° of abduction and flexion.

These comparative trials indicate that there is no statistical advantage of surgical treatment over conservative treatment, using these particular surgical methods. They should not be used to indicate that there is no place for surgery.

Recommended treatment

Where there is little physical demand on the shoulder, such as in patients in sedentary occupations and those with little sporting demand, it seems appropriate to manage the patient conservatively. In a small percentage of cases, where late difficulties arise, surgery can be considered at a late stage.

It is, however, possible to predict patients who are likely to have a poor outcome from conservative management. Those patients with very heavy manual jobs, particularly those with significant overhead work, and those who participate in throwing sports, should be considered for early intervention. Those for whom prolonged disability would incur serious financial difficulty may also be considered for early intervention. Those patients with a gross subcutaneous dislocation are also likely to have an unsatisfactory result.

Coracoclavicular disruption associated with fracture of the lateral end of the clavicle (Fig. 10.6) will frequently progress to painful non-union of the clavicle, even if the acromioclavicular complex becomes reasonably stable; these should be treated surgically, either by internal fixation or by the technique of Weaver and Dunn (1972).

The method of Weaver and Dunn, in line with their own recommendations, avoids second operations, complications of metal implants, and secondary osteo-arthritis. This is now a widely accepted method of repair, although several modifications have been described, including the use of a small piece of acromion taken with the end of the ligament, to attach to the clavicle.

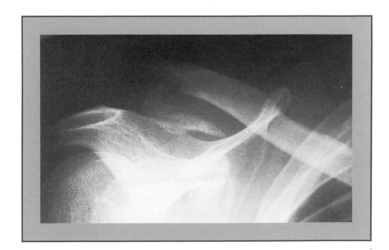

Figure 10.6 – *Coracoclavicular disruption associated with fracture of the distal clavicle.*

Excision of the distal end of the clavicle has been criticised as leaving the shoulder prone to tire easily. However, in the series of Warren-Smith and Ward (1987), 5 of the 10 patients who admitted to tiring easily, in response to direct questioning, denied any discomfort, and all considered that they had normal use of their shoulder. Several authors have reported high incidences of radiographic change in the distal clavicle, both with conservative management (Dias *et al.*, 1987) and following surgery (Paavolainen). With this in mind, the controlled excision of a small portion of the clavicle, to avoid late degenerative changes, may not seem as unacceptable as at first thought.

Temporary absorbable tape passed around the coracoid, or through the conjoint tendon, and then through or around the clavicle may also be used to support the repair in its early stages; this is recommended. However, non-absorbable tape should not be used as it can cheese-wire through the clavicle.

Juvenile patients

In juvenile patients, Grade-3 elevation of the distal clavicle may be the result of avulsion of the clavicle from its periosteal sleeve. In these cases, operative management is required to replace the clavicle back into its sleeve and to secure it there. In these patients, the coracoclavicular ligaments may be intact to the periosteum, and this simple measure may ensure an excellent result. Conversely, failure to replace the clavicle in its sleeve may result in the formation of a bifid end to the clavicle.

Late treatment

Patients with serious lasting disability should be considered for surgery. In these patients, there is usually an abnormality at the distal end of the clavicle, and resection of a small portion of the clavicle is probably wise. The Weaver and Dunn technique may again be employed.

Particular difficulties here may include the presence of ossification, or clavicular fragments, within the underlying scar tissue. The original coracoclavicular ligaments are usually impossible to identify, and secondary adaptations within the adjacent soft tissues may subject the repair to particular strain, especially with posterior dislocations of the clavicle. Particularly where the clavicle is clearly difficult to hold reduced, the use of a temporary support, such as bioabsorbable tape, is highly recommended.

Disease of the acromioclavicular joint

Osteoarthrosis

The most common pathology to arise in the acromioclavicular joint is degenerative osteoarthrosis. This is frequently of traumatic origin, but may be idiopathic. It may also be occupational in origin, or may follow specific pathology. Where the condition follows trauma there is often detectable instability, which is not the case with idiopathic or occupational arthrosis.

Traumatic osteoarthrosis is due to direct damage to the joint, and to abnormal movement at the joint due to the instability. Occupational arthrosis is probably due to repetitive movements, particularly if elevation and adduction are involved. These cause twisting and shearing at the joint, leading to deterioration of the articular disc and articular surfaces.

Whilst the pain arising at the joint itself may be the main problem, and presenting feature, degenerative change my be accompanied by osteophyte formation, and this may also present inferiorly and cause impingement on the rotator cuff (Fig. 10.7). Thus, acromioclavicular disease may present as impingement, with classical features of rotator-cuff disease, and pain radiating down the outer aspect of the upper arm. There may be either a high painful arc as described above, due to the disease at the joint, or this may run into the more classic 80–120° arc seen with impingement under the coraco-acromial arch. Thus there may be symptoms in both rotator cuff and acromioclavicular distribution.

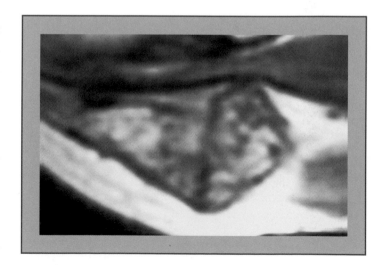

Figure 10.7 – *Close-up of MRI scan: osteophytes under the acromioclavicular joint causing gross impingement.*

Diagnostic injection

Diagnostic injection of the acromioclavicular joint with lignocaine is especially useful where there is difficulty distinguishing between acromioclavicular and subacromial pathology. The best way to locate the joint is to find the step at the distal end of the clavicle and enter the joint obliquely, from a slightly lateral direction, midway between the anterior and posterior margins of the clavicle. It should be remembered that the joint is usually orientated obliquely and is of small volume (rarely more than 1 ml). In some patients, the front of the joint may be more easily palpated and the joint thus entered from an anterior approach.

Rotator-cuff pathology

Where there is reasonable suspicion of cuff pathology, in addition to acromioclavicular arthropathy, a magnetic resonance scan is the ideal investigation.

With worsening osteophytosis, patients may present with frank rotator-cuff tears, caused directly by inferior bone spurs (Fig. 10.8). It must not be forgotten, in the treatment of proven cuff tears, that the source of the main pain may, nevertheless, be the acromioclavicular joint.

Infection

Infection in the acromiclavicular joint is unusual. It may be pyogenic, sometimes occurring after steroid injection.

Staphylococcus aureus is the most common organism. The erythrocyte sedimentation rate will be raised, and there will usually be localized evidence of infection. Tuberculous infection has been recorded and should be considered if there is unexplained swelling, which may be painless, especially if there is any history, past or present, of tubercle.

Rheumatoid arthritis

Rheumatoid arthritis in the shoulder may rarely involve the acromioclavicular joint alone, but is more commonly seen in combination with disease of the glenohumeral joint. It is a frequent source of pain, and it is most important to distinguish acromioclavicular joint pain from pain in the glenohumeral joint before undertaking shoulder replacement.

Osteolysis

Osteolysis of the distal clavicle is an unusual condition, which, in the absence of known trauma, occurs almost exclusively in relation to weightlifting. There is typical radiological lysis, sometimes almost like cyst formation at the tip of the clavicle, but without any sclerosis or osteophyte formation (Fig. 10.9). Microscopy reveals destruction of the distal end of the clavicle, including cartilage and bone, with no involvement of the acromion. There is usually chronic aching with well localized pain. Injection with local anaesthetic alone should help to confirm the diagnosis. If the condition fails to settle, then alternative causes of lysis should be considered and appropriate investigation undertaken.

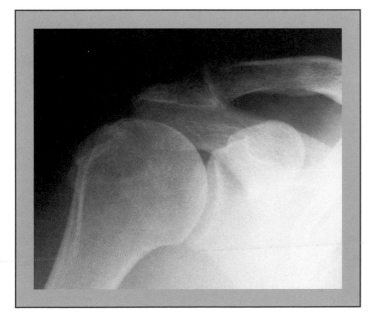

Figure 10.8 – *Acromioclavicular arthritis with osteophytosis and associated rotator-cuff tear.*

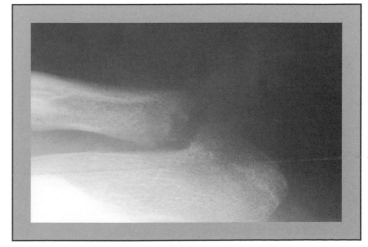

Figure 10.9 – *Osteolysis of the distal clavicle in a weight-lifter.*

Myeloma, hyperparathyroidism and infection should all be considered, especially if there is no history of weightlifting.

Osteolysis may respond to conservative treatment, particularly steroid injection, but if severe or persistent may require excision of the distal clavicle.

Post-traumatic osteolysis is not uncommon following injury to the acromioclavicular joint and should be treated by excision arthroplasty if symptomatic, and by stabilization of the joint if appropriate.

Cysts

Chronic cysts overlying the acromioclavicular joint are rare and are usually associated with underlying massive rotator-cuff tear, with erosion of the undersurface of the joint by the superiorly migrating humeral head.

Groh *et al.* (1993) described treatment of chronic cysts, associated with pain and limited movement, in four patients, by large humeral head hemiarthroplasty, with no operative treatment directed at the acromioclavicular joint or the cyst. At an average of 27 months following surgery, all four patients were pain-free, with no recurrence of the cyst.

Treatment of the painful acromioclavicular joint

Infection, malignant lesions, and metabolic problems should be treated along conventional lines and are not specifically covered here.

Once infection and malignancy have been excluded, treatment of the painful acromioclavicular joint may be conservative, using non-steroidal therapy (topical application is especially appropriate in this superficial joint) or physiotherapy in the form of ultrasound or interferential (exercises, and deep frictions are rarely helpful).

Further to these forms of treatment, steroid injection is frequently of value, but may be relatively short-lived in effect. Nevertheless, even short-lived benefit serves to indicate the likelihood, subsequently, of excision arthroplasty being of benefit.

Resection arthroplasty

Where symptoms become chronic, resection of the distal clavicle is the most commonly used surgical procedure for the relief of symptoms. This has typically been carried out as an open procedure, with resection of the distal 1–2 cm of the clavicle (the exact amount has been much discussed, but it is essential that the resection remains distal to the trapezoid ligament, to avoid destabilizing the joint). It is also essential to preserve or repair the acromioclavicular ligaments; this avoids leaving posterior instability, which would increase the likelihood of posterior abutment which can cause continuing postoperative symptoms.

Open surgery is best carried out through a sagittal skin-crease ('bra-strap' or 'sabre') incision, which leaves the least noticeable scar. The soft tissues over the joint consist of the deltotrapezius raphe, joint capsule and periosteum. These may be opened in a transverse (coronal) direction, creating a soft-tissue envelope, which is closed securely following the bone resection. The most distal soft tissue over the clavicle must be separated by sharp dissection because it will not 'strip' with a periosteal elevator. The distal clavicle is then resected using an oscillating saw.

It is wise to resect a little more from the posterior aspect of the clavicle, to avoid subsequent residual abutment against the medially inclining posterior acromion, and the oblique supero-inferior inclination of the joint should be appreciated in resecting the appropriate length.

The soft-tissue envelope is closed with strong mattress sutures, absorbable subcutaneous sutures and subcuticular monofilament, subsequently removed at 3 weeks. This leaves a better scar than absorbable skin sutures; a drain is unnecessary. As long as the joint is not destabilized, no specific restriction on activity is needed and the procedure can be carried out as a day-case.

Too great a degree of excision can cause tiring of the shoulder, even if the joint remains stable, and in a woman with heavy breasts, the bra-strap may cut into the gap, causing pain. Too inadequate an excision of bone can leave residual symptoms and regrowth of bone can occur following resection (Fig. 10.10), but rotator-cuff pathology is probably the main cause of persistent symptoms following resection of the distal clavicle alone. For this reason, excision of the distal clavicle is increasingly being carried out as an arthroscopic procedure. This can be carried out in isolation, by a direct approach only to the joint, but is usually carried out in combination with standard glenohumeral arthroscopy and subacromial bursoscopy. The latter gives the opportunity to evaluate the cuff and to carry out repair or decompression where appropriate.

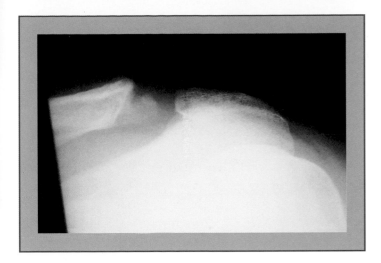

Figure 10.10 – *Regrowth of bone can occur following resection of the distal clavicle.*

Flatow (1995) describes a two-portal superior approach for direct arthroscopic resection of the acromioclavicular joint. With this technique he recommends that only 5–7 mm of bone need be removed. The larger amount of bone generally resected with open surgery is suggested to be necessary because of increased anteroposterior movement induced by disturbance of the stability of the joint at open surgery, by interference with the acromioclavicular ligaments.

Ciullo (1995) carried out arthroscopic resection of the distal clavicle in 230 patients and showed that 91%

were completely relieved of their pain. This was carried out by the three-portal technique at the same time as inspection of the glenohumeral joint and subacromial bursa. Three percent of patients developed heterotopic ossification.

Alternatively, an arthroscopy and arthroscopic decompression may be carried out, followed by open excision of the joint (taking care to preserve and close the soft tissues).

It should be borne in mind that degenerative change usually affects both sides of the joint, and excision of a small piece of distal clavicle and a small portion of medial acromion is often more logical than excision of the distal clavicle alone. This does not apply in clavicular osteolysis, but is especially important where osteophytes are present under the acromion.

Summary

The acromioclavicular joint is highly vulnerable to injury. The majority of injuries are of minor importance and heal well with conservative treatment. The art of treating the acromioclavicular joint is in knowing which injuries require surgical reconstruction, and which are best left alone. The Weaver Dunn operation is a highly versatile and simple procedure for the surgical treatment of both acute and chronic dislocation of the acromioclavicular joint.

CHAPTER 11

The patient with swelling at the sternoclavicular joint

C. Warren-Smith

Introduction

The sternoclavicular joint is usually an unobtrusive little joint. It is therefore alarming, both to the patient and the surgeon, when it suddenly swells up. This swelling may occur after trauma, when the joint is either dislocated or fractured, or the joint may become painful and swell up out of the blue. Both scenarios are unusual, and one can be life-threatening, so it behoves the surgeon to have an understanding of the underlying functional anatomy, presentation and modes of treatment.

As with the acromioclavicular joint, the sternoclavicular joint enjoys a virtually subcutaneous position, and swelling of the joint or expansion of the adjacent bone is apparent at an early stage of disease. A number of patients present, however, who complain of 'sudden swelling' of the joint, and in whom the swelling is a bony expansion. Several patients have claimed that the swelling has occurred overnight. Clearly this expansion could not have happened suddenly, so it is apparent that even visible swelling can arise insidiously and not be noticed by the patient until it becomes painful.

Pain can be accurately localized, to the joint itself, by the patient, and the joint can be directly examined for tenderness. Pain from the sternoclavicular joint often radiates along the course of the clavicle to the shoulder joint. The clinical history should be elicited in the standard form, as shown in chapter one.

To examine this joint best, the examiner should stand on a small platform behind the patient and put one hand over each sternoclavicular joint. This allows both joints to be palpated simultaneously, while allowing the patient a full range of movement.

Subluxation or dislocation of the joint, occurring with movement, is then readily appreciated, and may be compared with the opposite joint. Having compared the two joints, each can then be examined separately for instability, with one hand, while stressing the end ranges of movement with the other hand on the patient's shoulder.

Functional anatomy

The sternoclavicular joint lies between the upper outer part of the manubrium sterni and the medial end of the clavicle. It is the only direct connection between the shoulder girdle and the axial skeleton. It acts as the pivot point for all movements of the shoulder complex on the skeleton, and its ligaments also help to support the clavicle in its elevated position.

The sternoclavicular joint is a true synovial joint, between the sternal end of the clavicle, and the clavicular notch of the manubrium sterni and adjacent part of the first costal cartilage. It is a very shallow joint, which relies almost entirely on its ligaments for stability. These ligaments are strong and consist of the sternoclavicular ligaments anteriorly and posteriorly, the interclavicular ligament across the superior aspect of the manubrium from one clavicle to the other, and the costoclavicular ligament from the first rib to the clavicle (Fig. 11.1). The costoclavicular ligaments are also known as the rhomboid ligaments, and consist of two sheets of tissue arising from the first costal cartilages, and inserting into the rhomboid depression of the undersurface of the clavicle. There may be a bursa between the two layers. These ligaments are the fulcrum of movement for the medial end of the clavicle.

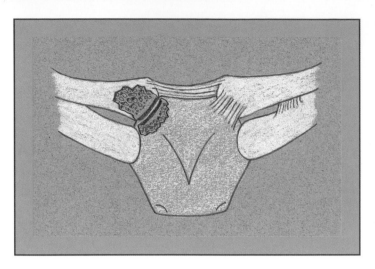

Figure 11.1 – *The sternoclavicular joint and its ligaments.*

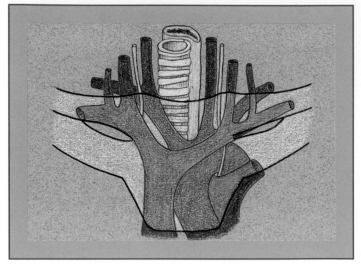

Figure 11.2 – *The posterior relationships of the sternoclavicular joint.*

Milch (1952) emphasized the importance of the rhomboid ligaments for the stability of the sternoclavicular joint. He stated that as long as the rhomboid ligament remains intact, dislocation of the sternoclavicular joint is an anatomic impossibility.

There is an intra-articular disc which arises from the superior aspect of the first rib, often inferior to the medial end of the clavicle, and inserts onto the upper part of the face of the clavicle, dividing the joint into two compartments.

The epiphysis of the medial end of the clavicle is one of the last to ossify; this may not occur until the age of 18 and Langen (1934) observed that complete anatomic maturity is reached between the ages of 25 and 30.

Movements at the joint include elevation and depression of the clavicle, protraction and retraction of the clavicle, and rotation. There are approximately 55° of elevation, 5° of depression, 30° each of anterior and posterior movement and 45° of rotation possible at the joint.

For the shoulder surgeon, the posterior relationships of the joint are of considerable importance; the great vessels, trachea, oesophagus and dome of the lung all lie close to the joint, and may be damaged or embarrassed by posterior dislocation of the clavicle (Fig. 11.2).

Investigation

Plain radiography

Examination of the joint by plain radiography is difficult. Probably the best view is a straightforward chest X-ray, which shows both joints moderately well, and allows reasonable comparison of bony contours. Bone quality is difficult to appreciate because of overlying structures. A variety of views can be attempted to throw the joint into prominence, but these are usually unsatisfactory. An anteroposterior (AP) view with a cephalic tilt of 40° may be useful to confirm displacement. Conventional X-ray tomography can be used to highlight the joints, and will often provide satisfactory information for initial diagnostic purpose.

Computerized tomography (CT) and magnetic resonance imaging (MRI) scanning

Undoubtedly the best imaging of the joint is by CT scan or MR scan. CT can give excellent appreciation of the bony anatomy and soft tissue contours (Fig. 11.3), and 3-D reconstruction may also be helpful (Fig. 11.4). For soft-tissue abnormalities and suspected malignancy, MRI scanning is ideal.

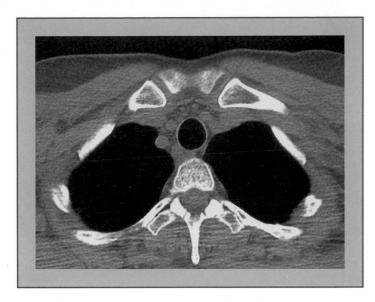

Figure 11.3 – *A CT scan of the sternoclavicular joints.*

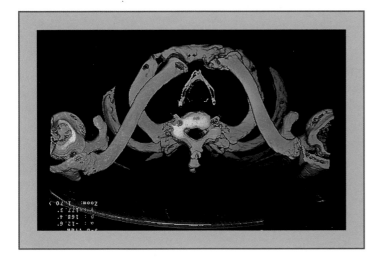

Figure 11.4 – *A three-dimensional reconstruction of the sterno-clavicular joint showing severely painful near-ankylosis following trauma.*

Traumatic swelling of the sternoclavicular joint

Trauma to the sternoclavicular joint is relatively rare, with an incidence of only 13 cases in 1603 shoulder injuries (Rowe, 1988). Nettles and Lindscheid (1968) retrospectively reviewed the notes of 60 patients, with anterior dislocation of the sternoclavicular joint, seen in the Mayo Clinic over 50 years; they noted that sternoclavicular dislocation represented only 1% of all dislocations. Furthermore, they found 57 patients with anterior dislocations (3 bilateral) and only 3 patients with posterior dislocations. Rowe further noted that in a review of 34 sternoclavicular dislocations, there were 30 superior (anterior) dislocations and 4 posterior dislocations; these also comprised 11 acute, 12 chronic (1 floating clavicle) and 11 recurrent (4 voluntary).

Because the sternoclavicular joint is protected by strong ligaments, displacement is relatively rare compared, for example, with the acromioclavicular joint. That the majority of dislocations are anterior is probably due partly to the general anatomy, and partly to the fact that the posterior sternoclavicular ligament is stronger than the anterior.

Trauma to the sternoclavicular joint is almost always indirect. Because of the close position of the ribs, and the strong superior interclavicular ligament, the commonest displacements are anterior and posterior. Injuries may consist of subluxation or dislocation of the joint alone, or may be associated with fracture. Fractures of the immediately adjacent clavicle may occur without injury to the joint, but with the overlying swelling may be difficult to separate from dislocation without imaging. For this purpose, straightforward CT scanning is unequalled (Fig. 11.5 and 11.6).

Nettles and Lindscheid (1968) found that the causes of the dislocations in their series were as follows: road accidents 15, falls 11, crush injuries 6, heavy lifting 4, and miscellaneous traumatic causes 13. Eleven were spontaneous, including three patients with bilateral dislocations.

Any dislocation may subsequently give rise to symptoms and this may be due to damage at the joint in the presence of an apparently normally reduced, stable joint, or due to persistence of some degree of instability. The joint may remain in a permanently subluxed or dislocated state, or may be associated with recurrent dislocation and spontaneous reduction with movement.

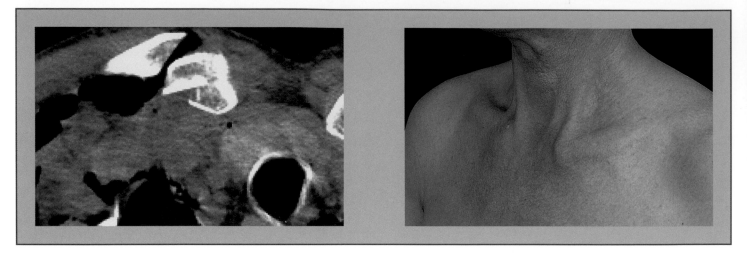

Figure 11.5 – *A CT scan showing fracture of the clavicle immediately adjacent to an intact sternoclavicular joint. A pneumothorax is also present. This patient went on to painless pseudarthrosis of the fracture and is shown in Figure 11.6.*

Figure 11.6 – *Painless pseudarthrosis of a fracture of the clavicle mimicking dislocation of the sternoclavicular joint.*

A word of caution

Before talking about treatment it is pertinent to say a few words about the use of pins in, or around, the sternum. It is a well recognized fact that pins may migrate from the medial clavicle, sternoclavicular joint or sternum. Clark *et al.* (1974) reported a case of fatal aortic perforation and cardiac tamponade, and Daus *et al.* (1993) reported a case of migration into the right ventricle. Cases have been recorded of migration into the neck, the mediastinum, the lungs and the heart. Several deaths are recorded, including one patient in whom the pin used was actually intracardiac at the end of the initial stabilization procedure (Smolle-Juettner *et al.*, 1992). Threaded pins are not immune from migrating. Even if the pin is bent at right angles, breakage can occur, with migration of a piece left behind.

The shoulder surgeon uses pins in this location at the patient's peril, and to his cost. If they must be used, they should be left out through the skin, bent at right angles close to the skin, and removed at the earliest possible time. The patient must be informed of the danger and instructed to watch the length of the pin at least daily and to report any change immediately. Furthermore, in order to minimize the risk of fatigue fracture the patient must be instructed not to elevate the arm above 90°.

As there is a well reported incidence of satisfactory results following conservative management of anterior sternoclavicular dislocation and following closed reduction of retrosternal dislocation, it is reasonable to avoid open surgery in most cases. Where surgery is indicated the ligaments should be repaired or substituted, and pins only used as a last resort, and for temporary stabilization only.

Because of the essential movements of the joint, not least those small movements that occur with respiration, arthrodesis of the joint is not an option. Stabilization of the joint or resection of the joint are the only surgical options. Resection of the joint should respect the rhomboid ligament.

Paediatric or immature injuries

As indicated above, the epiphysis appears late, at age 18, and fuses at about the age of 25. Before the medial epiphysis ossifies it is very difficult to tell between a sternoclavicular dislocation and an epiphyseal injury, but it is probable that most injuries to the region occurring before the appearance of the epiphysis on X-ray are, in fact, epiphyseal separations, as reported by Denham (1967).

Until the medial epiphysis actually fuses, epiphyseal type injuries can continue to occur. Most common is a Salter–Harris II injury. The epiphysis and a small portion of metaphysis are left attached at the joint, while the clavicle displaces. The periosteal sleeve ruptures and the medial end of the shaft protrudes. Lewonowski and Bassett (1992) have reported that posterior displacement of the clavicle can occur as an epiphyseal injury, as with actual dislocations.

Simple reduction may suffice, or if closed reduction is unsuccessful, then open reduction and repair of the periosteal sleeve will be required. This can be supplemented with direct heavy suture material across the epiphysis if desired, or even with a screw if there is a large metaphyseal fragment. These injuries are rewarding to recognize and treat.

Beware the so-called persistent dislocation in the immature situation. This may well represent an epiphyseal separation with subsequent callus formation and remodelling (Fig. 11.7). Attempts to reduce this will not be successful!

Anterior dislocation

Anterior dislocation is not a life-threatening condition. The rhomboid ligaments, the interclavicular ligament, and the intra-articular disc attachments are ruptured. Reduction may be easy, or may be blocked by malpositioning of the disc or other debris within the joint. However, the deforming upward force of the sternomastoid, together with the inherently

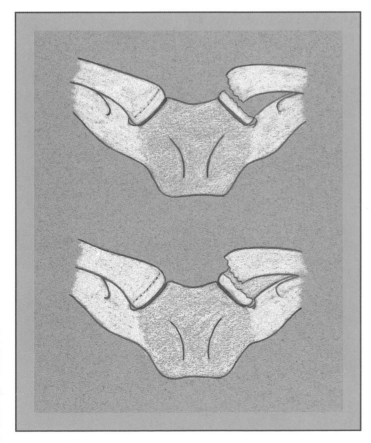

Figure 11.7 – *Epiphyseal separation and callus remodelling simulating persistent dislocation.*

unstable shallow shape of the joint, can lead to re-displacement.

Nettles and Lindsheid (1968) retrospectively reviewed the notes of 60 patients, seen in the Mayo Clinic over 50 years, and found 16 cases of anterior dislocation treated non-operatively with prompt reduction and figure-of-eight bandage. Of these, two were lost to follow-up. Eleven (78.5%) had no recurrence and no significant pain. Three had recurrence of dislocation. Of 30 patients presenting with chronic dislocation, 6 became lost to follow-up, but 16 had minimal or no symptoms on follow-up and only 8 had significant problems. Overall 69% of those treated by closed methods had satisfactory results and of 41 patients with chronic or recurrent dislocation only 11 (26.8%) had sufficient difficulty to warrant surgical intervention.

De Jong and Kaulesar Sukul (1990) reviewed 10 of 13 patients treated conservatively, at a mean of 62.9 months. Of these, nine patients had other serious injuries. Conservative treatment consisted of analgesics only, or sling or adhesive strapping. Seven patients had no complaints. One patient had an associated brachial plexus lesion, one had poor function, possibly associated with a glenohumeral dislocation, and one patient complained of pain around the joint on extreme abduction. They concluded that non-operative treatment gives very good results.

Although conservative management may be successful in the majority of cases, there is the occasional patient with persistent problems due to an unstable, or persistently dislocated joint. Where the instability is a minor subluxation only, with apparently intact rhomboid ligaments, treatment by steroid injection may initially be tried; this will avoid the need for surgery in a few cases. If unsuccessful, then resection of the medial 1 cm of the clavicle may be performed. Eskola *et al.*(1989) have reported that an excision of 2.5 cm gives an unacceptable result. A recent paper by Acus *et al.* (1995) reported the results of resection of the medial clavicle in 15 patients, in whom an average of 2.9 cm was resected (range 1–4 cm), reviewed at 4.6 years (range 1–14 years). Their results also show worse results when approximately 2–3 cm is resected, although interestingly excision of 3 cm or more is associated with a good result. Similarly, if the pain is arising at the medial end of the clavicle, being permanently displaced, but not unstable, then resection of the medial end of the clavicle is appropriate. Where, however, the sternoclavicular joint keeps dislocating and causing symptoms, stabilization by ligamentous reconstruction, to replace the damaged rhomboid ligaments, is appropriate.

Lowman (1928) described the use of a fascial sling for the correction of recurrent sternoclavicular dislocation; variations on this theme have been widely used and reported in small numbers (Fig. 11.8). The problem with the use of fascia is the need for a second operative site.

Jackson Burrows (1951) described the operation of subclavius tenodesis in which the tendon of the subclavius muscle is left attached to its insertion on to the first rib and its cartilage, but is detached from its muscle and passed through a drill hole in the clavicle. This avoids the need to drill through the manubrium. This is a satisfactory method if the tendon is found to be sufficiently stout.

Brown (1961) reported 10 cases repaired by ligament reconstruction, using the reflected sternocleidomastoid muscle, supplemented by a rush pin passed through the medullary cavity of the clavicle via a drill hole and across the joint into the manubrium. He specifically recommended the use of the rush pin and the use of a predrilled hole through the outer cortex only, as a way of avoiding the complications of wires discussed above; despite this, two pins broke at the level of the joint and one pin was misdirected and penetrated the pulmonary artery. Once again, if you want to keep your professional indemnity association happy you must never use pins around the sternoclavicular joint.

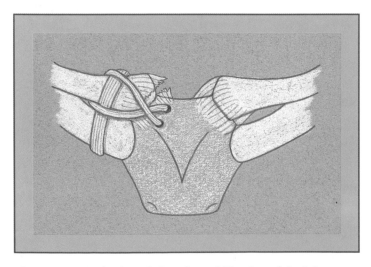

Figure 11.8 – *The fascial sling for stabilization of the joint.*

Omer (1967) suggested a medial clavicular osteotomy, in addition to the joint repair, to reduce the lever-arm effect of movements of the upper limb, which threaten to disrupt the joint in the early stages following repair. This allows some flexibility at the level of the rhomboid ligaments until the osteotomy unites. This ingenious manoeuvre has not gained wide acceptance.

For open surgery the joint is approached through as high a transverse incision as the surgeon feels is acceptable for the task. Scars directly over the sternoclavicular joint frequently lead to very thickened and often keloid scars. The higher up the neck, the better the cosmetic result. It is important to accurately close the platysma.

Gentle blunt retrosternal dissection allows palpation of the back of the sternum and allows for the placement of a guard for any drilling procedures. The joint may then be stabilized using strips of either fascia lata or artificial material across the joint itself, or by Jackson Burrows tenodesis, or by using the reflected clavicular head of the sternocleidomastoid. This latter approach also removes one of the deforming forces for redislocation.

Posterior dislocation

Posterior, or retrosternal, dislocation is usually caused by a direct posterior force on the clavicle near its medial end, or a fall on to the shoulder when the shoulder is hunched forwards. Atraumatic cases have, however, been recorded.

With retrosternal dislocation the normal prominence of the medial end of the clavicle is absent. If there is pressure on the major veins there may be venous congestion of the face and if there is pressure on the trachea there may be acute breathlessness. This is a potentially life-threatening situation. It is particularly common amongst jockeys and is known as 'a brush with death'. It should be considered in anyone who is breathless after a fall on to the shoulder and can truly be an emergency.

Retrosternal dislocation can be associated with tearing of the brachiocephalic vein; in a review of the literature Worman and Leagus (1967), noted that of 60 cases of retrosternal dislocation, there were 16 complications including 2 deaths. Computerized tomography scanning is advisable, time permitting, in all cases of suspected retrosternal dislocation.

Ideally, manipulative reduction should be undertaken where there are facilities for urgent open reduction, but in extremis should be undertaken without delay. The shoulders should be braced backwards, with a sandbag between the shoulder blades, to exert traction along the length of the clavicle, and the arm is then drawn downwards, using the fulcrum of the clavicle over the first rib to lever the medial clavicle superiorly and to allow it to reduce into joint. Buckerfield and Castle (1984) reported that six out of seven cases reduced in this manner were stable, and also noted that the literature suggests that the other method frequently quoted — of abduction and traction — is unsuccessful in 32% of cases. A figure-of-eight bandage is usually adequate to maintain reduction, but if it is not, an open stabilization should be undertaken, in view of the potential damage to retrosternal structures (Fig. 11.9).

Buckerfield and Castle also recorded that, in the English literature, the average age of patients with retrosternal dislocation was 18.6 years, indicating that the majority of injuries occur when the epiphyseal plate is still open; it is likely that a much higher proportion of retrosternal injuries are epiphyseal than has previously been recognised, and this may explain why the reductions are usually stable. Indeed, they questioned the frequency of open reduction previously reported to be necessary.

Where reduction is clearly unsuccessful, or where late presenting dislocation is associated with problems, an open approach to the joint and ligamentous reconstruction is appropriate in a similar manner to that described for anterior dislocation. Discussion with a thoracic surgeon before commencing acute cases, where damage to the great vessels may be suspected, is sensible.

In a few cases, where retrosternal dislocation has recurred, claviculectomy has been carried out (this has also been carried out for other reasons). Wood (1986) and Rowe (1988) both report surprisingly good results with claviculectomy.

Voluntary dislocation

Voluntary or habitual dislocations may occur. These are usually painless and may be bilateral; they will usually be atraumatic. General ligamentous laxity is often not present. Surgery is best avoided.

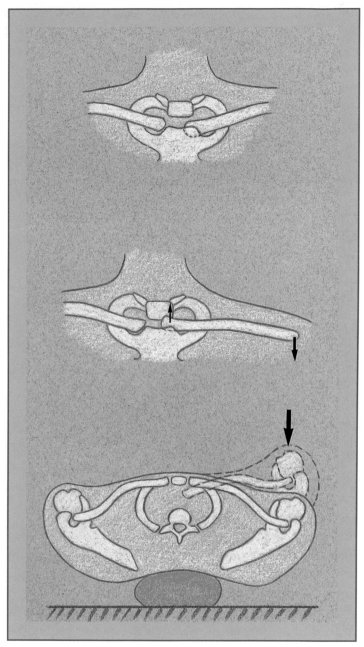

Figure 11.9 – *Manipulative reduction of retrosternal dislocation as described by Buckerfield and Castle (1984).*

Floating clavicle

Simultaneous sternoclavicular and acromioclavicular disruption may occur and this situation is commonly known as 'floating clavicle', or panclavicular dislocation. This is a rare injury and is usually, but not always, associated with severe trauma. Cases have been reported where treatment has been entirely conservative, with a satisfactory outcome, and others have remained symptomatic at one or both ends.

Beckman (1924) reviewed 15 cases of simultaneous sternoclavicular and acromioclavicular luxation, treated without surgery, and found that 10 obtained a good functional result. Sanders *et al.* (1990) suggested that the acromioclavicular injury should be treated as for an isolated injury, and the sternoclavicular joint disregarded even if it is unstable. They reported six cases, of whom four required acromioclavicular reconstruction because of persistent aching. Where the sternal end of the clavicle is retrosternal it should not be disregarded, but should be treated as a serious injury. Closed manipulation is unlikely to be successful and the use of a percutaneous towel clip, or open surgery, may be required.

Sudden swelling of the sternoclavicular joint without trauma

Diagnosis of the swollen sternoclavicular joint, presenting spontaneously in the middle-aged woman, is extremely taxing for the surgeon, and frustrating for the patient.

Osteoarthritis

Symptomatic degenerative arthritis is rare. This is probably due to the protective effect of the strong ligaments and limited movement at the joint. It is also due in part to the separation of the joint by the intra-articular disc. When significant degenerative arthritis does occur it is usually as a sequel to trauma and is unilateral. Otherwise, osteoarthritis is more common in men, and on the dominant side. Notwithstanding the rarity of a clinical problem, cadaver studies have shown that degenerative changes are common, usually commencing on the clavicular side of the joint.

Painful osteoarthritis may be associated with swelling of the joint, which will present anteriorly, due to the structures limiting posterior expansion, and may mimic anterior subluxation. Rest may help, as may anti-inflammatory drugs, but physiotherapy is of little value. Steroid injections may afford relief, at least in the short to medium term. For those where unacceptable symptoms persist, excision of the joint remains the most effective long-term treatment.

Infection

Both pyogenic and tuberculous infection may occur. This is usually unilateral. In pyogenic septic arthritis, the organism is usually *Staphylococcus aureus* or *Pseudomonas aeruginosa*, but a number of miscellaneous organisms have been reported. Pyogenic infection has been recorded, particularly in association with drug abuse. The joint will usually show the classical features of pyogenic infection, with pain a prominent feature. Destruction of the joint may occur with subsequent long-term symptoms (Fig. 11.10).

Tuberculous infection may be painless and patients may present with a long history which belies the actual diagnosis. With the rarity of the condition, and the insidious history, the possibility of tuberculosis may easily be overlooked. It should be suspected, especially in anyone with present or previous tuberculous disease (Yasuda *et al.*, 1995). Computerized tomography scanning or MR scanning may be supplemented with radio-isotope scanning to exclude the possibility of other bone or joint involvement. In addition to appropriate antibiotic therapy it is possible that the mass may need to be excised, including parts of the clavicle, sternum, and first rib. If there is bone as well as joint involvement, antibiotics should continue for 12 months.

Arthritides

Ankylosing spondylitis may affect the sternoclavicular joints and is usually symmetrical. There will usually be other features of the condition. Rheumatoid arthritis

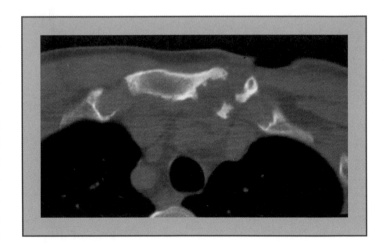

Figure 11.10 – *Destruction of the sternoclavicular joint following pyogenic infection.*

may affect the joint and will usually be associated with the involvement of other joints, and with raised sedimentation rate.

Idiopathic synovitis may occur with none of the features of a generalized arthropathy. This is usually unilateral. The sedimentation rate is normal, as are other blood tests. The joint is swollen and contains thickened synovium and granulation tissue. There may be destruction of articular disc and cartilage. The isolated swelling may give rise to the mistaken diagnosis of a subluxation. The condition rarely causes significant pain, nor disability, and biopsy is best avoided by confirmation of normal haematology and by MR scan if there is worry about other pathology.

Condensing osteitis

Osteitis condensans is an odd condition affecting the medial end of the clavicle. The condition is rare, but the differential diagnosis is malignant disease. It was first described by Brower *et al.* (1974) and is also known as aseptic enlarging osteosclerosis of the medial one-third of the clavicle (Fig. 11.11). Radiographs show enlargement of the medial end of the clavicle, associated with sclerosis, and varying obliteration of the medullary cavity, but no lysis. The sternoclavicular joint itself is

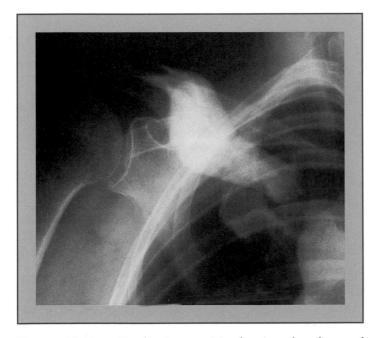

Figure 11.11 – *Condensing osteitis showing the abnormal fusiform swelling of the medial border of the clavicle.*

normal. Radio-isotope bone scans are generally abnormal. Computed tomography and MR scans show no abnormality of the surrounding soft-tissue planes.

The condition is commonest in women of late child-bearing age. Pain is usually modest and tenderness and palpable enlargement are generally only present in long-standing cases. There are no changes in the overlying soft tissues and there are no associated systemic symptoms. Movements at the sternoclavicular joint are not affected. Bilateral cases have not been reported. After some months or years, a firm fusiform swelling occurs adjacent to the sternoclavicular joint. Erythrocyte sedimentation rate may be mildly elevated, but biochemistry including alkaline phosphatase is normal. Culture from biopsy specimens shows no evidence of an infective aetiology. The aetiology of the disease is unclear. Histology shows an increase in thickness of normal trabeculae, and periosteal reaction may be present. It has been postulated that it is associated with repetitive mechanical stress at the sternoclavicular joint and simply represents a reaction to mechanical stress. Treatment with anti-inflammatory medication may be helpful. In refractory cases, excision of the medial end of the clavicle may be required.

As long as the clinical and radiographic features are typical, extensive investigation are probably unnecessary, as long as the condition is monitored (Kruger *et al.*, 1987). Where there is any doubt as to the nature of the condition biopsy should be undertaken.

Miscellaneous

A normal anatomical variation of the medial end of the clavicle may occur, in which there is thinning of the bone in the region of the rhomboid fossa. When this is well defined it may simulate a bone tumour (Treble, 1988).

Tietze's syndrome generally involves the medial ends of the ribs and the costal cartilages. The 2nd rib is that most commonly affected. There is painful, non-suppurative swelling of the costochondral junctions and there may be hypertrophy and excess calcification of the costal cartilages. Periosteal reaction of the medial end of the rib may occur, particularly on the superior aspect. Actual enlargement of the first rib can also occur, and rarely the sternoclavicular joint itself may be directly involved. This condition usually occurs in the 2nd–4th decades of life in both sexes.

Sternoclavicular hyperostosis is a rare condition in which there is symmetric enlargement of the medial clavicles, together with synostosis of the sternoclavicular joints (Fig. 11.12). The sternum itself may become widened and thickened. This is commonest amongst Japanese people in the age group 30–60 and there is a strong association with pustulosis plantaris (Chigira *et al.*, 1986). It has been suggested that there is a bacteroid aetiology with focal infection elsewhere causing both the pustulosis and the hyperostosis. Tonsillectomy is one of the more successful ways of treating this condition! Cases have also been reported in association with venous congestion of the upper part of the body, due to bilateral occlusion of the subclavian veins.

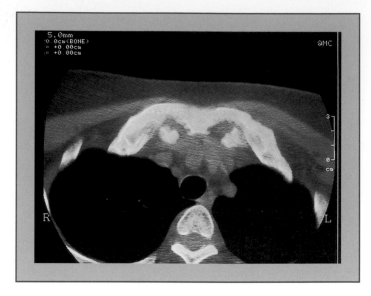

Figure 11.12 – *Sternoclavicular hyperostosis. Bony fusion can be seen between the manubrium and the clavicle and first rib.*

Summary

Swelling of the sternoclavicular joint is unusual, and as such can be highly alarming, both to the patient and the treating surgeon.

Posterior dislocation is very rare but can be life-threatening. Anterior dislocation is commoner and often recurrent.

There are a small number of quite bizarre conditions which lead to the insidious onset of marked swelling and pain in the middle-aged female. The diagnosis of these conditions is difficult, and often inconclusive, and they remain difficult to treat, and all too often impossible to cure.

CHAPTER 12

Management strategies for two- and three-part proximal humeral fractures

P. Schranz

Introduction

Fractures of the proximal humerus account for 5% of all fractures in the population as a whole. Seventy-five percent of these occur in patients over the age of 60 and they are three times more common in females (Lind *et al.*, 1989). In the elderly, in particular, they are the second most common fracture after proximal femoral fractures (Buhr & Cooke, 1959). Whereas there is a well-defined strategy for dealing with fractures of the proximal femur in the elderly, treatment for proximal humeral fractures tends to be made up 'on the spot'. The aim of this chapter is to help the surgeon to choose an appropriate management plan for his patients, based upon an understanding of the behaviour of different fracture types and also the limitations imposed by the elderly patient with osteoporotic bone.

The vast majority of proximal humeral fractures are undisplaced, or minimally displaced, and do not need surgical treatment. In order to plan sensible treatment for the smaller group of displaced fractures we need to define the type of fracture that we are dealing with, so we should spend a little time discussing classification.

Classification

The most widely used classification system for proximal humeral fractures is that proposed by Neer (1970b) who classified fractures according to the presence or absence of displacement of one or more of the four major fragments. Neer identifies a minimum displacement group, defined as displacement no greater than 1 cm or angulation no more than 45°. The displaced fractures are then classified according to the number of segments involved, and named according to the segment that is maximally displaced (Fig.12.1). Neer's classification became popular because it attempted to relate fracture classification to prognosis; a two-part fracture having a better prognosis than a three- or four-part fracture. However, a number of authors have reported difficulties with interobserver reliability using this classification. Sidor *et al.* (1993) reported on a series of 50 fractures of the proximal humerus using a trauma series of scapular anteroposterior, scapular lateral and axillary radiographs and five observers (four orthopaedic surgeons and one skeletal radiologist). This study revealed agreement between observers in only 30 % of the fractures.

In a similar study, Brien *et al.* (1995) used two radiologists and two orthopaedic surgeons to analyse a series of 28 fractures. The overall agreement between pairs of observers was 65%.

Some of the difficulties experienced by surgeons using the Neer classification stem from confusion with terminology. The classification attempts to provide a guide to prognosis by distinguishing between undisplaced and displaced fractures. The classification refers to the different *segments* of the proximal humerus (articular segment, greater tuberosity, lesser tuberosity, shaft). Fractures are then divided into *groups* based on the presence of displacement of a fracture segment. Regardless of the number of segments fractured, all undisplaced or minimally displaced fractures are

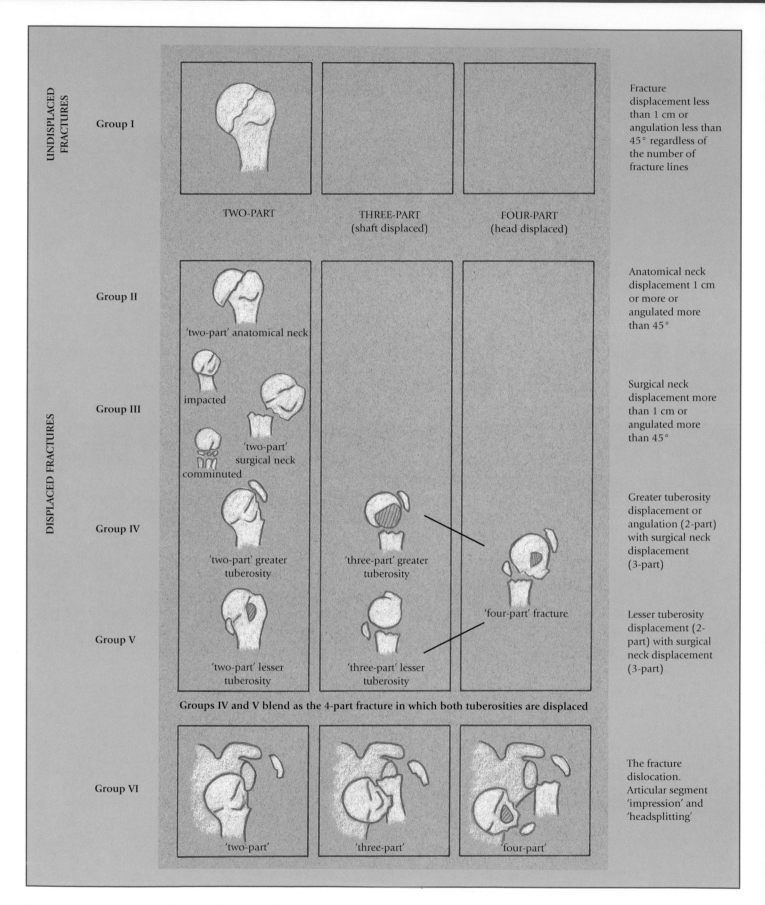

Figure 12.1 – *Neer's classification of proximal humeral fractures. (Reproduced with permission from Journal of Bone & Joint Surgery.)*

classified as Group I. In this group, no segment was displaced more than 1.0 cm or angulated more than 45°. The remaining groups are named according to the segment that is mainly involved in the displacement, with a final group encompassing fracturedislocations.

The main area of difficulty with reproducibility of this classification system has been determining the degree of displacement and angulation of individual fracture fragments. In a recent paper Bernstein *et al.* (1996) found that even when utilizing computerized tomography (CT) scanning it proved difficult to determine the number of segments fractured and the degree of displacement of these segments.

Despite these limitations the Neer classification remains in widespread use and provides us with a common language.

The AO Classification of fractures, whilst comprehensive, allowing fractures of the upper humerus to be classified into one of 27 patterns, suffers from similar problems with interobserver reliability. Siebenrock and Gerner (1993) used five shoulder surgeons to classify 95 fractures of the proximal humerus using the Neer and AO classification systems. Unanimous agreement only occurred in 26% using Neer's classification and 38% using the AO classification.

In order to classify the fracture, a trauma series of anteroposterior, lateral and axillary radiographs are essential. The shoulder is a particularly difficult area for our radiographers to image and it is up to the treating surgeon to insist on good quality views. A trip down to the X-ray department, while the trauma series is being performed, will help the surgeon to understand the difficulties faced by the radiographers. It is also a good opportunity to applaud good films when they emerge. If classification is difficult, despite good quality films, then the use of CT scanning will help to identify the number of fracture fragments, although determining the degree of displacement may still be a problem as discussed earlier.

Scoring

When comparing the results of different forms of treatment of displaced fractures of the proximal humerus, it is essential that we all speak the same language and all assess shoulder function in a similar way.

Neer's scoring system (1970) is weighted heavily towards pain and a functional range of movement such that any patient with significant pain, despite good restoration of anatomy and reasonable function, is graded a failure.

The University of California at Los Angeles (UCLA) Shoulder-Rating Scale again strongly emphasizes pain and function, with a maximum of 10 points for each category. It gives less importance to flexion range and strength (5 points maximum each) and patient satisfaction (5 maximum) giving a maximum possible score of 35 points.

Stableforth (1984) proposed a simplified assessment of results based on restoration of function as he felt that elderly patients made fairly simple demands on their shoulders.

The Hawkins Rating Scale (Hawkins *et al.*, 1986) scores the ability to perform 11 tasks and the average of the 11 scores is determined for an overall score. A score of 3.5 or greater is classified as good, 2.5–3.4 points as fair and < 2.5 points as poor.

The American Shoulder and Elbow Surgeons (ASES) rating system (Bigliani, 1991) assesses pain, range of motion, strength and stability. All criteria are weighted equally with a score from 0 to 5. In addition a detailed functional assessment is carried out evaluating the patient's ability to perform 15 functional tasks.

In the UK, the functional scoring system devised by Constant and Murley (1985) is widely used. This system combines a number of subjective and objective parameters and is weighted more heavily for range of motion than pain, activities of daily living, or power.

The reader must therefore be cautious in his interpretation of clinical results based on different scoring systems, as a case judged a failure by one scoring system may do better when scored using a different system.

The shoulder scoring systems discussed above are summarized in Table 12.1.

Table 12.1 Shoulder scoring systems.	
Neer	1970
UCLA	1970s
Stableforth	1984
Constant	1985
Hawkins	1986
American Shoulder and Elbow Surgeons	1991

Undisplaced fractures (Neer Type I)

Although this chapter will concentrate on displaced fractures, 85% of proximal humeral fractures are undisplaced, or minimally displaced, and do not require operative intervention. However, these patients should still receive the surgeon's attention in the fracture clinic as they will need guidance, reassurance and advice.

These fractures are usually stable and require short-term immobilization for comfort. Although collar 'n cuff immobilization under a shirt is often used, it can allow inferior subluxation and distraction at the fracture site so a commercially available shoulder sling such as Polysling (Seton) is preferable. The patient should be counselled that it is common to have night pain for the first 3 days due to haematoma, and reassured and encouraged to start gentle movements of the limb as soon as comfort permits — generally within the first 2 weeks. These fractures unite within 6–8 weeks, at which time formal physiotherapy may accelerate the return to normal function.

A number of series report good or excellent results in around 90% of cases after early functional treatment (Clifford, 1981; Mills & Horne, 1985; Young & Wallace, 1985; Kristiansen & Christensen, 1987). Clifford (1981) pointed out that the patients who were rested for longer in a sling required a more prolonged period of physiotherapy to regain a satisfactory result. These patients need to know the likely timescale of recovery and need to be encouraged not to lose heart as it may take as long as 6 months before the final range of movement and functional outcome is achieved.

Displaced two-part fractures

Two-part anatomical neck fractures (Neer Type II)

These fractures are rare and account for 0.8% of upper humeral fractures. (Szyszkowitz *et al.*, 1993). The concern with these fractures is the viability of the humeral head. The blood supply to the anterior two-thirds of the humeral head is from the arcuate artery — a branch of the anterior circumflex humeral artery. The posterior one-third is supplied by the posterior circumflex humeral artery, with perforators from the metaphyseal periosteum. The risk to the head is dependent on the degree of displacement of the head

and the amount of medial metaphysis on the proximal fragment. The larger this metaphyseal component, the greater is the likelihood of some retained blood supply from the posterior circumflex maintaining viability of the humeral head. If displacement is greater than 1 cm then hemiarthroplasty is likely to be the preferred option; in younger patients with good bone stock and minimal displacement, internal fixation using AO cancellous screws may be attempted. Even though the head is likely to have been rendered avascular, Hawkins (1993) suggests that blood supply transmitted through the undisturbed tuberosities may prevent avascular necrosis.

Two-part surgical neck fractures (Neer Type III)

In two-part fractures, the humeral shaft is displaced medially and anteriorly by the pull of pectoralis major, latissimus dorsi and teres major (Fig.12.2), Closed reduction of this fracture is usually achievable, but maintaining the reduction is more of a problem. In their small series, Young and Wallace (1985) found 100% incidence of re-displacement after manipulation alone.

Kristiansen and Christensen (1987) obtained good or excellent results using Neer's criteria in over 80% of cases using non-operative techniques. Whilst this may be the case, there is a worryingly high incidence of late displacement and so, unless there are compelling anaesthetic reasons for not proceeding further, some form of stabilization is usually required after closed reduction, though opinions vary as to the precise technique used.

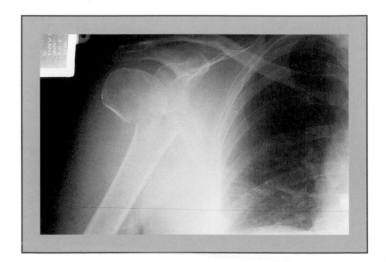

Figure 12.2 – *A displaced two-part fracture.*

Methods of fixation: two part fractures

There are many techniques and implants available and a range of fixation methods have been reported. This provides the surgeon with a number of options depending on the quality of the bone and soft tissue, the surgeon's assessment of the individual patient and the surgeon's comfort with what can be highly demanding technical exercises.

The young motorcyclist with good bone stock and multiple injuries is going to need a stable shoulder, rigidly fixed to allow the use of crutches. The elderly osteoporotic patient needs the minimum fracture stability necessary to allow some early functional movement, without compromising the fracture reduction.

Percutaneous techniques

Although theoretically these techniques have the advantage of causing minimal soft-tissue disruption and are said to be relatively quick to perform, many an experienced shoulder surgeon has struggled for hours attempting percutaneous wiring. There is ample potential for disastrous complications, particularly nerve injury, pin migration and infection.

It is essential with any closed technique to be able to image the upper humerus in two planes. Reduction and imaging techniques should be rehearsed before draping the patient to allow the necessary adjustments to be made. Supine or lateral positioning may be used according to personal preference. Remember that if you are using a radio-lucent arm board, the point of attachment of the arm board to the table is usually made of metal and invariably lies directly across the field of view.

K-wires

Kocialkowski and Wallace (1990) recommend obtaining reduction by traction with the humerus in maximum elevation. In their series two to four K-wires were inserted from the anterior humerus. Kocialkowski and Wallace reported a 41% incidence of K-wire migration. Their series also reported a 23% incidence of pin-track infection and early removal of the wires (4 weeks) was recommended.

Threaded pins

The use of threaded pins eliminates some of the problems of K-wire migration. Jaberg *et al.* (1992) described a technique using three threaded pins. In their series of 48 patients, reduction was obtained by a combination of longitudinal traction with the arm in 70° of abduction combined with posterior pressure on the humeral shaft. While this position is being maintained, a single anterior pin is inserted through the shaft into the centre of the humeral head, then two further pins are inserted from a lateral position entering above the deltoid insertion to avoid injury to the radial nerve. Beware of entering the deltoid too proximal though, as the axillary nerve is situated fairly close by. Seventy percent of patients in their series were assessed as good or excellent. By cutting the pins short, and allowing them to lie subcutaneously, the pin-track infection rate was kept down to 10%. The author's experience with this technique is limited. The greatest practical problem was getting the pins to enter the humeral shaft at an acute enough angle to end up centrally in the head (Fig.12.3). Jaberg suggests maintaining the humeral head slightly medial to the shaft to encourage central pin placement.

External fixation

Percutaneous external fixation allows greater stability of the fracture site and will therefore permit earlier mobilization.

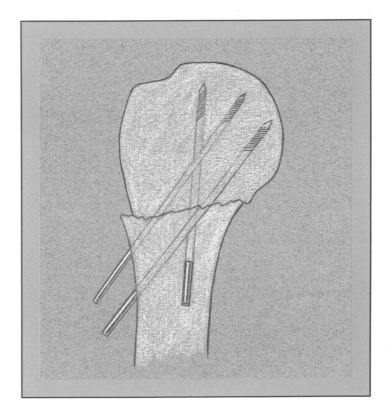

Figure 12.3 – *Threaded-pin fixation.*

Kristiansen (1989) describes the use of the Hoffman external fixator in a series of 28 fractures, the majority of which were two and three-part fractures. He reported 68% good or excellent results with five cases of pin-track infection and loosening (17%). The cases of loosening occurred in patients with severe osteoporosis and the technique is not recommended in such cases.

In view of the risk of axillary and radial nerve damage, it is safer to apply the fixator using an open technique, directly visualizing the bone rather than relying on a stab incision and crossed fingers. This really negates its advantages.

Open techniques

Rush pins

This technique has been available for over 50 years and remains popular. This intramedullary technique avoids the problems associated with fixation of fractures in osteoporotic bone. Weseley *et al.* (1977) report on a series of 16 fractures treated with Rush pins, from a total series of 700 proximal humeral fractures. Weseley recommends using the semiclosed technique described by Rush. This involves two incisions: one small incision over the greater tuberosity to allow entry of the Rush pin, and a second small incision in the deltopectoral groove to allow palpation and reduction of the fracture using the finger. Unfortunately, the paper does not report on functional results although in 10 cases the Rush pins were removed after union. It is preferable in all but the very frail, unfit patient, to plan elective removal of the Rush pins at around 12 weeks provided union has occurred.

Robinson and Christie (1993) described excellent or satisfactory results in 16 out of 23 patients (69%). They describe the use of two prebent pins inserted through the greater tuberosity and used a tension-band wire through the eye of the pin to prevent upward migration. The pins were removed at union, in a large majority of cases in their series, to relieve minor shoulder discomfort.

Zifko *et al.* (1991) describes the use of flexible intramedullary pins that incorporate curves at their proximal and distal ends. After reduction of the fracture, the pins are inserted in a retrograde fashion through a triceps-splitting incision. An 8 mm hole is made in the posterior distal cortex proximal to the edge of the olecranon fossa and three to five pins are inserted and tapped home. Unfortunately, the complication rate in this series was significantly high. In 31% of cases the fracture displaced within the first 2 weeks. Pin migration leading to humeral head perforation occurred in 25% of cases.

Mouradian device

Mouradian (1986) describes the use of a modified Zickel supracondylar rod, now known as a Mouradian nail. This device consists of a curved intramedullary rod that accepts two cancellous screws through the proximal end. It is inserted through a hole made in the greater tuberosity after reduction of the fracture. The proximal cancellous 'locking' screws are inserted after impaction of the fracture. The author recommends immobilization for 2 weeks (Fig. 12.4). In his series of 31 fractures, including two-, three- and four-part fractures, this device appeared to be most effective in treating two-part fractures, achieving a mean Neer score of 87, with no non-unions.

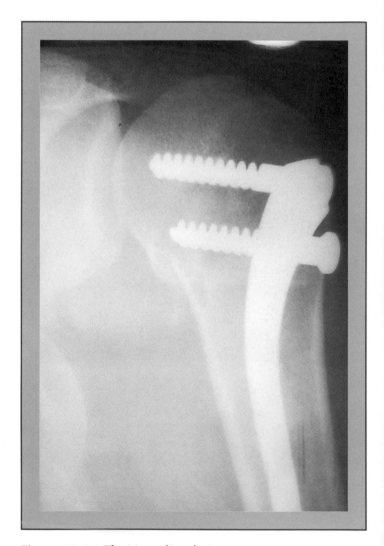

Figure 12.4 – *The Mouradian device.*

Tension-band techniques

The use of tension-band techniques in the proximal humerus allows stable fixation even in the presence of osteoporotic bone. Hawkins *et al.* (1986) describe the use of two tension-band wires inserted through the proximal fragment and tendinous part of the cuff. This really is a versatile technique and the reader is encouraged to study Hawkins' description of the technique in detail. In order to gain strong purchase on the osteoporotic bone, Hawkins recommends that the tension band passes through the tendon as well as the underlying bone, obtaining purchase on the cuff. Hawkins recommends the use of a 14 gauge colpotomy needle (Fig. 12.5). This author has found that a 14 gauge intravenous cannula with the plastic sheath removed, or alternatively a Toohey needle borrowed from the anaesthetic room, works equally well though it is important to choose wire that is able to pass easily through a 14 gauge hole. In addition, care should be taken to minimize the amount of kinking of the wire as it is otherwise difficult to pass this through the second hole in the humeral shaft.

Cornell *et al.* (1994) modified this technique by using a 6.5 mm AO cancellous screw to provide lag screw fixation. This is then supplemented by the use of two tension bands. They reported union in all cases within 12 weeks and 62% scoring good function on the Hawkins' scale.

AO plating

In younger patients, with adequate bone stock to allow screw purchase, rigid internal fixation using AO screws and plates will allow early return of a functional range of motion. However, if plates and screws are used in elderly osteoporotic bone the end result will be disastrous. The AO T-plate utilizes 6.5 mm cancellous screws in the humeral head. The plate is rigid, bulky and not easy to

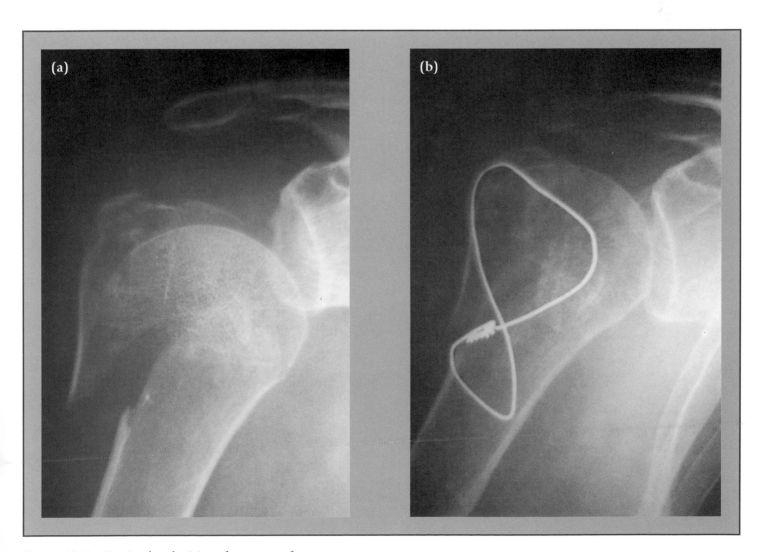

Figure 12.5 – *Tension-band wiring of a two-part fracture.*

mould. If accurate placement of the plate is not possible then the smaller cloverleaf plate modified by Esser (1994) is an ideal alternative. This plate is low-profile and can be sited lateral to the bicipital groove, not interfering with the blood supply to the head. It allows placement of multiple small-fragment screws in the head increasing the strength of proximal purchase, and the plate is easily contoured (Fig. 12.6).

Robinson and Christie (1993) reported a significant difference in results of plating similar two-part fractures when different age-groups were compared. Mean Neer scores of 89 were obtained in the under 50s group and a mean score of only 51 in the over 60s. This latter group had a high incidence of fixation-failure due to loosening of the screws in the humeral head.

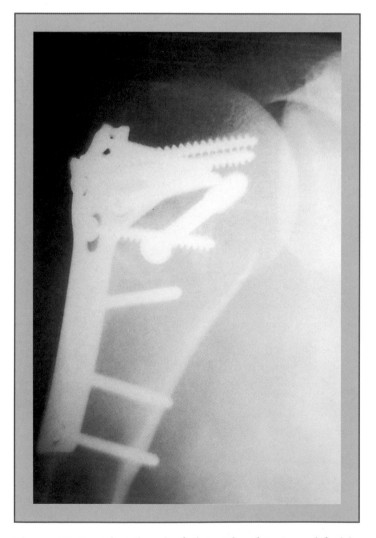

Figure 12.6 – *The Cloverleaf plate. The plate is modified by snipping off one wing and the superior flange to allow application without impingement on the biceps tendon or acromion.*

Syszkowitz *et al.* (1993) reported on a large series of 143 fractures treated by internal fixation, using AO principles. Their series consisted of 36% AO Group-A fractures, 33% Group-B fractures and 21% Group-C fractures. They reported 52% satisfactory results overall. Syszkowitz and his team concluded that AO-plate fixation is a demanding technique that requires a wide exposure and has a real danger of causing avascular necrosis of the humeral head, subacromial impingement and screw loosening. In view of these problems they recommend the use of the low-profile cloverleaf plate, or minimal internal-fixation techniques such as tension band wires.

The AO semi-tubular plate can be modified by flattening one end and bending it to a right-angle. This allows it to be used as a blade plate using tension band principles. A reconstruction plate works just as well (Fig. 12.7). This technique offers the advantages of rigid fixation gaining good proximal purchase without the problems sometimes associated with screws in the humeral head.

Two-part greater tuberosity fractures

Displaced fractures of the greater tuberosity are essentially avulsions of the rotator cuff. This results in a longitudinal tear between the supraspinatus and the subscapularis. Displacement of the fragment may be superior as well as posterior, depending upon which portion of the cuff remains attached to it. The greater tuberosity fragment usually retracts proximally beneath the acromion. Standard anteroposterior radiographs alone may underestimate the amount of displacement and should be supplemented by axillary views (Flatow *et al.*, 1991). The aims of surgery should be to restore the greater tuberosity fragment to its bed as well as to repair the tear in the rotator cuff. As there is no underlying disturbance to the blood supply of the head, provided the displaced fracture is reduced and fixed and the cuff tear repaired, the prognosis is excellent. In Flatow's series 100% excellent or acceptable results were achieved. Unreduced greater tuberosity fractures cause disability in abducting the arm, weakness in the cuff as well as the direct effect of impingement of the fragment beneath the acromion.

Displaced greater tuberosity fractures may occur in association with anterior dislocation. If the tuberosity fragment reduces, after reduction of the dislocation, then the fracture may be treated by immobilization. If, however, there is residual displacement of 1 cm in any plane then open reduction should be performed.

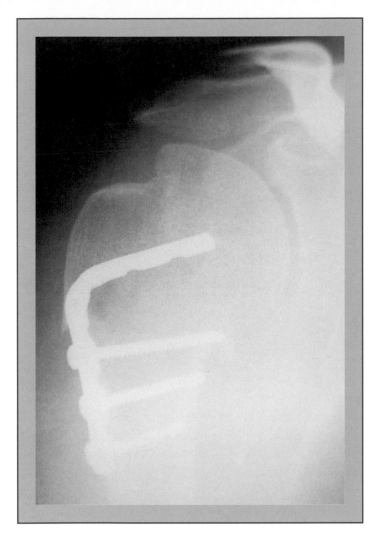

Figure 12.7 – *'L' plate fixation. In this case a reconstruction plate was used.*

Surgical technique

The greater tuberosity can be approached through a small deltoid-split incision, placed in the line of the transacromial approach, provided the split does not extend more than 4 cm distal to the acromion, to avoid damaging the axillary nerve. The retracted greater tuberosity fragment is retrieved from beneath the acromion and held with tissue forceps or stay-sutures. Great care should be taken when retrieving this fragment as the use of heavy grasping forceps may result in the tuberosity fragmenting. Occasionally, there is only a thin shell of bone attached to the supraspinatus and once it is brought into view it is safer to grasp the fragment with transosseus stay-sutures. There are a number of reported techniques for fixing the reduced fragment in place. Flatow *et al.* (1991) used non-absorbable sutures passed through the fragment and through the bony bed. In younger patients with good bone stock, large AO cancellous screws may be used. Care should be taken to site the screws such that they do not cause subacromial impingement on shoulder elevation. Alternatively, a tension-band wire may be used either through the greater tuberosity or through the cuff. This may be passed through a drill hole in the proximal shaft. In practice it is difficult to site this hole and pass the wire through, so the author recommends passing the tension band around a cortical screw inserted through the upper humerus, taking care to site the screw and wire away from the axillary nerve. The surgeon must ensure good bicortical purchase with his screw otherwise there is a real danger of the fixation loosening.

Displaced two-part lesser tuberosity fractures (Neer Type V)

This is the rarest group of fractures and may occur in isolation or in association with a posterior humeral head dislocation. Treatment is essentially reduction of the dislocation, which may result in reduction of the lesser tuberosity fragment. Any residual displacement of the lesser tuberosity does not appear to have significant functional implications (Neer 1984).

Displaced three-part fractures

Three-part humeral fractures involve a fracture of the surgical neck as well as an avulsion fracture of one of the tuberosities. These fractures are usually displaced and are highly unstable, due to the pull of the muscles on the intact tuberosity, causing internal rotation of the head in greater tuberosity detachment, and external rotation with abduction of the head in lesser tuberosity avulsions.

Conservative management

The results following conservative management of displaced three-part fractures are variable. Results vary from 47% satisfactory results (Rasmussen *et al.*, 1992), 52% good results (Leyshon, 1984) to 64% satisfactory results in Kristiansen and Christensen's series (1987).

Neer (1970(b)), in his classic work, painted a bleak picture of conservatively treated three-part fractures, with no patients scoring excellent or satisfactory results after conservative management. The inability to control the humeral head makes closed management of these fractures extremely difficult and this method should only be reserved for patients who are either medically unfit for surgery, or have very limited functional goals.

Surgical options

Before embarking on surgical treatment of these complex fractures the surgeon must be able to accurately define the fracture pattern. We have mentioned earlier the difficulties with some of the classification systems available. If the surgeon is unable to definitively classify the fracture on plain radiographs, then CT images should be obtained to allow proper preoperative planning. It is also important that the surgeon confirms that he has his full surgical armamentarium available before the case starts, as he may have to resort to one of several options, including the possibility of hemiarthroplasty, depending on how the case progresses.

Make sure that you have appropriately trained assistants and brief the operating-room staff on your plan of action and fixation options. It is essential that there is no undue pressure on the surgeon to rush this type of case. If you tell the whole team that the case is likely to take at least a couple of hours, then they can make sure that sufficient protected theatre time is available. Do not be tempted to tell them that you just plan to 'whizz a few wires in, it should not take long....'.

The blood supply to the humeral head fragment is likely to be at least partly jeopardized by this injury and care must be taken during any operative procedure to preserve whatever blood supply may be left. The *goals of surgery* should therefore be to use the minimum amount of intervention necessary to reduce the head into the glenoid and secure sound enough fixation to allow relatively early rehabilitation. Ensure that your exposure allows access to the injured area without undue tension applied to the soft tissues. Remember, minimal fixation does not necessarily mean minimum exposure (Table 12.2).

Results of surgical treatment

Percutaneous threaded-pin fixation

Jaberg *et al.*'s technique (1992) described earlier on in this chapter may also be used to treat three-part fractures, utilizing two further pins inserted in a retrograde direction through the greater tuberosity and into the medial cortex of the shaft. Jaberg recommends that these greater tuberosity pins should be removed 3 weeks after surgery. In Jaberg's series all eight patients with three-part fractures had excellent or good results.

Table 12.2 Methods of fixation.

Percutaneous techniques
    K-wiring
    Threaded pins
    External fixator
Open techniques
    Rush pins
    Mouradian device
    Tension-band wiring
    T-plate
    Cloverleaf plate
    L-plate

External fixation

Reduction of these unstable fractures using external fixation requires the use of temporary pins to obtain purchase of the humeral head and greater tuberosity. Once these two fragments are reduced onto the shaft the external fixator is applied. Kristiansen's series (1989) included 14 three-part fractures and he reports only 43% excellent or satisfactory results. This technique is difficult enough to master in two-part fractures. Unless the treating surgeon has experience and confidence in external fixation techniques, this method is *not recommended* as a first choice for three-part fractures.

Mouradian device

This device, described earlier, has been used to re-attach the two major fragments, i.e. the humeral head and shaft, together. The greater tuberosity is then reduced and held in place with non-absorbable sutures. In Mouradian's series of 10 three-part fractures, the average postoperative Neer score was 80, i.e. satisfactory, although there were two failures.

Tension-band wiring

This technique has the advantages of allowing rigid enough fixation to allow early mobilization without the impingement problems of screws and plates. Hawkins *et al.* (1986) technique, using two tension-band wires has been described earlier and is a useful technique to master.

In his series of 15 patients with three-part fractures, 8 patients (53%) scored 3.5 or greater on the Hawkins' functional scale. The results do not indicate individual

Neer scores; however, analysis of his data suggests that 12 out of 15 patients (80%) would have obtained satisfactory Neer scores. All fractures united and there were no failures of fixation. There were two cases of avascular necrosis.

Cornell (1994) described his modification of Hawkins' technique and used a 6.5 mm AO cancellous screw to secure the impacted humeral head to the shaft. He then recommended using two tension-band wires to stabilize the tuberosity fracture and give greater stability to the shaft fracture. In his small series, there were five three-part fractures with four out of five scoring 3.5 or greater, i.e. good on the Hawkins' functional scale.

Plates and screws

In the younger patient with good bone stock, absolute stability may be achieved using a T-plate, a small condylar plate or a modified cloverleaf plate. The need to achieve rigid fixation to allow early mobilization must be balanced by the real risk of potential damage to the already vulnerable blood supply to the humeral head in these three-part fractures. Specifically, the area of the bicipital groove should be avoided when plating these fractures in order to avoid damage to the arcuate artery as it leaves the anterior humeral circumflex artery.

Szyszkowitz *et al.* (1993) in their large series reported 52% satisfactory results after internal fixation. They concluded that plate fixation in proximal humeral fractures is a very demanding technique associated with multiple complications if performed without regard to specific osteosynthesis techniques. Complications of surgery include avascular necrosis, subacromial impingement, especially after using a T-plate, nerve lesions, and plate and screw loosening.

If it is possible to achieve sufficient stability with less invasive fixation techniques such as tension-band wiring then plate fixation may be avoided. There are, however, some situations where these previously discussed techniques may not be suitable. In cases of metaphyseal comminution, a bridging plate such as a T-plate may be useful. The T-plate is bulky, however, and may cause impingement on humeral elevation if not positioned low enough down on the greater tuberosity. It is also very rigid and if not contoured appropriately, fracture displacement may occur as the screws are tightened.

The cloverleaf plate has a number of advantages and is to be recommended in preference to a T-plate. The plate should be modified, as described by Esser (1994), by shearing off the superior and anterior arms of the plate, allowing the plate to be contoured along the proximal humerus and allowing multiple screw purchase in the humeral head. The plate is positioned laterally on the upper humerus and so avoids crossing the bicipital groove and does not threaten the arcuate artery. The plate is designed for the smaller 4.0 cancellous screws proximally and small-fragment 3.5 mm cortical screws on the shaft. The screws are less likely to cause problems with impingement than the larger 6.5 mm cancellous screws used with the AO T-plate. Esser reported good or excellent results in all 24 patients with three-part fractures in his series. The modified AO semitubular plate, described earlier in this chapter, may be used in three-part fractures. The flattened flange allows purchase of the humeral head without screws. It may be combined with the use of a tension-band wire to re-attach the greater tuberosity fragment (Schai *et al.*, 1995).

Hemiarthroplasty

Hemiarthroplasty is required in cases where there has been significant comminution or depression of humeral-head fragments. Its use in four-part fractures will be discussed in the following chapter. Neer (1970(b)) also advocated the use of his prosthesis in selected cases of displaced three-part proximal humeral fractures. It may have to be resorted to in the elderly if a tenuous repair is obtained after attempted internal fixation. The principles of the technique have been described earlier in this book and technical aspects of its use in trauma will be discussed further in the following chapter.

Hawkins and Kiefer (1987) stress the importance of tension-band wiring the tuberosities to the shaft and encourage the use of autogenous bone graft from the head, to aid union between the tuberosity and the shaft.

Fracture-dislocations

Dislocations may occur in association with two-, three- or four-part fractures of the proximal humerus. The majority of these are anterior dislocations. Treatment should be directed initially at the reduction of the dislocation by closed or open means. The pull of the attached muscles on the proximal fragment may make closed reduction less than straightforward and if there is any difficulty you should not hesitate to open the shoulder. Once the dislocation has been reduced, an assessment of the degree of stability should be carried out and if residual displacement of fragments occurs then operative treatment is required on similar lines to the options detailed in this chapter. Prognosis in these fracture-dislocations is related to the Neer grade, i.e. a two-part fracture-dislocation has a better prognosis than a three- or four-part fracture-dislocation (Fig. 12.8).

It is important to discourage overenthusiastic, early active rehabilitation of these fracture-dislocations, as fixation failure may lead to further instability at the joint.

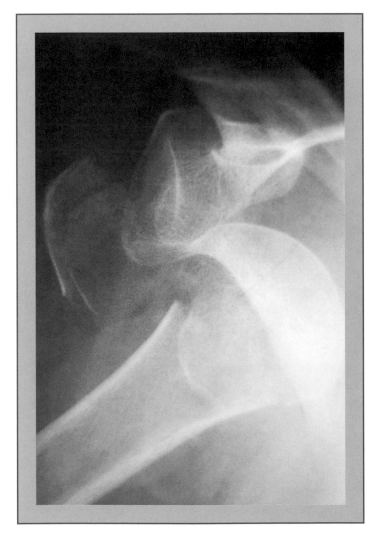

Figure 12.8 – *Fracture-dislocation.*

Complications

Avascular necrosis

The incidence of avascular necrosis of the humeral head varies with fracture type, from a negligible amount in the undisplaced Group-I fractures, to around 90% in displaced four-part fractures. The incidence in three-part fractures varies from 6% (Neer, 1970b) to 25% (Kristiansen & Christensen, 1987). Despite this it appears that avascular necrosis in the upper humerus does not inevitably lead to humeral head collapse and joint destruction. Lee and Hansen (1981) suggest that posttraumatic avascular necrosis in the upper humerus is followed by rapid revascularization by creeping substitution. They recommend that, wherever possible, the humeral head should not be discarded as it may be revascularized without collapse. This is discussed further in the next chapter. (Table 12.3)

Non-union

Non-union in proximal humeral fractures is relatively uncommon. The precise incidence is not known but there have been around 100 cases reported in the last 30 years (Jupiter and Mullaji, 1994). The majority of non-unions occur in displaced two-part fractures. Nayak *et al.* (1994) used modified Rush rods and tension-band wiring to supplement bone grafting, while Jupiter and Mullaji (1994) used a 90° blade plate. The author has used a modified cloverleaf plate with bone graft in this situation to good effect. The

Table 12.3 Complications.
Avascular necrosis
Non-union
Nerve injury

principles of treatment are preservation of soft-tissue attachments, rigid fixation of the fragments and cancellous bone grafting.

Nerve damage

The incidence of nerve damage in association with fractures or fracture dislocations of the upper humerus varies between 21% and 45% (De Laat *et al.*, 1994). De Laat's series was a prospective study of 101 patients who sustained either a primary shoulder dislocation (44) or a humeral neck fracture (57), the majority of these fractures being two-part surgical neck fractures. All fractures were treated conservatively by immobilization. Electromyograph testing was carried out on all patients with a clinical suspicion of nerve injury and the results showed axonal degeneration in 31 (54%) fractures. Axillary nerve involvement occurred in 37% of cases, the suprascapular nerve was involved in 29% of cases and the radial nerve in 22% of cases. The study revealed that clinical testing of sensation did not seem to have any diagnostic significance, as the presence of sensory loss was not associated with a higher incidence of motor lesions and many patients with normal sensation had motor lesions. The prognosis of these nerve lesions is generally good and in De Laat's series the majority of their cases recovered to MRC Grade 4 power in less than 4 months. However, the presence of an undiagnosed nerve lesion may account for some of the lack of progress of some of our patients and it is important to persevere with physiotherapy and encouragement while the nerve lesion recovers.

Summary

Proximal humeral fractures are common in the elderly population. Although the majority of upper humeral fractures are undisplaced and may be treated conservatively, there is still a great deal of uncertainty as to the best way of managing displaced two- and three-part fractures. A wide range of surgical treatment options are given in this chapter and no single technique is appropriate for all fractures. The surgeon needs to make an assessment of the patient, the type of fracture and the surgeon's level of expertise before embarking on a surgical approach to these fractures. Tension-banding techniques should be used in preference to rigid-plating techniques in all but the youngest of patients. The potential for disaster after operative intervention is particularly high even in the most experienced hands. Operative shoulder surgery in upper humeral fractures should therefore be a planned procedure rather than a rushed onslaught. If the fracture pattern suggests that the necessary expertise is not readily available then resist the temptation to dive in. At the end of the day, a malunited, conservatively treated fracture may be easier to salvage than an infected non-union after failed surgical treatment.

CHAPTER 13

The four-part fracture: rebuild or replace?

P. Schranz

Introduction

Four-part fractures of the proximal humerus are complex fractures to treat. Neer and others have demonstrated that displaced four-part fractures or fracture-dislocations have the worst prognosis of all proximal humeral fractures. The debate about treatment options for these fractures has gone on for over 20 years and continues to this day. To some, these fractures may appear impossible to treat and you may be tempted to do nothing in the hope that the patient will somehow sort out the problem for you. Unfortunately, trussing up your patient in a sling and prescribing analgesics and physiotherapy is not good enough. It has been tried on numerous occasions and the consensus found in the orthopaedic literature is that there is little place for conservative management in the treatment of these complex fractures. There is also a misconception that these fractures occur mainly in elderly patients with relatively low functional demands. In Neer's original series (1970(b)) his patients had an average age of 55 years and he made the point that the majority of these were in their most productive years. Neer (1970(b)) reported 100% failure in his series of 38 four-part fractures treated conservatively. Rasmussen (1992), Leyshon (1984) and Stableforth (1984) reported similarly disappointing results, with pain a persisting problem. Stableforth's series did identify a subgroup with impacted, minimally displaced four-part fractures that fared somewhat better.

So nature is not likely to solve our problems for us. We need to understand what makes four-part proximal humeral fractures such a problem in order to plan our treatment strategy.

The problem

The main problem is that we have a fracture with four fragments, one of which — the humeral head — is very likely to have become avascular. You will recall from the previous chapter that the main source of blood supply to the humeral head is the arcuate artery — a branch of the anterior circumflex humeral artery. In addition, blood supply reaches the humeral head along the medial periosteal route from the posterior circumflex humeral artery, as well as through the tuberosities, which in turn receive some supply through their attached muscles. The blood supply to the proximal humerus is shown in Figures 13.1a&b. All these sources of supply are destroyed in a displaced four-part fracture and Neer considered the results of head-conserving surgery to these fractures to be so poor (100% failure in his cases) that he advocated prosthetic hemiarthroplasty as the primary treatment of choice. This line of reasoning is sound and is the one we use every day in our management of displaced subcapital fractures of the hip in the elderly, although, even in the hip, less radical surgery is routinely practiced on the continent of Europe.

Some would argue that there is no debate, we should just carry out primary hemiarthroplasty on all these fractures. After all, the literature would to an extent support this rationale. There is no doubt that Neer's results following hemiarthroplasty are excellent with only one complication — an infection in 32 cases. Even Neer, however, states that 'the typical result was satisfactory but imperfect and the recovery period was prolonged'.

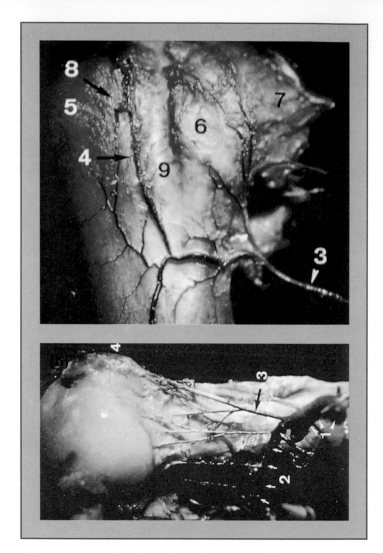

Figure 13.1 – *Blood supply to the proximal humerus (Gerber, 1990). (a) Anterior aspect of the humeral head. Anterior circumflex humeral artery [3], anterolateral branch of anterior circumflex artery [4], greater tuberosity [5], site of entry of anterolateral branch into bone, continuing as the intra-osseus arcuate artery [8]. (b) Anteromedial aspect of the humerus. Axillary artery [1], posterior circumflex humeral artery [2], anterior circumflex [3], insertion of subscapularis [4]. (Reproduced with permission from J Bone Joint Surg).*

Schai *et al.*'s multicentre analysis (1995) of displaced four-part fractures concluded that the results of humeral head-preserving surgery were significantly worse than the results following primary prosthetic replacement. Schai *et al.* observed total humeral head necrosis in 10 out of 13 cases where humeral head-conserving surgery was performed. In Schai's series, those patients with primary prosthetic replacement achieved higher Constant scores than cases treated non-operatively or by internal fixation. In addition, he reported that cases which subsequently

underwent prosthetic replacement, following initial osteosynthesis, had slightly lower functional scores than patients undergoing primary prosthetic replacement.

Is there ever a case for internal fixation?

There is little doubt that prosthetic hemiarthroplasty has been the mainstay of treatment for these displaced fractures. Neer's figures are excellent, with in excess of 90% good or excellent results. These results have not been matched by any other series and figures of 60–80% are more usual. However, although the results of hemiarthroplasty have been gratifying in terms of relieving pain, the final functional results have not been uniformly acceptable. It is therefore appropriate that we examine other operative treatment options. Can we afford to preserve the humeral head? Neer did not seem to think so. He reported uniformly poor results with internal fixation. The reported reasons for failure in his series were collapse or resorption of the humeral head in 50% of his cases and the head was discarded during surgery in the remaining 50%.

Should we routinely discard the humeral head in these cases, writing it off as avascular? This would be logical if the humeral head behaved like the femoral head in a displaced subcapital fracture. There is no doubt that the humeral head is, or does become, avascular in the majority of these fractures. Does this inevitably mean that the humeral head is non-viable?

Lee and Hansen (1981) suggest that, although avascular necrosis does occur in these fractures, the humeral head is quickly revascularized by creeping substitution, which prevents humeral head collapse, unlike in the femoral head. Kofoed (1983), however, suggested that after a four-part fracture-dislocation the humeral head did not totally revascularize for 9 months. Taking Lee and Hansen's suggestion into account it is possible that Neer's figures for operative treatment of four-part fractures may have improved had he not discarded the humeral heads at the time of surgery. Schai *et al.*'s study reported that cases where partial necrosis of the humeral head occurred had functional scores that did not differ significantly from cases with normal radiological appearance of the humeral head.

So, although total necrosis of the humeral head is likely to lead to significant symptoms, if we are able to encourage even part of the humeral head to preserve its blood supply, the end result may be less disappointing.

If we study the attempts of a number of surgeons to conserve the humeral head in displaced four-part fractures the results are variable although encouraging. Rigid internal fixation using AO T-plates has proved to be unsatisfactory. Rigid internal fixation using plates and screws almost inevitably results in avascular necrosis, although this may not necessarily result in humeral head collapse as discussed earlier.

Sturzenegger *et al.* (1982) reported the results of treatment of 27 multifragment fractures by open reduction and internal fixation. His series reported 60% good or excellent results following internal fixation and he emphasized the use of minimal internal-fixation techniques. His incidence of avascular necrosis was 22% overall, with a lower incidence of 10% in cases treated with minimal internal fixation using tension-banding techniques. Szyszkowitz *et al.* (1990) reported a higher failure rate of 60% in four-part fractures, using AO plates and screws in the majority of his cases; although in his paper he reports a total of 20% excellent results after internal fixation and uses this as an argument for not proceeding directly with hemiarthroplasty.

Less invasive techniques of fixation seem to produce somewhat better results. Darder *et al.* (1993) have recently described their results of open reduction and internal fixation of 35 patients with displaced four-part fractures, using tension-band techniques. Darder reported 64% excellent or satisfactory results using Neer's criteria. Significantly, there was no case of loss of reduction in this series and an incidence of avascular necrosis of 27% after a mean follow-up of 7 years. Of these, the majority were in cases of fracture-dislocation and only 2 cases progressed to humeral head collapse. The technique adopted involved a fairly large exposure, but minimal metalwork. Through an extended deltopectoral incision, the fracture was exposed by opening the clavipectoral fascia, using the long head of the biceps as the key landmark to aid reduction. Once the humeral head was elevated and the tuberosities were reduced, fixation was carried out using two intramedullary modified K-wires and tension-band wiring. The 3 mm K-wires were modified with a flattened proximal end which had a hole in it to accommodate a wire. A shorter K-wire was inserted through the lesser tuberosity into the shaft — a longer K-wire was inserted through the greater tuberosity. The wires were inserted such that they crossed within the medullary canal. A tension-band wire was then inserted through the holes and through drill-holes in the humeral shaft 5 cm distal to the fracture. When tightened, this construct appeared stable enough to allow early passive-mobilization exercises at 48 hours, with graduated exercises at 14–21 days.

The Mouradian device, described in the previous chapter, has been used successfully in the treatment of four-part fractures. Mouradian (1986) reported an average Neer score of 81 in his series of seven patients treated with his device. He does admit to having selected younger healthy patients (average age 46) whom he judged to be reliable. He recommends hemiarthroplasty in patients over 60 years of age.

The four-part valgus impacted fracture

Jakob *et al.* (1991) described a variant of the displaced four-part fracture that was associated with a lower incidence of avascular necrosis (Fig. 13.2). In this fracture type, classified as C2.2 and C2.1 using the AO Classification, the humeral-head fragment impacts into valgus and, provided there has been no lateral or posterior displacement, Jakob suggests that there may be sufficient soft-tissue attachments to the humeral head to prevent avascular necrosis. This is borne out by the relatively low incidence of avascular necrosis of 26% in his series of 19 valgus four-part fractures treated operatively. Remember that in the upper humerus, avascular necrosis does not necessarily equate with failure and collapse. Though once collapse has occurred, the inevitable sequelae follow (Fig.13.3).

Jakob advocates the use of minimal internal-fixation techniques once reduction has been achieved using closed or open techniques. In the majority of cases in his series, open reduction was performed through a deltoid-split incision and the valgus head was elevated into the reduced position, using a bone punch or laminar spreaders. Kirschner wires or screws were used to maintain the reduction and the tuberosities were then reduced and fixed with screws or wires. Jakob reported 74% good results using this technique.

Resch *et al.* (1995) reported on their series of 22 patients with valgus impacted four-part fractures. Resch excluded any patients with any lateral displacement of the humeral head and advocated a careful elevation and

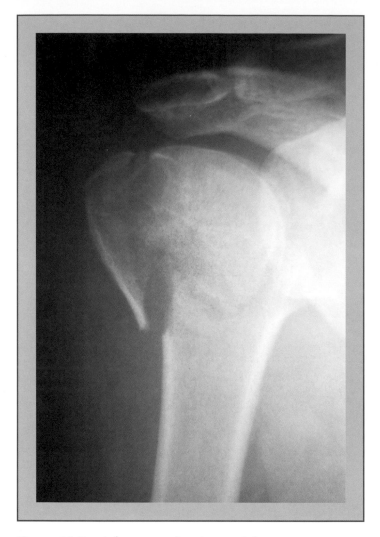

Figure 13.2 – *A four-part valgus impacted fracture.*

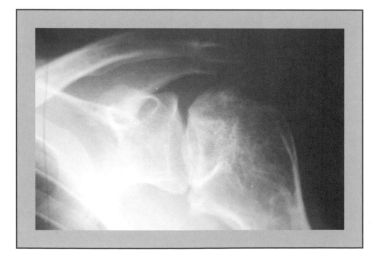

Figure 13.3 – *Avascular necrosis with humeral head collapse.*

reduction of the impacted humeral head. Resch used percutaneous K-wires to maintain the head reduced, and augmented this with autologous cancellous bone graft to fill the defect. The tuberosities were then reduced and fixed to each other and to the shaft, using multiple transosseous sutures. His cases were immobilized in an abduction plaster cast for 10 days prior to commencing an exercise programme. Resch recommended removal of the K-wires at 6 weeks. Resch's results, admittedly in a group of relatively younger patients (mean age 50), revealed an avascular necrosis rate of only 9%. Resch reported an average loss of 32° of abduction when compared to the contralateral joint, with an average loss of 26° flexion and 18° external rotation. The average functional score compared with the contralateral side was 84%.

In both these series, the authors emphasize that there must be no lateral or posterior displacement of the humeral head as this would increase the risk of avascular necrosis.

Esser's (1994) technique of using a modified cloverleaf plate has produced surprisingly good results in these difficult fractures. This technique relies on early operative fixation, most patients in this series were operated upon within 3–8 hours of their initial injury. Esser stressed limited exposure and careful soft-tissue dissection as well as accurate contouring of the cloverleaf plate (Fig. 13.4). In his series, Esser achieved an excellent result in his eight cases of four-part fracture, with fair results in his two cases of four-part fracture-dislocation.

There does therefore appear to be some justification for preserving the humeral head in selected patients with four-part proximal humeral fractures. It is important to look specifically for the valgus impacted fracture, as illustrated above. In the younger patient, an attempt should be made to preserve the head using minimal internal-fixation techniques, as in over two-thirds of cases the results are likely to be satisfactory.

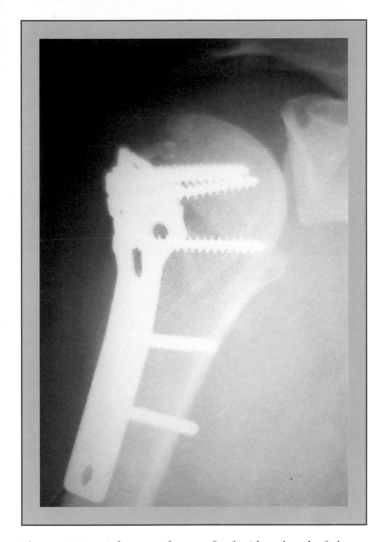

Figure 13.4 – *A four-part fracture fixed with a cloverleaf plate.*

Hemiarthroplasty

Despite the techniques described above there will be occasions when it will prove impossible to preserve the humeral head. Primary arthroplasty is mandatory in head-splitting fractures or depressed fractures of the humeral head. Arthroplasty is also indicated in the elderly osteoporotic patient with poor bone stock. Hemiarthroplasty will also be required, as a salvage procedure, in cases where humeral head-conserving surgery has failed.

There is no doubt that hemiarthroplasty provides gratifying pain-relief in the majority of patients. Tanner and Cofield's paper (1983) revealed satisfactory pain relief in all 16 acute cases and in 90% of chronic cases,

this latter group was essentially a group with persisting symptoms following malunion of four-part fractures and fracture-dislocations. Functional analysis revealed that all patients were able to perform most tasks associated with the activities of daily living, although 25% were unable to use the arm at shoulder level.

These figures contrast with a rather depressing account of the results of prosthetic replacement by Kraulis and Hunter (1977) who report 9 failures out of 11 cases and concluded that 'It appears that prosthetic replacement of the humeral head does not offer the patient any advantage when compared with other reported methods.' This may have been a somewhat pessimistic conclusion, especially considering the small series studied, but may reflect what may be encountered in district general hospitals where cases requiring hemiarthroplasty occur relatively infrequently.

Stableforth (1984) is more encouraging. In this prospective study 11 out of 16 cases (69%) were pain-free after hemiarthroplasty, with 14 out of 16 cases (88%) independent for activities of daily living at 6 months. Stableforth emphasizes the importance of physiotherapy, sometimes continuing for several months, and stresses that as improvement may continue for 12–18 months, the patients' mental alertness and determination to improve may be of more importance than the individual's age.

Goldman *et al.*'s series (1995) of 26 patients reported good pain relief in 73% of cases. However, a similar percentage of patients also reported difficulty with some functional tasks, such as lifting and using the arm at shoulder level.

Range of motion after hemiarthroplasty is less predictable and often a little disappointing. In Goldman *et al.*'s series, range of forward elevation averaged 107°. Rietveld *et al.* (1988) analysed the effect of range of motion on the final clinical result. His team studied 14 patients with hemiarthroplasty for four-part fractures using Neer scoring, videofluoroscopy and electromyograph recordings during abduction. Rietveld showed a direct relationship between range of motion and the clinical result, with 10 patients scoring satisfactory or better and 4 failures, with an average Neer score of 76. All patients were independent for eating and toilet hygiene, but only 50% were able to use the arm in an overhead position or comb their hair.

In addition, Rietveld showed a relationship between the 'humeral offset' and the clinical result. The humeral offset is the horizontal distance between the geometric centre of the humeral head and the lateral edge of the greater tuberosity. This humeral offset affects the efficiency of the lever arm of the supraspinatus and the deltoid, especially in the 30–60° arc of motion. Those cases with excellent results had a humeral offset that approached normal. As the humeral offset diminished, the action of the supraspinatus was altered to produce a compressive force at the glenohumeral joint while the deltoid produced upward migration of the humeral head with a resultant loss of glenohumeral abduction. This may in part explain why the results of hemiarthroplasty for osteoarthritis are better than for trauma as in the former there is little bone loss and the normal humeral offset is more easily maintained (Fig. 13.5).

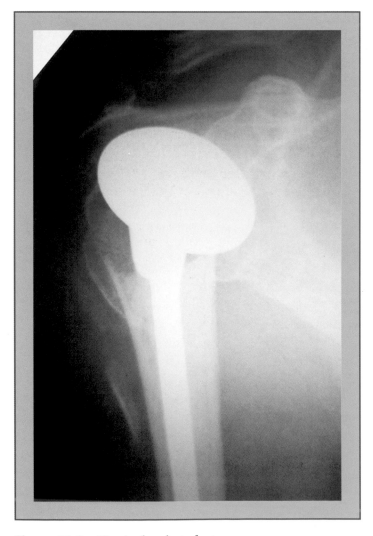

Figure 13.5 – *Hemiarthroplasty for trauma.*

How do we improve the results of hemiarthroplasty for trauma?

We have already discussed the importance of restoring a normal humeral offset at the time of surgery in order to maximize the efficiency of the supraspinatus and deltoid. Compito *et al.* (1994) examined the factors associated with success and failure of arthroplasty in acute trauma. In their paper, based on the results of nine series of four-part fractures treated by primary hemiarthroplasty, 80% of cases achieved satisfactory or better results. A significant number of patients in these series had problems with pain, stiffness and functional disability.

Compito's series identified a number of factors that were pivotal in determining success or failure after hemiarthroplasty.

Factors adversely affecting outcome after hemiathroplasty are summarized in Table 13.1.

Preoperative factors affecting outcome

Associated injury to the brachial plexus or peripheral nerves occurs in between 6% and 27% of patients with 4-part fractures. The majority of these closed injuries will resolve and may be treated expectantly. However, nerve lesions do diminish the patient's ability to cooperate with rehabilitation programmes. This may compromise what may otherwise have been a technically satisfactory result.

Perioperative factors

Failure of fixation of the greater tuberosity will lead to a poor result with impingement, weakness of elevation and pain. This was the single greatest cause of failure in

Table 13.1 Factors adversely affecting outcome after hemiarthroplasty.

Pre-operative	Nerve or brachial plexus injury
Perioperative	Inadequate fixation of greater tuberosity
	Incorrect soft-tissue tension
	Insufficient humeral offset
	Incorrect version of prosthesis
Postoperative	Uncooperative patient
	Inadequate/inappropriate rehabilitation
	Pericapsular calcification
	Unrepaired cuff tear

Compito's series. Hawkins and Switlyk (1991) stress the importance of using bone graft from the humeral head to encourage union. Although the Neer II prosthesis has holes within the proximal flange, Hawkins counsels against using wire through the flange as there is a tendency for the wire to break at this point. He recommends attaching the tuberosities directly to the shaft, and to each other, using No 2 non-absorbable suture or wire and supplementing this with cancellous bone graft from the humeral head.

The use of uncemented prostheses has been associated with a high incidence of loosening (Hawkins & Switlyk, 1991; Compito *et al.*, 1994). Routine cementing of the prosthesis is now recommended. This also allows accurate determination of the humeral offset and the correct soft-tissue tension without the risk of pistoning of the prosthesis.

Postoperative factors

One factor that consistently affects the final outome after hemiarthroplasty is the extent of the patient's cooperation with the rehabilitation programme (Hawkins & Switlyk, 1991; Compito *et al.*, 1994). Patients who are unable, or unwilling, to play a full part in their rehabilitation are likely to end up with a stiff, useless and probably painful shoulder after surgery. Some might suggest that these patients may possibly do better treated non-operatively, although in addition to loss of function these patients are likely to end up with some pain and it may be better to accept limited goals and carry out a hemiarthroplasty purely as a pain relieving operation. Careful patient selection is ideal, although admittedly it is sometimes difficult to predict patient's compliance with a future rehabilitation programme at the time of the initial consultation.

Pericapsular calcification may occur in between 14% (Neer, 1970(b)) and 36% (Kraulis & Hunter, 1977) of patients. This complication is seen more often if surgery has been delayed, especially beyond 10 days, and its onset may limit the final range of movement and therefore the final functional result.

Associated cuff tears will naturally compromise the clinical result. These should be recognized and repaired at the time of surgery, but these are more commonly encountered in Group-IV fractures involving the greater tuberosity alone.

Surgical technique

The technique of hemiarthroplasty has been described in chapter nine but a number of areas should be emphasized, with particular reference to the trauma situation.

The approach

These operations are difficult enough without us making things more difficult for ourselves with inadequate surgical exposures. The use of an extended deltopectoral approach is to be encouraged. Further access may be obtained by releasing the deltoid *distally* and tenotomizing the pectoralis major. A wide approach is necessary to allow gentle manipulation of soft tissues and reduce the risk of further damage, especially when trying to retrieve a dislocated humeral head from the depths of the axilla.

In these cases it may be safer to carry out a coracoid osteotomy after predrilling to allow exposure and preservation of the brachial plexus.

The key to the dissection is the long head of the biceps. First identify it distally in relatively normal territory, then trace it proximally. It will lead to the lesser tuberosity medially and the greater tuberosity laterally. The humeral head may not be visible and will be found on a deeper plane. It should be removed carefully, but not discarded as it provides a useful source of bone graft. Heavy non-absorbable sutures should be placed around the tuberosities at the tendon–bone junction.

The humeral shaft can be delivered through the wound by extension of the arm and should be handled gently to avoid a humeral-shaft fracture.

Unlike in prosthetic replacement for arthritis, precise neck section using cutting jigs is not possible. The surgeon is faced with a ragged delivered proximal-humeral shaft and strives to recreate some semblance of normality. The prosthesis should be placed in 30° of retroversion, using the transepicondylar plane at the elbow as a reference. The fin of the prosthesis will come to lie just posterior to the bicipital groove in this position. In cases of fracture dislocation, the humeral version should be adjusted by 5–10° away from the direction of the dislocation, i.e. anteverted in posterior dislocation and retroverted in anterior dislocation. The prosthesis should be inserted to maintain the humeral offset, as discussed earlier, and should not be inserted too far down the shaft. There should be enough room distal to the head of the prosthesis to allow the tuberosities to be placed below the level of the head. If this is not done, there will be impingement on abduction. It is a little difficult to check the soft-tissue balance with two freely mobile tuberosities. It is useful to gauge the amount of tension required to reduce the tuberosities beneath the prosthesis, as if this is excessive the joint will be 'overstuffed' and the repair may fall apart on adducting the arm, or at the very least the final range of motion will be disappointing.

It is advisable to pass multiple non-absorbable sutures or wires through predrilled holes in the humerus prior to cementing. Once a trial reduction has been carried out and the appropriate depth of insertion of the prosthesis estimated, the shaft may be prepared for cementing. Distal plugging, drying of the canal and pressurization of the cement are desirable and are carried out as described in the chapter on shoulder replacement. The tuberosities may then be secured to the shaft, and to each other, with bone graft from the head to aid union. The rotator interval should be closed and an assessment of the stability of the tuberosity repair should be made. This will dictate the pace and limits of postoperative rehabilitation. If there is concern about the strength of the repair, the arm may be supported in a position of slight elevation and forward flexion.

Rehabilitation

The results of joint arthroplasty are dictated by the success of the rehabilitation programme. We have seen how a poor range of motion is associated with a poor functional result. The rehabilitation programme should allow early return of range of motion within the limits dictated by the surgeon. These limits can only be determined by the surgeon at the time of the operation. The rehabilitation programme is therefore, to some extent, individualized for each patient. The early phase, commencing on the first postoperative day, aims to restore passive range of motion both in abduction, forward flexion and external rotation. The surgeon should demonstrate to the patient and the physiotherapist that he is confident enough with the stability of his fixation to passively elevate the arm to 90°. Once the patient can see that it is achievable by the surgeon, he will not resist the efforts of the physiotherapist to achieve the same range. Once the tuberosities have united, usually within 6–8 weeks, active assisted elevation using pulleys may start. At 3 months stretching exercises for the cuff are introduced

together with isometric cuff exercises. Provided the patient has regained near normal motion at the glenohumeral joint and the integrity of the tuberosity repair is confirmed, strengthening exercises may begin. Stretching exercises remain a feature of late rehabilitation and should continue for up to 12 months after surgery to regain as much motion as possible.

The programme will fail and a good result will be jeopardized if the patient does not cooperate, from the outset, with this long and demanding rehabilitation programme. It is vital therefore that, from the outset, the patient should understand that they are in for a good few months of very hard work if they wish a shoulder with excellent function rather than a shoulder that is simply 'all right'.

Complications

The majority of complications related to the operative treatment of displaced four-part fractures of the humerus are predictable and preventable. Remember the *Six Ps (Prior Planning and Preparation Prevents Poor Performance!)*

Overenthusiastic attempts at closed reduction of these fractures may cause nerve injury or fracture comminution. Poor patient selection may result in prolonged attempts at rigidly fixing osteoporotic bone with predictably disastrous results.

In Compito *et al.*'s series, multiple causes of failure occurred in 83% of cases but the most common cause of failure in her series was detachment of the greater tuberosity.

Prosthesis loosening should no longer be a problem now that routine cementing of the prosthesis is accepted.

Malposition of the prosthesis, commonly inadequate restoration of height with inadequate reduction of the tuberosities, leads to weakness and impingement. Problems with incorrect version of the prosthesis need to be anticipated at the time of cementing and a trial reduction at the time of surgery is advisable.

The incidence of ectopic bone formation is related to the delay between injury and surgery, so adequate time needs to be made available on trauma lists or shoulder lists for these fractures to be dealt with expeditiously.

Finally, even the best operation is only as good as the rehabilitation programme that follows it.

Summary

Four-part fractures of the proximal humerus are a serious problem for the patient and the surgeon. We have seen how, in selected cases, it is possible to preserve the humeral head, particularly in the younger patient with good bone stock and in the case of the valgus impacted four-part fracture.

We have discussed prosthetic replacement and its role in relieving pain. We have discussed the factors that may prejudice a good result after arthroplasty and have outlined some guidelines to minimize technical errors. This type of surgery is demanding and there is a definite learning curve. It is useful if cases requiring arthroplasty are referred to colleagues who have expressed a particular interest in the shoulder and shoulder trauma.

CHAPTER 14

Fractures of the clavicle: neglected or abused?

P. Schranz

Introduction

The clavicle provides the only bony connection between the upper limb and the thorax through its articulations at the sternoclavicular and acromioclavicular joints as well as through the costoclavicular and sternoclavicular ligaments. The clavicle acts as a strut, holding the scapula and upper limb away from the thorax, especially in abduction. This allows the glenohumeral joint to be orientated in a plane that facilitates the positioning of the hand in space. The clavicle is mobile in three planes and allows transmission of force along its shaft (compressive), around its longitudinal axis (rotational) and translational movements, the clavicle pivoting around the costoclavicular ligament. It is not surprising, therefore, that the clavicle is vulnerable to injury either at the articulations or along its length. Nordqvist and Petersson (1994) reported the incidence of clavicular fractures as 4% of all fractures. In their study of the Malmo population, the incidence was reported as 64/100 000 and the incidence is rising.

Classification

Allman (1967) classified clavicular fractures, according to their location, into mid-shaft fractures (Group 1), lateral-end fractures (Group 2) and medial fractures (Group 3).

Allman Group 1 fractures are the most common. In Nordqvist's series this group comprised 76% of all clavicular fractures. Allman subdivides this group into Group 1A — undisplaced midshaft fractures — the majority occurring in children, and Group 1B displaced midshaft fractures, occurring in adolescents and young adults. Comminuted midshaft fractures (Group 1C) occur most frequently in young adult males and are associated with high-energy injuries.

Group 2 fractures involve the lateral end of the clavicle and comprised 21% of Nordqvist's series. Allman (1967) subdivided this group into Type A — undisplaced fractures and Type B — displaced fractures.

Neer (1984) describes three subgroups of lateral clavicle fracture (Fig. 14. 1). The Type-I fracture occurs lateral to the coracoclavicular ligament. It is a stable fracture and is usually undisplaced, or minimally displaced, as the clavicular shaft is still tethered down by the intact ligament. The Type-II fracture is unstable. The fracture occurs through a slightly more medial plane than does the Type-I fracture and the underlying coracoclavicular ligament is ruptured, allowing the medial fragment to displace superiorly (Fig. 14.2). The Neer Type-III fracture is an intra-articular fracture of the lateral clavicle within the acromioclavicular joint.

Allman's Group-3 fractures, involving the medial end of the clavicle are relatively uncommon, comprising 3% of clavicular fractures in Nordqvist's series. These fractures occured predominantly in elderly men.

The AO alphanumeric classification of fractures designates the clavicle as **91.2-** followed by the subgroups **A,B,C** denoting extent of comminution and hence energy level.

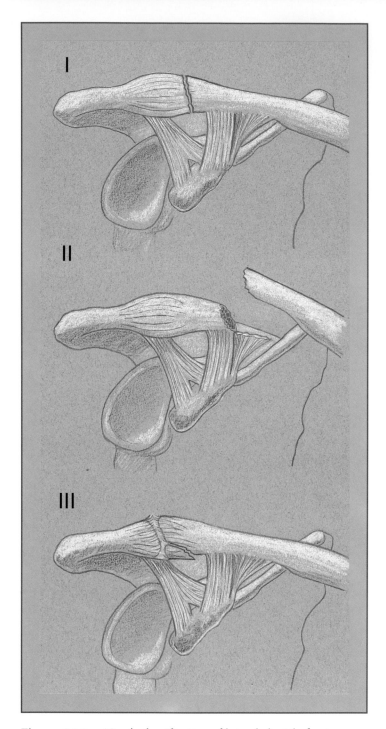

Figure 14.1 – *Neer's classification of lateral clavicle fractures.*

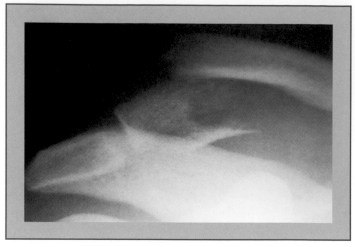

Figure 14.2 – *Neer Type II lateral clavicle fracture.*

Mechanism of injury

Clavicle fractures occur as a result of a fall on to the point of the shoulder (Post, 1988; Stanley *et al.*, 1988). It is tempting, as Allman did in 1967, to suggest that each fracture type results from a different mechanism of injury. Neer (1984) suggested that fractures of the lateral clavicle may be due to a blow to the top of the shoulder. There is a misconception that a fall on to the outstretched hand is a common cause of a fractured clavicle. Stanley *et al.*, (1988) analysed the mechanism of injury in a series of 150 consecutive patients presenting with a fractured clavicle and found that 87% of patients had fallen on to the shoulder, 7% had sustained a direct blow on the point of the shoulder and only 6% had fallen on to the outstretched hand. In an analysis of the forces involved in clavicular injury, Stanley *et al.*, (1988) demonstrated that the 'critical buckling load' could be exceeded by a force equal to body weight and concluded that, regardless of the fracture type, the most likely mechanism of injury was a fall onto the point of the shoulder. Stanley also commented, that in cases where patients give a clear history of a fall on to the 'outstretched hand', that it is likely the individual falls and the shoulder makes contact with the ground, inducing a compressive force on the clavicle, resulting in a fracture (Table 14.1).

Table 14.1 Mechanism of injury.	
Fall onto shoulder	87%
Direct blow to shoulder	7%
Fall onto outstretched hand	6%

Diagnosis

The history of a fall on to the point of the shoulder should immediately raise suspicion of a clavicular fracture. The subcutaneous nature of the bone allows ready access to the gentle examining surgeon. In the typical low-energy fall, provided the skin is not being compromised by a sharp bone spike, management is straightforward. In the high-energy injury, the index of suspicion should be higher and a comprehensive history and examination is mandatory. As well as the clavicle itself, attention should be paid to the acromioclavicular and sternoclavicular joints to assess possible dislocation. The chest should always be examined to exclude underlying rib fractures or pneumothorax. The root of the neck and the upper limb should be examined for evidence of underlying neurovascular compromise, especially in high-energy injuries. X-rays in two views should be obtained to assess the degree of displacement.

Treatment

The vast majority of clavicular fractures are managed perfectly adequately conservatively. Conservative management does not equate with neglect, in fact in many ways conservative management of fractures in general is more time-consuming and labour intensive than operative management.

The aim of conservative treatment is to keep the patient comfortable while allowing the clavicle to unite in as near to an anatomical position as possible. In practice, the vertical and posterior displacement of the two main fracture fragments is easier to control than the shortening. One of the ways to guarantee malunion of the clavicle is for junior medical and nursing staff to confuse *collar and cuff* immobilization with a *broad arm-sling*. The two are *not* interchangeable. Collar and cuff immobilization is inappropriate for the management of clavicular fractures as there is no support for the lateral

fracture fragment. The weight of the arm will serve to distract the fracture site and only make the patient more uncomfortable and the deformity worse. A properly applied broad arm-sling, regularly adjusted, will support the weight of the arm and will reduce the tendency of the lateral fragment to displace. The use of disposable foam shoulder immobilizers (e.g. Polysling) provides a cheap comfortable alternative. However, the foam does stretch with time and these do need to be tightened regularly otherwise they will be no better than collar and cuffs.

Figure-of-eight bandages do not provide any additional advantage over broad-arm slings. In order for them to be effective they need to be tightened regularly, on a daily basis and in some cases may then cause symptoms due to local compression around the fracture site. Andersen *et al.* (1987) reported that simple slings caused less discomfort and his series did not demonstrate any difference in the final functional and cosmetic outcome.

Post (1988) advocated the use of plaster of Paris shoulder spica casts for active or uncooperative adolescents or adults. Although this may be a technique to resort to in individual isolated cases, it is, in my opinion not a viable proposition for the vast majority of patients that we deal with.

The clavicle is a subcutaneous bone and the skin overlying the fracture may be jeopardized by the medial fracture fragment or occasionally by a rotated central comminuted fragment. The pressure on the skin may be reduced by nursing the patient supine, using a single pillow with a small bolster between the shoulders. The fracture may then be treated by immobilization in a sling. However, if the tenting recurs, and the area of skin overlying a fragment is liable to ischaemic necrosis, the surgeon must intervene to relieve the pressure on the skin. One option is to treat the patient with bed rest for around 3 weeks until the fracture shows early union. This, I suspect, is not likely to be tolerated by the majority of our patients, though it may be useful for some individuals, especially if a good cosmetic result is essential and a surgical scar unacceptable.

Neviaser (1987) recommends avoiding surgical treatment for prominent subcutaneous fragments, provided the skin is not compromised by ischaemia, as he suggests that the fracture will remodel over time. However, if the treating surgeon judges that there is a real danger of skin compromise, then open reduction is required.

Most clavicular fractures go on to unite uneventfully and many patients discard their slings long before their 6-week review. It is, however, important to confirm clinical and radiological union at this stage to avoid missing the early signs of delayed or non-union. Too vigorous early physiotherapy at this stage has been responsible for a number of non-unions in my experience. Indications for operative treatment are displayed in Table 14.2.

Open fractures

Open fractures of the clavicle are usually the result of high-energy trauma. The fractures are often comminuted and the open skin wound is frequently a Grade-1 puncture wound from within out. These injuries require thorough wound irrigation and excision followed by stabilization of the fracture to allow the underlying soft tissues to heal. There are a number of surgical options, all with their own particular advantages and drawbacks. The favoured technique is internal fixation using AO-reconstruction plates, other reported techniques rely on intramedullary fixation, using Steinmann pins or long screws, and the use of external fixators.

As the soft tissues are likely to have already been significantly disrupted at the time of the injury, care must be taken at surgery not to further jeopardize the soft tissues by needless strong retraction or wide periosteal stripping.

Neurovascular compromise

Neurovascular complications occur uncommonly. A number of authors have reported cases of injury to the brachial plexus in association with clavicular fractures (Howard & Shafer, 1965; Miller & Boswick,1969; Bartosh *et al.*, 1992; Poigenfürst *et al.*, 1992). Associated injury to

---

Table 14.2 Indications for operative treatment.

Open fractures
Fractures with neurovascular compromise
Polytrauma
Displaced Type-II lateral fractures
Floating shoulder

---

underlying vessels has also been reported (Tse *et al.*, 1980; Poigenfürst *et al.*, 1992). These injuries occur in high-energy trauma and are usually associated with fractures of the medial-third of the clavicle (Bartosh *et al.*, 1992). The brachial plexus injury may occur as a result of direct pressure from the medial fracture fragment. However, it is important not to miss underlying cervical spine injuries or traction injuries of the brachial plexus. A careful history and examination may provide clues but if there is any doubt, providing the patient's general condition does not preclude it, then a magnetic resonance imaging (MRI) scan of the cervical spine and brachial plexus may localize the area of injury. This has important implications when it comes to discussing prognosis, as a severe traction injury of the brachial plexus with root avulsion is likely to have a far worse prognosis then local brachial plexus injury due to direct pressure. Clearly the suspicion of a brachial plexus injury demands consultation with a specialist centre at the earliest opportunity.

Polytrauma

In multiply injured patients especially with a combination of upper- and lower-limb injuries, early stable fixation of clavicular fractures is essential if these patients are to be encouraged to mobilize using crutches. In the case of multiple fractures of the upper limb, stabilization of the clavicle will allow early mobilization of the shoulder, elbow and forearm. This is particularly the case when clavicular fracture occurs in combination with a fracture of the proximal humerus or the glenoid (floating shoulder). All the benefits gained by stabilizing a proximal humerus fracture will be lost if the physiotherapist is unable to move the humerus due to pain arising from the concomitant fracture of the clavicle that has remained untreated.

Displaced Type-II lateral clavicle fractures

Neer's (1984) classification of lateral clavicle fractures has already been described. While the Type-I, undisplaced, stable injury is adequately treated conservatively, there is controversy about the best way to treat the displaced, unstable Type-II lateral clavicle fracture. Neer originally advocated the use of transacromial Kirschner wires to stabilize lateral clavicular fractures (Neer, 1968). However, this method of stabilization has not met with universal approval and is probably best avoided. Kona *et al.* (1990), in a retrospective review of 19 patients managed using this technique, reported a high incidence of complications with a 32% non-union rate and a 26% infection rate.

The reported incidence of non-union of Type-II fractures treated conservatively is around 30% (Edwards *et al.*, 1992). Edwards' series comparing the results of conservative versus operative treatment comes out strongly in favour of operative stabilization of these fractures. In his series of 23 cases treated operatively with a coracoclavicular screw, 100% union was achieved, compared with 25% union in the non-operated cases. Ballmer and Gerber (1991) in their small series reported satisfactory union without complication.

If a coracoclavicular screw is used, it is recommended that the screw is removed under local anaesthetic after radiological consolidation of the fracture site 6–9 weeks after surgery. The use of the AO 4.5 mm malleolar screw is recommended as it has a relatively large head and is easily palpable through the skin, allowing it to be removed under local anaesthetic.

Neviaser (1987) also advises open reduction of these fractures and recommends the use of cerclage wires to maintain reduction.

Nordqvist *et al.'s* large series (1993) looked at the natural history of conservatively treated lateral clavicle fracture in a group of 110 cases followed up for a mean of 15 years. Their paper confirmed a 30% rate of non-union, although the majority of these were asymptomatic, suggesting that a 'wait-and-see' approach may be appropriate.

Lateral clavicle fractures are difficult to treat. The fragments are usually very small, sometimes too small to obtain secure fixation using screws and plates and although the initial intra-operative X-ray may appear satisfying, fixation failures do occur. The use of a modified cerclage wire passed through drill holes in the bones may allow sufficient purchase of the fracture fragments to maintain apposition until union.

If the fragment is small, or there is concern about the bone quality, then Nordqvist's wait-and-see approach may be the preferred option. Late reconstruction in the form of a Weaver–Dunn stabilization may be useful if symptoms persist.

Special situations

In selected cases where malunion will seriously interfere with function, such as where the individual needs to carry loads on a shoulder harness (e.g. military personnel, parachutists, mountaineers, divers), open reduction and internal fixation may be the preferred option, although careful siting of the fixation device will be required to avoid irritation.

Surgical treatment: the options

Surgical treatment options are summarized in Table 14.3.

Internal fixation

The 1990s approach to the use of internal fixation is to aim to achieve stable fixation of the fracture in a functional position with minimal damage to the underlying soft tissues. The accepted opinion until recent years has been that internal fixation is associated with an unacceptably high incidence of complications. However justified this criticism may have been at the time, to a large extent the reasons for these complications can be explained. Inadequate fixation techniques, poor respect for soft tissues, neglect of bone grafting and the problems of infection, are all likely to yield a predictably poor result. The territory around the clavicle should be treated with respect, but the treating surgeon should not be discouraged from operating on these fractures. In the acute situation dissection in this area is relatively straightforward provided due care is taken. Although the majority of clavicle fractures unite perfectly adequately when treated conservatively, there are circumstances, previously highlighted, where internal fixation of clavicular fractures is indicated and indeed benefit both the patient and surgeon.

Surgical technique

Preoperative planning of the fixation technique is essential. The surgeon should confirm that he has the necessary instruments and the appropriate implants to carry out the planned procedure. The surgical tactic should be explained to all members of the operating-theatre team. It takes less than a minute to tell the theatre sister what you plan to do and what equipment you require.

Table 14.3 Surgical options.
Internal fixation
External fixation
Intramedullary fixation

The patient should be anaesthetized and placed in a semireclining position. It is not essential for the arm to be draped free although this may aid manipulation of the fracture fragments. The patient's head should be turned away from the injured side and the neck laterally flexed gently away from the site of surgery. This allows access to the superior aspect of the clavicle when drilling. The use of two disposable U-drapes is a satisfactory way of draping and avoids the need for elaborate head towelling. The iliac crest should routinely be prepared and draped to allow the possibility of graft harvesting should it be required.

For male patients an infraclavicular horizontal incision is preferred. Female patients may prefer an S-shaped incision sited close to the necklace line. This allows sufficient access once the edges are undermined and yields an acceptable cosmetic result. In both sexes, the area to avoid is the area of skin inferior to the medial one-third of the clavicle, as incisions in this area are more prone to keloid formation. Once skin and platysma are divided the supraclavicular nerves should be sought and protected around nylon slings. Usually the middle and medial nerves are both encountered during the procedure and attempts to preserve them should be made. However, preoperatively the patient should be warned about the possibility of numbness in the infraclavicular region. Occasionally, the middle nerve interferes with placement of the plate or comes to lie directly over the plate, in which case it is probably better to sacrifice it. Each of the two main fracture fragments should be exposed only enough to allow reduction. The use of pointed reduction forceps will allow the fracture fragments to be gently realigned and clavicular length to be restored. Do not attempt to anatomically reduce the smaller comminutions, as they may become stripped of their blood supply. It is sufficient to realign them gently using a dental hook and 'ligamentotaxis' by gentle distraction of the main fracture fragments. On no account should instruments be inserted blindly inferior or posterior to the fragments in view of the proximity of the great vessels and brachial plexus. Once clavicular length has been restored it is usually possible to obtain initial lag-screw fixation using a 3.5 mm cortical screw. Placement of the plate depends, to a certain extent, on the fracture pattern. In some cases anterior placement of the plate is possible, although more often a superior placement is more straightforward. The plate should be accurately contoured prior to placement, as otherwise loss of reduction will occur. The siting of the initial lag screw should have taken into account the placement of the plate, alternatively the lag screw may be removed after contouring the plate and a longer lag screw inserted through the plate. Extreme care must be taken when drilling in this area. The surgeon is advised to use his drill as one would use a reamer, gently advancing and withdrawing until the far cortex is breached, avoiding overpenetration. The use of a tri-fluted drill with an oscillating drill bit is ideal if available.

The choice of implant depends upon the nature of the fracture and local availability. Although in relatively simple fractures standard 3.5 mm AO dynamic compression plates (DCPs) may be used, the 3.5 mm reconstruction plate, with its lower profile and its ability to be contoured in two planes, to fit the S-shaped clavicle more easily, is the preferred implant (Fig. 14.3). Recently the use of the AO low-contact dynamic compression plate (LCDCP) has been reported (Mullaji and Jupiter, 1994). This plate allows ease of contouring with uniform plate bending, greater biocompatibility and a smaller contact area with the underlying bone, leading to less disruption of the underlying blood supply.

In the presence of a high-energy injury, causing comminuted fragments or significant periosteal stripping of the major fragments due to the initial injury, cancellous bone grafting should be considered and indeed is recommended. The small amount of cancellous graft required can usually be harvested from the iliac crest using a percutaneous trephining technique, leading to low morbidity at the donor site. The wound is

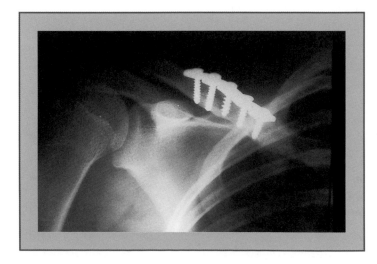

Figure 14.3 – *AO reconstruction plate comminuted clavicle.*

then closed over suction drainage, ensuring that the platysma is closed as a separate layer. Until wound healing has occurred the arm should be immobilized in a shoulder sling. Early functional range of movement is allowed, but this should be restricted to movement below shoulder level for the first 6 weeks to reduce the likelihood of implant failure and non-union.

Poigenfürst *et al.* (1992) reported their results in a very large series of 122 fresh fractures treated using AO techniques, using either the 3.5 mm DCP or the 3.5 mm reconstruction plate. They report a 7.3% superficial infection rate and a non-union rate of 4%. Bone grafting was not used routinely in this series. There were four re-fractures following plate removal and it is recommended that plates should not be routinely removed.

The use of smaller, 2.7 mm, AO DCP has been reported. Schwarz and Höcker (1992) analysed their results following plating of 36 fresh clavicular fractures. They reported no infections. Four failures were reported, three non-unions and one re-fracture after removal of the plate. In this series, bone grafting was not used and had it been one could postulate that the non-union rate may have been lower.

External fixation

External fixation of the clavicle has been used to stabilize clavicular fractures successfully. Schuind *et al.* (1988) report their results using a Hoffmann external fixator, using 3 mm threaded pins inserted after pre-drilling. Their series of 20 fractures all united. There were two cases of pin-track infection. It must be emphasized that the surgeons used an open technique, the external fixator pins inserted under direct vision once the fracture had been openly reduced. The fixators were removed at an average of 51 days after surgery. This technique may be useful in specific situations of grossly contaminated open wounds, but I would not advocate its routine use in closed fractures.

Intramedullary fixation

The potential for disastrous complications following the use of intramedullary Kirschner wires in this region have led to the abandonment of this technique in favour of more effective and safer techniques discussed earlier. Even in the relatively safer area of the Type-II lateral clavicle fracture the use of Kirschner wires is no longer recommended (Kona *et al.*, 1990). Neviaser (1975) has reported the successful use of an intramedullary Knowles

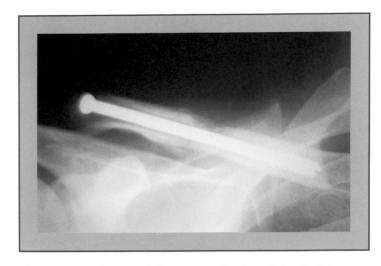

Figure 14.4 – *Intramedullary screw fixation of the clavicle.*

pin, but the technique is not in widespread use and one must question whether fixation with this device is stable enough to allow early mobilization (Fig. 14.4).

Non-union

The incidence of non-union in conservatively treated clavicle fractures varies between 0% (Stanley & Norris, 1988) and 1.9% (Marsh & Hazarian, 1970). In operatively treated fractures, using AO techniques, the incidence is higher at 4% (Poigenfürst, 1992). The majority of clavicular non-unions occur at the middle one-third of the clavicle. At this point the clavicle is tubular with a thick cortex, has very little cancellous bone and is devoid of muscle attachments, creating the ideal environment for non-union. It is unusual for clavicle non-unions to be asymptomatic, with 75% of non-unions presenting significant symptoms (Foy & Fagg, 1990). These symptoms may vary from pain after heavy work to symptoms of neurological or vascular compromise due to compression of the brachial plexus or subclavian vessels between the pseudarthrosis and the first rib (Fig. 14.5).

Diagnosis

The diagnosis should be suspected in patients complaining of residual symptoms of pain 12 weeks after treatment of the clavicular fracture. Suspect it especially in cases of high-energy trauma affecting the middle one-third of the clavicle. The physical findings on examination may be subtle. There will be pain over the clavicle at the extremes of abduction and adduction. In slimmer individuals it may be possible to detect motion

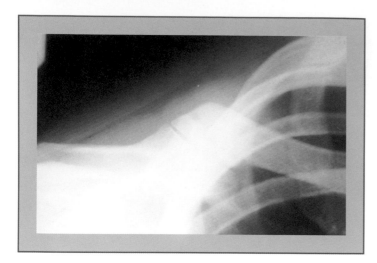

Figure 14.5 – *Clavicle non-union.*

between the two main fracture fragments by moving the medial and lateral clavicular shaft in opposite directions. This relative motion may be palpable over the non-union as the arm is elevated. X-rays may prove difficult to interpret as, although in the atrophic non-union the diagnosis may be straightforward, it is difficult to distinguish the appearance of a united clavicle from the exuberant callus found in hypertrophic non-union. Oblique views may assist in this situation. It is also sometimes useful to screen the pseudarthrosis under image intensifier to confirm that there is movement at the fracture site.

Treatment

Except in the case of the frail, elderly patient who makes very little demands on their clavicle, the majority of clavicular non-unions require surgical treatment.

The aim of surgery is to encourage union of the clavicle in a functional position. In cases where there has been significant bone resorption and shortening, an intercalary tricortical graft may have to be interposed to restore length. The use of supplementary cancellous bone graft, in most cases, is recommended apart perhaps in cases of hypertrophic non-union where compression applied across the pseudarthrosis is theoretically all that is required. However, the amount of soft-tissue stripping that necessarily occurs at the time of surgery, to allow exposure of the fracture ends and reduction with restoration of length, is likely to compromise the blood supply to the fracture ends further, so a biological boost in the form of a cancellous bone graft is a wise adjunct.

The technique in widest use is the use of a plate and graft and this will be described in detail. Other techniques will be discussed briefly but the approach is similar.

The plate and graft technique involves a similar approach to that described earlier. Extreme care must be taken as there is usually gross distortion of the anatomy around the pseudarthrosis. The principle to be recommended is to stay close to bone throughout. Identify a relatively normal part of the clavicle first and work your way gently towards the site of the pseudarthrosis, using a fine scalpel and a narrow periosteal elevator. Try to identify the junction between callus and normal bone as this will help to align the two fracture ends. It is often necessary to excise some of the excess callus to allow decompression of underlying structures. If this callus is judged to be of good quality it may be used to supplement cancellous grafting at the end of the procedure. Occasionally, it is necessary to perform an oblique osteotomy at the adjoining surfaces of the pseudarthrosis to allow apposition and lag-screw fixation. Pay particular attention to the positioning of the lag screw, bearing in mind the intended placement of the plate. A 3.5 mm AO reconstruction plate is the preferred implant (Fig. 14.6). If this is not available then the 3.5 mm AO DCP may be used, though it is a little more bulky and more difficult to contour. At least three screws should be inserted in each fragment. A superior placement is most efficient biomechanically, as the plate will behave as a tension-band plate and should withstand both bending and torsional forces (Jupiter & Leffert, 1987). On no account should the periosteum or

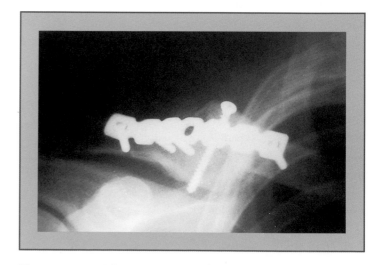

Figure 14.6 – *AO reconstruction plate to clavicle non-union.*

fascia posterior or inferior to the clavicle be breached, as this will endanger underlying vessels and nerves. The area posterior and inferior to this periosteal/fascial layer should be considered *'tiger country'*. Once the plate is in place, cancellous graft should be laid around the anterior, superior and inferior surfaces of the fracture. Closure is as described earlier. The shoulder should be immobilized for a period of 3–6 weeks, depending upon the rigidity of the initial fixation. Therefore the operating surgeon should specify his postoperative instructions in the operating notes to prevent all the surgeon's good work being undone by too vigorous early physiotherapy. Fixation is usually sound enough to allow early pendulum movements. For the first 3 weeks following surgery a sling should be worn for comfort and active exercises above shoulder height should be avoided until signs of union are observed.

Jupiter and Leffert (1987) reported a union rate of 93.7% using a plate and graft. Jupiter suggest that the extent of displacement of the fracture fragments may be a factor in the development of a non-union, implying a greater amount of initial damage to soft tissues (Table 14.4).

Manske and Szabo (1985) in their small series reported a 100% union rate using a similar technique to that of Jupiter and Leffert. Eskola *et al.* (1986) reported similarly gratifying results, with union in 94% of cases. Their series, however, also demonstrated that this surgery is not without risk and they described a 17% complication rate with one unfortunate patient sustaining a pneumothorax, air embolus, brachial plexus injury and injury to a subclavian vein. It behoves us to acknowledge that this is potentially dangerous surgery, and a careful planned approach to surgery in this region cannot be overemphasized.

Table 14.4 Operative treatment of non-union.

Authors	Union rate (%)
Manske and Szabo (1985)	100
Eskola *et al.* (1986)	94.0
Jupiter (1987)	93.7
Boehme *et al.* (1991)	95.0
Capicotto *et al.* (1994)	100

A number of authors have described techniques combining intramedullary fixation with cancellous grafting. Capicotto *et al.* (1994) treated 14 cases of non-union using an intramedullary threaded Steinmann pin. This was drilled in an antegrade fashion out of the lateral fragment of the clavicle, exiting posterior to the acromioclavicular joint, and then drilled retrograde across the reduced fracture site. Cancellous graft was then packed around the pseudarthrosis. The threaded pins were removed once union occurred. Capicotto *et al.* reports a 100% union rate, but in 50% of patients there was tenderness at the lateral edge of the Steinmann pin.

Boehme *et al.* (1991) advocate the use of a modified Hagie pin supplemented by bone grafting. In their series of 50 patients a union rate of 95% was achieved. This technique utilizes a Hagie pin which is a threaded rod with fine pitch at one end and a coarse pitch at the other. Their technique is performed through a curved vertical incision along Langer's lines. The fracture ends are exposed and the intervening scar tissue is excised. The intramedullary canals of the medial and lateral fragments are reamed out, remaining within the clavicle medially but exiting posteriorly in the lateral fragment. The modified Hagie pin is then advanced, coarse threads leading, across the fracture gap and into the medial fragment. A nut is applied to the threaded lateral end of the Hagie pin, allowing some compression at the fracture site. In the majority of their cases, osteoperiosteal rib graft was laid across the non-union. Boehme recommends removal of the Hagie pin once union has occurred.

Middleton *et al.* (1995) report success with their technique of partial excision of the lateral clavicular fragment in jockeys with non-unions. This sounds a little bizarre; however, the six jockeys presented in their paper had sustained repeated injuries to the same clavicle after falls while horse-racing and this technique did allow the individuals to return to full activity without any apparent adverse effects. In this particular group of high-demand individuals, who required a permanent solution to their repeated non-unions, this somewhat unorthodox treatment worked well. For the rest of our patients with symptomatic non-union of a clavicular fracture, AO plating with supplementary cancellous grafting is the preferred option.

Summary

Clavicle fractures are common. They usually occur as a result of a fall on to the point of the shoulder. Conservative treatment, using a broad arm-sling is effective in the majority of low-energy, minimally displaced fractures. Specific indications for operative fixation have been discussed. AO-plate fixation supplemented by cancellous bone grafting is the recommended method of choice for both primary surgical treatment in selected cases and in treatment of symptomatic non-union.

CHAPTER 15

The fractured scapula

P. Schranz

Introduction

The scapula is a flat blade of bone suspended in muscle which covers over 80% of its surface, with an articulation at its lateral pole, a spine and two apophyses — the acromion and the coracoid. Scapular fractures are relatively rare, occurring in 0.5–1% of all fractures. (Hardegger *et al.*, 1984). Unlike the humerus or clavicle that are sometimes fractured after relatively trivial injuries,

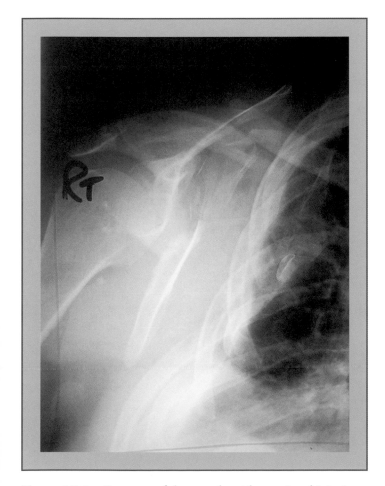

Figure 15.1 – *Fractures of the scapula with associated injuries.*

it takes a great deal of energy to fracture the scapula. This should alert you, the surgeon, to be on the lookout for serious associated injuries whenever you encounter a scapular fracture. Because they occur most commonly after high-energy trauma, with a number of associated injuries, delay in diagnosis is not uncommon (Armstrong & Van der Spay, 1984) even though patients usually have physical signs of injury in the region of the scapula. The relatively subtle signs are overshadowed by more extensive obvious injuries to the chest or limbs (Fig. 15.1) Patients with scapular fractures, even if isolated injuries, should be admitted to hospital overnight and followed-up the next day with a chest X-ray to rule out late pneumothorax or pulmonary contusion.

Classification

Fractures of the scapula can be divided into extra-articular fractures of the body, scapular neck, acromion and coracoid and intra-articular glenoid fractures. Hardegger *et al.* (1984) describes eight different types of fracture; these are classified regionally (Fig. 15.2).

Extra-articular fractures
Scapular body fractures
Fractures of the body of the scapula account for 65–90% of scapular fractures (Nordqvist and Petersson, 1992). Because the body is embedded in the depths of large muscles, fractures of the body occur relatively infrequently and when they do occur they are a result of high-energy trauma. They are therefore frequently comminuted and displaced. The area fractured most frequently is the fossa of the subscapularis. The muscle sandwich that surrounds the scapula does tend to prevent extreme displacement of the fragments and, due to the abundant blood supply, these fractures tend to unite without too much encouragement. Nordqvist

239

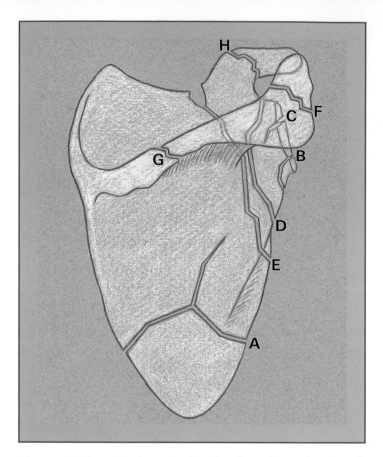

Figure 15.2 – *Hardegger's classification. (Reproduced with permission from Journal of Bone & Joint Surgery.)*

reviewed the long-term results of patients with scapular body fractures and confirmed that conservative management is appropriate in virtually all cases. In Nordqvist's series, 78% of patients reported a satisfactory or good result, with relatively minor residual disability. Most patients were able to return to work within 6 weeks of injury unless they were limited by an associated injury. Only four patients out of this series of 129 cases had to change jobs as a result of their injury. In cases of extreme displacement of the lateral margin of the body in the so-called burst fracture (Hardegger *et al.*, 1984) there may be penetration into the joint impeding movement. In these cases the fragment requires reduction or removal (Fig. 15.3a,b).

Scapular neck fractures

The next most commonly encountered fractures are those of the anatomical or surgical neck. These usually occur as a result of direct trauma. Isolated extra-articular fractures, such as these, do well treated conservatively, although Ada and Miller (1991) found that displaced fractures of the scapular neck do

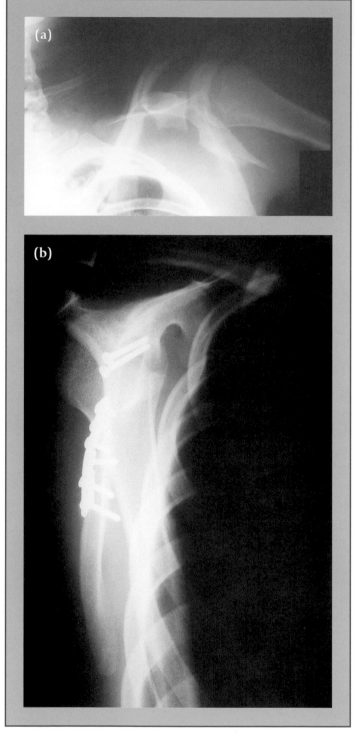

Figure 15.3 – *(a) and (b). Fractured scapula body and glenoid fracture.*

sometimes result in significant disability. Nordqvist and Petersson (1992) recorded unsatisfactory results in 32% of their cases. Malunion in this region may cause an irritating grating at the scapulothoracic articulation. In general, however, these fractures may be left well alone.

Extra-articular fractures of the scapular neck, in association with clavicular fractures, or disruption of the coracoclavicular ligament, give rise to a floating shoulder. In this situation there is no restraint on the amount of fracture displacement. In order to prevent gross displacement and malrotation of the fragments, it is advisable that at least the clavicle fracture should be stabilized primarily (Hersovici *et al.*, 1992). Other authors (Leung & Lam, 1993) recommend stabilization of the scapula, as well as the clavicle, to prevent residual medial displacement of the scapular neck. Displacement and rotation leads to alteration of normal muscle tension around the glenohumeral joint and functional loss (Hardegger *et al.*, 1984). Another variant in this region is the 'stove-in shoulder'. In this variant, the fracture is a relatively stable impacted fracture, similar to a central fracture dislocation of the hip. Oni and Hoskinson (1992) report satisfactory results following conservative management of this type of injury.

Fractures of the coracoid

These are rare fractures, sparsely reported in the literature. Coracoid fractures may occur in isolation or as part of an injury complex involving glenoid fractures, glenohumeral dislocations, acromioclavicular injuries or clavicular fractures. Eyres *et al.* (1995) proposed a classification into five types (Fig. 15.4). They suggest that Types I, II and III are avulsion injuries, due to traction, whereas the more significant Types-IV and -V fractures probably occur as a result of shear forces across the root of the coracoid.

Eyres recommends internal fixation of displaced Type-IV and -V fractures using cancellous screws through a deltopectoral approach, using direct visualization of the reduction of the glenoid surface through a split incision through the subscapularis (Fig. 15.5a,b).

Ogawa *et al.* (1997), in the largest reported series so far, of 67 patients with coracoid fractures, propose a simpler classification of these fractures into two types. Type-I fractures involve the base of the coracoid and occur proximal to the attachments of the coracoclavicular ligaments. Type-II fractures occur towards the tip of the coracoid, distal to the attachments of the coracoclavicular ligaments. The authors describe an association with acromioclavicular dislocation. Ogawa *et al.* regard the isolated Type-II fracture as a stable injury and recommend conservative treatment. When Type-I fractures occur in association with

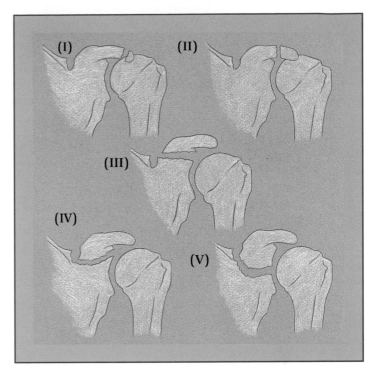

Figure 15.4 – *Fractured coracoid — classification (see text). (Reproduced with permission from Journal of Bone & Joint Surgery).*

associated injuries, resulting in a disruption of the scapuloclavicular link, stabilization of the coracoid fracture using a malleolar screw is recommended.

Acromion process fractures

Injuries to the acromion process are rare. In contrast to the acromioclavicular joint, injured frequently both on and off the sports field, acromion injuries contribute only 9% of all fractures of the scapula (Armstrong & Van der Spuy,1984) (Fig. 15.6) One of the largest series in the literature is by Kuhn and Blasier (1994) who reviewed a series of 27 fractures of the acromion process presenting over a 15-year period. Acromion fractures may occur following direct trauma, may be due to muscular forces causing avulsion injuries, or may occur, in the absence of acute trauma, as stress fractures. Hall and Calvert (1994) report a case of acromion stress fracture occurring in a golfer.

Kuhn classified acromion fractures into five distinct types:

Type-I fractures are minimally displaced, with subtype IA avulsion fractures occurring as a result of deltoid muscle contraction. These fractures usually heal after a short period of immobilization, though non-union has been reported (Kuhn & Blasier, 1994). They are caused

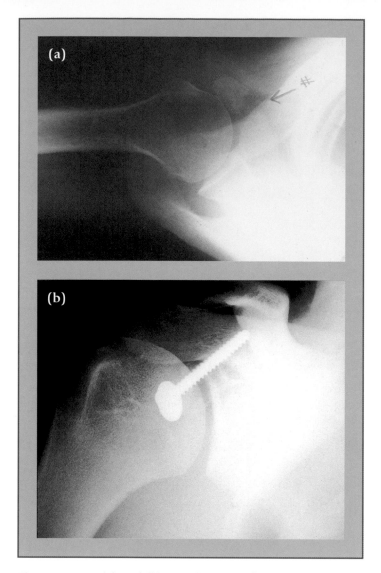

Figure 15.5 – *(a) and (b). Fixed coracoid fractures.*

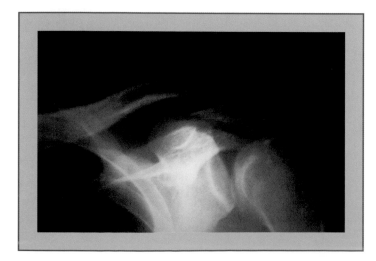

Figure 15.6 – *Acromion process fracture.*

usually either by a direct blow to the acromion, or in association with upward displacement of the humerus (Armstrong & Van der Spuy, 1984).

Type-IB, minimally displaced, fractures occur as a result of direct trauma to the acromion. Conservative treatment usually results in union, although Kuhn suggests that the use of crutches for concomitant lower-limb trauma may delay union.

Type-II fractures are displaced but do not encroach upon, or reduce the height, of the subacromial space. In Kuhn's series the majority of these fractures united satisfactorily after sling immobilization.

Type-III fractures encroach upon the subacromial space, either by the fragment displacing inferiorly or by an associated glenoid fracture displacing superiorly. If allowed to unite in a displaced position, these fractures give rise to significant loss of shoulder movement due to impingement and rotator-cuff injury.

Stress fractures of the acromion can be associated with rotator-cuff pathology or rheumatological conditions, and may lead to non-union. The overall incidence of non-union in Kuhn's series was 30%.

As in other parts of the scapula, fractures of the acromion often occur in association with other injuries such as rib fractures, spine fractures or brachial plexus injuries. They should therefore not just be looked upon as interesting oddities but also as signs of serious underlying injury.

Fractures of the scapular spine

These relatively uncommon fractures make up 6–11% of all cases of scapular fractures reported in large series (Armstrong & Van der Spuy, 1984; Ada & Miller, 1991). They may occur in association with scapular body fractures. Comminuted scapular spine fractures are disabling. In Ada and Miller's series (1991), of 148 scapular fractures, 10 patients had comminuted scapular spine fractures. Fifty percent of these had shoulder weakness, 75% had rest pain and more than half had night pain felt mainly in the subacromial region. Ada postulates that symptoms are due to dysfunction of the rotator cuff caused either by direct muscle damage, by the fragments in the more comminuted fractures, or indirect rotator-cuff impairment due to surrounding haemorrhage around the cuff.

Stress fractures of the scapular spine have been reported in lorry drivers (Ho *et al.*, 1993). The mechanism is probably repetitive direct loading of the scapular spine by loads being lifted on and off lorries.

Non-union of the scapular spine occurs occasionally and can be symptomatic (Ada & Miller, 1991; Robinson & Court-Brown, 1993). Treatment by internal fixation supplemented by bone grafting is advised.

Glenoid fossa fractures

Intra-articular fractures involving the glenoid form 6–10% of scapular fractures. Only about 10% of these are significantly displaced. Goss (1992) puts these figures into perspective when he points out that displaced glenoid fractures comprise only one of every 10 000 fractures. Rare though they may be, they are displaced intra-articular fractures and if these fractures are neglected they may give rise to considerable problems from posttraumatic osteoarthritis or instability. The surgical treatment of these displaced joint fractures is not easy and a well thought out surgical tactic can only be planned once the nature and extent of the fracture is identified.

Plain radiographs are best supplemented by computerized tomography (CT) images, to help appreciate the number of fracture fragments and the extent of displacement of the articular surface (Fig. 15.7).

Three dimensional CT images in this situation are a valuable adjunct in planning treatment.

Classification

Ideberg (1984) described a classification for fractures of the scapula involving the glenoid (Fig. 15.8). Six main fracture types are described with associated subgroups. The fracture complexity increases down the group.

The fracture pattern is dictated by the direction of the application of force from the lateral aspect of the humerus on to the glenoid.

Type-I glenoid rim fractures

This group of fractures are quite commonly encountered. They are true fractures of the glenoid rim rather than the labral avulsion sometimes seen after anterior dislocation of the shoulder. These rim fractures occur when the humeral head is driven directly on to the rim, rather than a rotatory dislocating force that would otherwise avulse the labrum and give rise to a dislocation.

When the force is directed somewhat anteromedially, the anterior rim is involved and gives rise to a *Type-Ia*

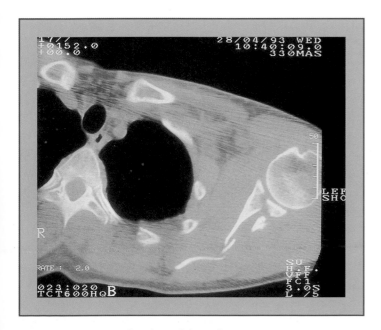

Figure 15.7 – *CT of a glenoid fossa fracture.*

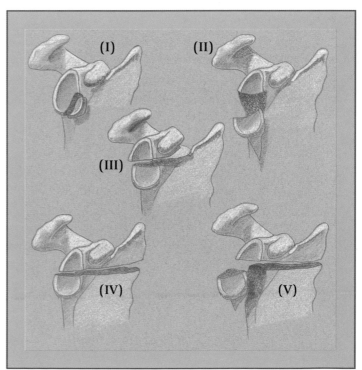

Figure 15.8 – *The Ideberg classification of glenoid fractures.*

fracture. If the force is directed posteromedially, part of the posterior rim is fractured off and a *Type-Ib* fracture occurs.

Type-II fractures

In these fractures the force through the head is directed inferiorly. This causes a fracture of the glenoid rim exiting at the lateral border of the scapula, allowing an inferior fragment to separate and displace. The concomitant inferior subluxation of the humeral head further increases the displacement of the inferior fragment.

Type-III fractures

When the force through the head is directed more superiorly the glenoid fracture exits through the upper half of the scapula, giving rise to a superior fragment that will include the coracoid process. This fracture line occurs at the epiphyseal line that passes through the upper part of the glenoid and separates two separate ossification centres — the dorsal scapula and the ventral coracoid. These fractures may occur in association with disruption of the superior suspensory complex (coracoid process, coracoclavicular ligaments, clavicle, acromioclavicular joint and acromion).

Type-IV fractures

In this group the force through the head is directed at the centre of the glenoid fossa. The humeral head then acts as a blunt chisel and causes a central transverse fissure fracture through the centre of the glenoid which exits at the medial border of the scapula.

Type-V fractures

The above fracture patterns may exist in combination with each other, giving rise to a number of subtypes of Type-V fractures. All the combinations contain a primary fracture line described in the Type-IV fracture. In the *Type-Va* fracture the primary fracture is associated with a second fracture-line exiting inferiorly (Type IV and II). The *Type-Vb* fracture pattern is a combination of the primary transverse fracture together with a superior fracture fragment (Type IV and III). The *Type-Vc* fractures are more complex fractures with a transverse fracture line (iv) an inferior fracture (ii) and a superior fracture (iii). These are immensely high-energy injuries and are associated with a high incidence of neurovascular damage.

Type-VI fractures

This is a group of severely comminuted 'bag of bones' fractures caused by extreme violence.

Pre-operative considerations

These fractures are extremely high-energy injuries and attention needs to be paid to associated life-threatening injuries before concentrating on the glenoid fracture. Airway problems should have been addressed, cervical spine injury excluded and major haemorrhage controlled either by direct pressure to a bleeding vessel, laparotomy to address a bleeding viscus or external fixation to control bleeding from a pelvic fracture.

Because of the very high incidence (15–55%) of associated chest injuries (haemo-pneumothorax, pulmonary contusion), chest drainage prior to surgery is advisable, as the surgery is prolonged and there is a real danger of a tension pneumothorax arising following assisted ventilation during the anaesthetic.

Treatment options

If after adequate imaging the glenoid fractures are felt to be minimally displaced, i.e. less than 4 mm separation, it is reasonable to opt for non-surgical treatment using a sling for comfort and range of motion exercises once the pain subsides. However, a further X-ray should be taken at 10 days to ensure that late displacement does not go unnoticed.

The results of conservative management of displaced intra-articular fractures of the glenoid are poor (Ada & Miller, 1991). Over the past 10 years there have been a number of publications advocating open reduction and internal fixation of displaced glenoid fractures (Goss, 1992; Hardegger *et al.*, 1984; Kavanagh *et al.*, 1993; Aulicino *et al.*, 1986; Leung *et al.*, 1993; Bauer *et al.*, 1995). Like the acetabulum, however, the results of inadequate restoration of congruency after open reduction and internal fixation are equally disappointing. Bauer (1995), in his review of patients conducted an average of 6 years following open reduction and internal fixation, found that the only poor result occurred in a patient with a residual 2 mm displacement at the glenoid articular surface. This means that if we are going to attempt an open reduction and internal fixation of a displaced intra-articular fracture of the glenoid, that it should be undertaken with the careful planning and precision.

The approaches

Anterior

Type-Ia fractures of the anterior glenoid rim should be approached through a standard anterior deltopectoral approach. The patient is positioned in the beach-chair position with a 1 litre bag of fluid along the medial border of the scapula and the head supported on a head ring or neurosurgical headrest. The shoulder is prepared using antiseptic solution and the prepared area is extended down to the wrist, axilla and across the front of the chest, extending up the neck. I prefer to use two disposable U-drapes to encircle the operating field, thereby avoiding the need for a head towel. The forearm is draped in a towel and stockinette and is supported either by the side of the body or out on an arm table, according to preference.

A deltopectoral incision is made extending inferiorly from just above the tip of the coracoid process. The cephalic vein is retracted laterally as its tributaries reach it from the lateral side. The conjoint tendons of coracobrachialis and the short head of biceps are retracted medially to reveal subscapularis. Identify the axillary nerve at this point and be aware of its proximity to your operative field. The subscapularis muscle is divided between stay-sutures 1–2 cm from its lateral border and is reflected off the capsule using a periosteal elevator. Once the capsule is exposed this may be incised as a separate layer and reflected to expose the anterior part of the glenoid rim. Particular care must be taken to avoid injury to the axillary nerve. Remember that, in the presence of acute trauma, the normal anatomy may become distorted so it is wisest to positively identify the axillary nerve before introducing any deep retractors or internal fixation devices.

Posterior

All remaining fracture types (except Type-VI which are unreconstructable) are best approached through a posterior approach or its posterosuperior variant. This approach may be relatively unfamiliar to some readers and it is well worth spending a little time revising the anatomy of the region. If access to an anatomy laboratory is available, the opportunity to practise the approach prior to attempting surgery in this region is invaluable.

Although the prone position may be used, it is advisable to use the lateral decubitus position, as access may be required from the front as well as the back. The arm is draped free and supported on a draped armboard or Mayo table. Several variants of skin incision have been described. Some authors opt for a curved incision running parallel to the spine and the medial border of the scapula (Muller *et al.*, 1991), alternatively a straight bra-strap incision may be preferred. What is important is that the skin incision allows adequate exposure of the underlying muscles without the need for strong retraction.

The posterior part of the deltoid muscle is sharply dissected off the scapular spine and is gently reflected downwards and laterally. Wallace (1991) advises against dissecting too deeply along the scapular spine otherwise infraspinatus may be elevated along with deltoid. Once the deltoid is reflected downwards and laterally, the neurovascular bundle containing the axillary nerve and the posterior circumflex humeral artery, should be identified and preserved, exiting from the quadralateral space. Next the plane between the infraspinatus and teres minor is identified and the two muscles are separated. This allows limited access to the posterior capsule. If greater access is required the infraspinatus muscle is divided 1 cm from its lateral insertion. It is then separated off the underlying posterior capsule and is reflected medially and superiorly. Positively identify the suprascapular nerve entering it after it winds around the base of the scapular spine and enters the muscle on its deep surface medially. Make sure that your assistant is well aware of the presence of both of these nerves and is warned to avoid strong traction in this situation. The capsule and the lateral edge of the scapula then come into view and an arthrotomy will allow good access to the posterior glenoid, especially if the humeral head is retracted away.

This approach allows good access to posterior rim fractures together with fractures of the inferior glenoid (Type-II and -Va). In order to gain access to the superior part of the glenoid and the base of the coracoid process, the *posterosuperior approach* is recommended (Goss, 1992). In this extension of the posterior approach, the skin incision is carried cranially over the trapezius. The trapezius muscle is split in the line of its fibres allowing access to the underlying supraspinatus. Access to the superior glenoid cavity and the base of the coracoid can be obtained by splitting the supraspinatus tendon in the line of its fibres.

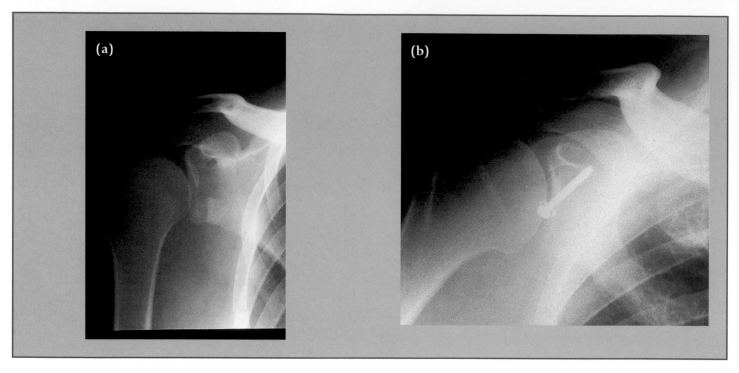

Figure 15.9 – *(a) and (b). Glenoid rim fractures.*

Fixation techniques

Type-I fractures

The aim of operative fixation in these fractures is to control instability and to keep the humeral head concentrically reduced on to the glenoid. Goss (1992) states that instability is likely to occur if there is 10 mm displacement of the fragments or if the anterior 25% or posterior 33% of the glenoid is involved. For simple anterior or posterior rim fragments, lag screw fixation using 3.5 mm or 4.0 mm screws is sufficient (Fig. 15.9a,b). When using lag screws to fix antero-inferior glenoid fragments, avoid overpenetration of the drill or screws, as the suprascapular nerve may be injured.

In cases where the anterior rim fracture is comminuted, Goss recommends excision of these fragments and their replacement by a tricortical bone block from the iliac crest that is internally fixed in place to reconstitute the anterior glenoid buttress. Allograft may provide a suitable alternative (Fig 15.10a,b).

Type-II fractures

These inferior fragments may be quite large and give rise to inferior glenohumeral instability when they displace. The bone along the lateral border of the scapula inferior to the glenoid is thick, good quality bone and will allow fixation of the fragment with small-fragment lag screws, supplemented, if fixation is inadequate, by a contoured 3.5 mm reconstruction plate or one-third tubular plate to provide buttressing.

Type-III fractures

The posterosuperior approach described above gives access to these fractures and will allow reduction under direct vision and fixation using lag screws. Additional stabilization of the disrupted superior suspensory complex may be required. Techniques for stabilizing this area are discussed in the chapter on the acromioclavicular joint.

Type-IV fractures

These transverse fractures through the centre of the glenoid may be reduced and fixed using either lag screws inserted from above or, alternatively, cerclage wires may be passed around or through the scapular neck. Reconstruction or semitubular plates may be used if applied in the relatively good quality bone of the scapular neck, but the siting of these plates is quite critical as it is easy to drift into the paper-thin scapular body which does not allow secure screw purchase.

Type-V fractures

These complex fractures pose the greatest challenge to the treating surgeon and should be approached with caution. A combination of techniques may be required

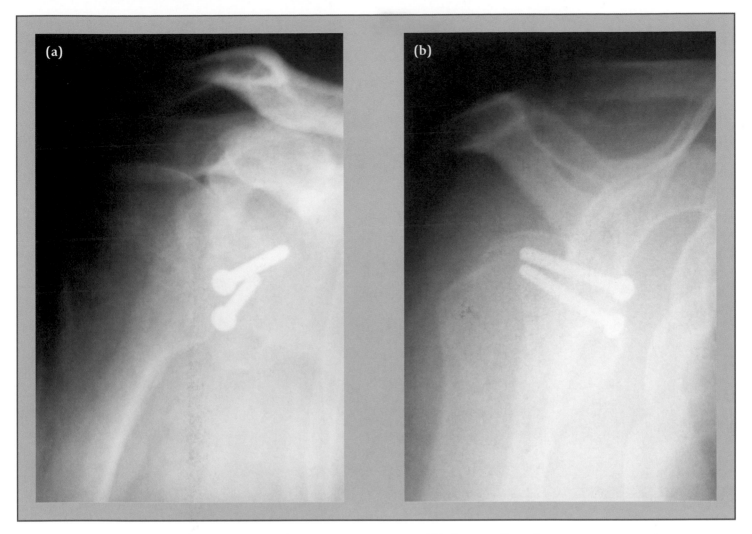

Figure 15.10 – *(a) and (b). Excision comminuted anterior rim — tricortical block using allograft.*

to stabilize these fractures. Lag screws should be used to reduce the superior or inferior secondary fracture-fragments whilst cerclage wires or small fragment plates control the transverse fracture.

Aftercare

The nature and pace of rehabilitation after these fractures depends on the degree of stability that was achieved intra-operatively and the strength of fixation. Simple fractures, rigidly fixed, may be treated by relatively early progressive range of motion exercises, after a short period of immobilization in a shoulder sling. Regular X-rays and close follow-up will reassure the patient and the surgeon that the fixation is not being jeopardized by the pace of the rehabilitation programme. In the more complex fractures, or in patients with poor bone quality where there may be some doubt as to the rigidity of fixation, the shoulder

should be immobilized in a shoulder spica for the first 3 weeks, following which the fracture is likely to be stable enough to allow immobilization in a sling and resumption of a progressive range of motion exercises.

At 6 weeks, all external support may be discarded and active functional movement should be encouraged. Early on in the rehabilitation of these fractures patients need to be advised that it may take anything up to 12 months before the final functional result is obtained. These patients should be kept under regular review to allow the surgeon to keep motivating the patient throughout this prolonged rehabilitation period.

Results of operative treatment

There were few publications on operative fixation of intra-articular glenoid fractures prior to the early 1980s. The early publications dealt with isolated case reports

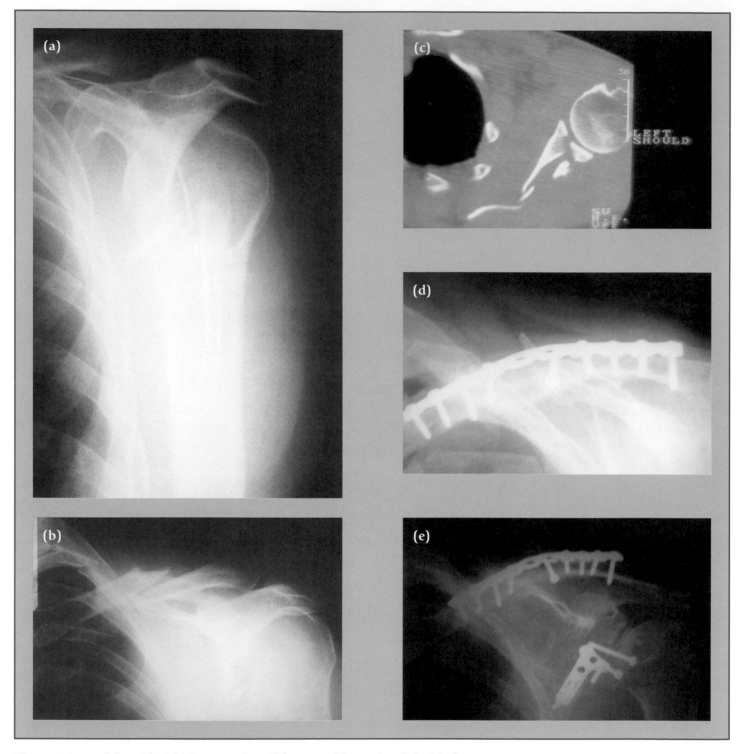

Figure 15.11 – *(a) to (e). A high energy glenoid fracture with associated clavicle fracture.*

and it was only in the mid 1980s that larger series of cases were available for peer review.

Hardegger *et al.* (1984) reported a series of 37 scapular fractures treated operatively over a 14-year period. These included 11 fractures of the glenoid rim and 12 fractures of the glenoid fossa. The subgroups of intra-articular fractures were not analysed separately, but the author quoted 79% good to excellent results overall.

Goss (1992) provided a very elegant description of the treatment of glenoid fractures and concluded that 'the functional end-result and the avoidance of post-traumatic glenohumeral instability or degenerative joint disease after operative treatment of markedly displaced fractures of the glenoid rim (Type I) and fossa (Types I through V) depends on the adequacy of the reduction, the quality of the fixation, and the rigour of the postoperative rehabilitation program'. Goss pointed out the lack of studies in the literature that reported functional outcomes after operative treatment of these displaced fractures.

Just over a year after Goss's paper appeared, two other papers by Kavanagh *et al* (1993) and Leung *et al.,*(1993) reported on small series' of displaced intra-articular glenoid fractures treated operatively.

Kavanagh *et al.'s* paper reported on nine displaced glenoid fractures with an average follow-up of 4 years. In this series, all patients were immobilized for 6 weeks postoperatively in a spica cast with the arm in 45° of abduction. Kavanagh reported fracture-healing at 3.5 months, with no patient reporting pain with daily use. Two patients had 'barometric' shoulders with aching evident when the weather changed. Range of motion was surprisingly good, despite the prolonged immobilization, with an average of 167° active abduction and 171° of flexion. Strength was reported as normal in seven patients, with mild weakness in the remaining two patients. There were no reported problems with loosening of implants and the only complication reported was a single patient with heterotopic bone. This patient had an associated closed head injury and surgery had been delayed by 5 days.

Leung *et al.'s* paper (1993) reported on 14 displaced intra-articular glenoid fractures. Leung's follow-up was an average of 30.5 months and he reports an average time for healing of 8.5 weeks, with no non-unions or infections. Fifty percent of his patients had no pain on activity while the remaining 50% reported slight pain on use. Range of motion achieved was good, with 64% regaining over 150° of abduction and flexion and the remainder achieving over 120° of abduction and flexion. There were no poor results in this series, with all patients resuming employment within a year of injury.

Figure 15.11 illustrates a typical high-energy intra-articular glenoid fracture that occurred after a fall from a bicycle. The injury was associated with a comminuted fracture of the clavicle, a haemopneumothorax and fractures of the upper three ribs. The patient was resuscitated, a chest drain was inserted prior to surgery and the clavicle fracture treated operatively using a reconstruction plate and cancellous bone graft. The patient was then turned prone and the glenoid fracture stabilized through a posterior approach. The patient regained a functional pain-free shoulder within 6 months.

Summary

Scapular fractures are high-energy injuries with a high incidence of serious associated injury. Initial treatment must be directed at dealing with the immediately life-threatening injuries. Computerized tomography scanning with 3D-imaging may be required to determine the fracture pattern and degree of displacement. The majority of fractures involving the body, spine and apophyses can be managed non-operatively. Displaced intra-articular fractures of the glenoid require open reduction and internal fixation. Grossly displaced fractures of the neck may also require stabilization. Rehabilitation should be supervised, progressive and include functional activities. It may take up to 12 months for the final functional result to be achieved.

CHAPTER 16

Paralysis and dystrophy around the shoulder

T. Bunker

Introduction

A wide range of diseases present at the shoulder clinic. In every clinic the shoulder surgeon is faced with cases of impingement, a variety of cuff tears, dislocations and subluxations, old fractures, malunions, non-unions, contractures, rheumatoid arthritis, osteo-arthritis, and secondary arthritis. Additionally, the shoulder surgeon is faced with rarer neurological disorders. Such disorders include suprascapular nerve entrapment and fascioscapulohumeral (FSH) dystrophy. In some cases effective treatments for these conditions are available, they include decompression of nerves, grafting of nerves, transferring muscles and fusion of joints.

Reviewing the last 1687 referrals to my shoulder clinic, 93 were for neurological disorders (Table 16.1). Three conditions accounted for two-thirds of these cases. The main three diagnoses were referred pain from the cervical spine, winging of the scapula, and thoracic outlet syndrome (TOS). The second league of diagnoses were brachial plexus injury, stroke shoulder, FSH dystrophy, neuralgic amyotrophy, suprascapular nerve-entrapment syndrome, syringomyelia, accessory nerve palsy, axillary nerve palsy, tetraplegia shoulder and dystonia. Curios were multiple sclerosis, polio and backpacker's shoulder. For each of these conditions we shall consider the functional anatomy, clinical presentation, examination, differential diagnosis and treatment.

Table 16.1 Neurological problems encountered in the shoulder clinic.

Referred pain from the cervical spine
Winging of scapula
Thoracic outlet syndrome
Brachial plexus injury
Stroke shoulder
Fascioscapulohumeral dystrophy
Neuralgic amyotrophy
Suprascapular nerve-entrapment syndrome
Syringomyelia
Accessory nerve palsy
Tetraplegia shoulder
Dystonia
Polio
Multiple sclerosis
Backpacker's shoulder

Referred pain from the cervical spine

Pain caused by irritation of the cervical spine nerve roots may be difficult to differentiate from true shoulder pain.

Neck pain accounts for the largest group of patients attending the shoulder clinic with neurological pain.

Clues as to the referred nature of the pain are the quality, radiation and associations of the pain. Pain referred from the neck may have a burning nature. The radiation is usually from the neck to the shoulder whereas true shoulder pain is based on the shoulder, but may radiate up into the trapezius. Neck pain often radiates into the occiput. The distal pattern of pain is different; shoulder pain radiates to the insertion of the deltoid muscle, lateral aspect of the elbow, radial border of the wrist and, very occasionally, the base of the thenar eminence. If the patient describes pain radiating distal to the radial border of the wrist, you must have a high index of suspicion that this is referred pain. Neurological symptoms may occur with shoulder subluxation, but again should alert the surgeon to the possibility of the patient having referred pain from the neck.

If the history alerts you to the possibility of the pain originating from the neck, you must be extra alert and observe the patient's neck movement during the interview, and before they suspect that an examination has started.

On examination observe the posture of the neck, be alert for spinal tenderness, paraspinal spasm, and tenderness over the assembling supraclavicular brachial plexus. Look at the full range of neck movement, the speed and quality of movement, end-point pain and pain on overpressure.

Objective physical signs are unusual in patients with neck pain. Norris and Watt (1983) recorded a neurological deficit in only 10 of 63 patients with soft-tissue injury of the neck; 10 had altered sensation, 6 had weakness and only 1 had a diminished biceps jerk. However, if alerted to the possibility of neck pain a full neurological examination should be undertaken as described in chapter one.

Neck pain is not exacerbated by shoulder movement and rarely leads on to shoulder stiffness. How to investigate and treat neck pain is beyond the remit of this book.

Winging of the scapula

Of the true neurological disorders of the shoulder, loss of thoracoscapular control leads the field (Fig. 16.1).

The scapula has a number of functions. Firstly, it acts as a stable base for glenohumeral movement. Secondly,

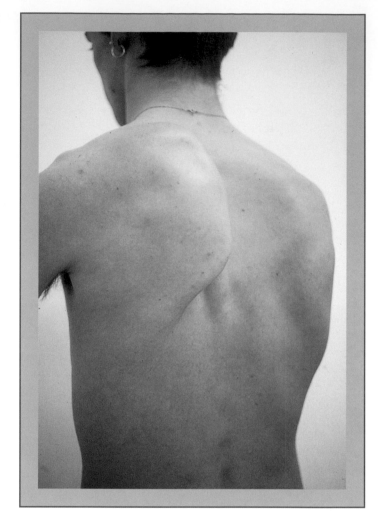

Figure 16.1 – *Winging of the scapula.*

it acts in synchrony with the glenohumeral joint and is responsible for one-third of the global range of shoulder movement. Thirdly, it adds to the stability of the glenohumeral joint by moving in harmony to maintain the resultant forces within the arc of the small glenoid surface. Fourthly, it acts as a shock absorber, soaking up the peak-loads sustained by the arm.

Since one-third of shoulder movement originates from the scapula, a loss of scapular control leads to a marked deficit in shoulder movement. If all scapular control has gone, such as is the case in FSH dystrophy, the scapula will actually move the wrong way as the deltoid muscle powers-up (reversed scapular rhythm), leading to a tremendous deficit in shoulder function, far in excess of the one-third that it should provide.

Seven muscles attach the scapula to the thorax: trapezius, serratus anterior, levator scapulae, the two rhomboids, pectoralis minor, and the omohyoid. The latissimus dorsi muscle has a partial attachment to the inferior tip of the scapula, but scapular stability is not its major function. The omohyoid is an often neglected muscle because its action upon the scapula is so small.

Of the above muscles, the trapezius and serratus anterior are by far the most important. Weakness or paralysis of either of these large muscles will lead to loss of scapulothoracic control, commonly seen as winging of the scapula.

Trapezius

The trapezius muscle acts to suspend, elevate, retract and rotate the scapula. It is supplied by the spinal accessory nerve. The spinal accessory nerve is the 11th cranial nerve. It travels a most circuitous route; its fibres start in the accessory nucleus which lies within the cervical spinal cord, extending from the 2nd to 6th cervical segments. The fibres then pass up through the foramen magnum into the skull and then out of the jugular foramen to exit the skull again. The nerve enters the sternomastoid muscle, which it supplies, and emerges into the posterior triangle of the neck at the junction of the superior and middle thirds of the sternomastoid. Crossing the posterior triangle the nerve then disappears under the anterior fold of the trapezius supplying four branches to the upper trapezius (Fig. 16.2). It then lies on the deep surface of the trapezius, to pass caudally, supplying the rest of the muscle.

The major risk to this nerve is the scalpel. The nerve is highly vulnerable to inexperienced surgeons at this point for it is closely related to the posterocervical lymph nodes. These lymph nodes, when swollen, appear irresistable to the budding biopsy skills of physicians and young surgeons, with inevitable consequences. The nerve may be deliberately sacrificed during radical dissection of the neck. The nerve may be cut during knife or 'glassing' fights, by blunt trauma, traction injury from 'whiplash' or brachial plexus traction injury. It is rare for the nerve to be damaged by neuralgic amyotrophy or radiation neuritis.

Clinically, the patient presents with pain, a drooped shoulder, facial numbness or paraesthesia, and weakness of elevation of the arm. The facial numbness and paraesthesiae are usually caused by concomitant injury to the transverse cervical and great auricular nerves, which emerge alongside the spinal accessory from the posterior margin of sternomastoid. Wasting of trapezius may be apparent. The scapula may wing because the

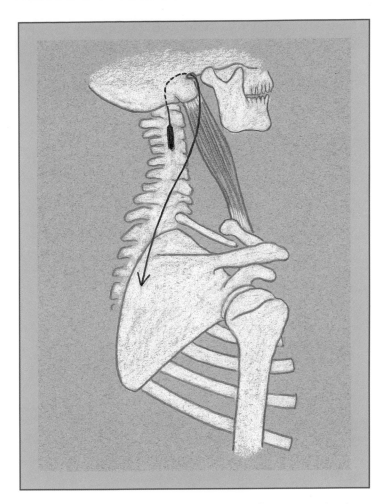

Figure 16.2 – *The spinal accessory nerve takes a most circuitous course to the trapezius.*

trapezius can no longer hold down the medial border of the scapula to the chest wall.

On examination the posture of the shoulder is assymetric, being lower than on the normal side. A scar is often present in the posterior triangle of the neck. The trapezius muscle is weak, as tested by the shoulder shrug. The scapula is rotated and wings.

If the nerve has been divided by surgery or a knife-wound, and is recognized, then it should be explored and repaired. Muscle transfers are far less successful than immediate nerve repair. However, the diagnosis is often delayed and repair is not possible. The favoured muscle transfer is the Eden–Lange operation. This has superseded the Dewar-type fasciodesis which tended to stretch out in the long term. The Eden–Lange transfer involves transfer of levator scapulae to the mid point of the spine of the scapula, and transfer of the rhomboids to the infraspinatus fossa. Bigliani *et al.* (1985) reported functional improvement with pain relief in six of seven cases.

Serratus anterior

The commonest cause of winging is weakness or paralysis of the serratus anterior muscle, secondary to a palsy of the long thoracic nerve.

The long thoracic nerve is formed from the anterior primary rami of C5 and C6; in more than half of patients there is a contribution from C7, and in one-third from C4. The nerve assembles within scalenus medius and then passes down posterior to the plexus over the first rib and on to serratus anterior giving branches to each digitation. It is quite a small nerve being only 2 mm in diameter.

The function of the serratus anterior muscle is to hold the scapula against the chest wall during pushing, punching and elevation of the arm. It is tested by asking the patient to press forwards against a wall (a standing press-up).

The long thoracic nerve may be injured during surgery, particularly during lymph node harvest (for staging carcinoma of the breast), during transaxillary excision of the first rib, with traction lesions of the brachial plexus, and sometimes from pressure of crutches or lying comatose with pressure against the chest wall (Saturday night palsy). However, one of the commonest causes is neuralgic amyotrophy.

Vastamaki and Kampilla (1993) examined the cause of serratus anterior palsy in 197 patients. In the largest group (35%) palsy was thought to be due to strenuous work or sports. Twenty-six percent of cases occurred as a result of local trauma, 11% of cases followed after surgery in the vicinity of the nerve, 6% of cases were associated with infections, 5% of cases occurred after anaesthesia and 17% of cases were unaccounted for. The median age of patients in this huge study was 29 years. Kaupilla (1993) felt that the majority of serratus anterior palsies were caused by pressure on the nerve by the lower angle of the scapula. Frostick (1996) has recently proposed surgical decompression of the long thoracic nerve in patients with winging, and suggests that the nerve is compressed subfascially during its course down the muscle.

Three-quarters of patients will recover in 12 to 18 months. The question is what to do for the remaining quarter with residual winging? Post (1995) describes transposition of the sternal head of pectoralis major to the inferior pole of the scapula using a coiled and sutured fascia lata graft. He states that this is an excellent operation for correcting scapular winging.

Neuralgic amyotrophy

This intriguing condition presents with severe shoulder and arm pain. This is often preceded by an influenza-like illness, generalized muscle aching and fever. Within days of the onset of pain there is marked weakness of the shoulder girdle. The pain then fades, but the patient is left with shoulder-girdle weakness, often involving serratus anterior, and causing winging and weakness of abduction and elevation of the arm. The prognosis for recovery is good, with 36% recovered at 1 year and 89% by 3 years.

The condition was first noticed by Spillane (1943) in soldiers during the Tobruk campaign of 1943, and there are similarities with 'Gulf War Syndrome'. In both cases service personnel were affected in a desert campaign. In both cases these personnel had been recently immunized. In both cases soldiers were treated with insecticides to prevent tick infestation. Dichloro-diphenyl-trichloro-ethane (DDT) and organophosphorus insecticides are both known causes of peripheral neuropathy. In both cases the patients suffered from a vague arthralgia, muscle aching and weakness.

In the cases described in the Tobruk campaign half of the sufferers were in hospital during the onset of the illness, 14 % had recently been immunized and a quarter gave a history of an influenza-like illness.

Recently human parvovirus 19 has been implicated in the aetiology of neuralgic amyotrophy (Flowers & Cowling, 1993). The condition commonly affects the deltoid, spinati, biceps and triceps as well as serratus anterior. Sensory changes occur in two-thirds of cases. The right arm is affected more commonly than the left, and men are affected more than women. Electromyograph (EMG) studies show fibrillation potentials and positive waves. The condition goes by a large number of differing names, such as brachial neuritis, brachial plexus neuropathy, and Parsonage–Turner syndrome, all of which add to the confusion. Differential diagnosis should include peripheral neuropathy from any cause (Table 16.2) Peripheral neuropathy may stem from toxic causes (arsenic, lead, mercury, alcohol, isoniazid, DDT and organophosphorus poisons such as sheep dip),

Table 16.2 Causes of peripheral neuropathy.

- Toxic
  - Arsenic
  - Lead
  - Mercury
  - Alcohol
  - Isoniazid
  - DDT
  - Organophosphorus
- Metabolic
  - Diabetes
  - Uraemia
  - Porphyria
- Deficiency
  - Vitamin B
  - Alcohol poisoning
- Radiation
- Infective
  - Leprosy
  - Diptheria
  - Tetanus
  - Polio
  - Parvovirus

metabolic causes (diabetes, uraemia, porphyria), deficiency syndromes (vitamin B, alcohol poisoning), radiation, neuritis, and infections (leprosy, diptheria, tetanus; polio, parvovirus).

The treatment of neuralgic amyotrophy is to await resolution. Most cases of isolated paralysis of serratus anterior will resolve spontaneously within 12 months. However, painful, chronic, disabling winging caused by an isolated serratus anterior palsy can be treated with a transfer of the sternal head of pectoralis major to the inferior pole of the scapula, using a fascia lata graft. This has superseded the transfer of pectoralis minor. Post (1995) reported excellent results in eight patients and describes the technical minutiae which must be followed to achieve a successful result from pectoralis major transfer.

Fascioscapulohumeral dystrophy

Fascioscapulohumeral dystrophy is an autosomal dominant disease with wide expression. Patients present from the ages of 13 to 30 usually with gross symmetrical wasting and weakness of scapulo-thoracic control. The dystrophy affects the facial muscles, trapezius, levator scapulae and the rhomboids, serratus anterior, biceps and triceps. The deltoid appears to be spared, or may even hypertrophy leading to a 'superman' appearance. Although this is a progressive muscular dystrophy, life expectancy is normal. When the patient attempts to elevate the arm the scapula rotates internally, instead of externally. Abduction may thus be severely limited to 40–60° only. This is associated with marked fatiguing. The diagnosis should be confirmed by a neurologist because other more generalized forms of muscular dystrophy can mimic FSH dystrophy.

If the scapular weakness is severe then scapulothoracic fusion should be considered. The Copeland–Howard fusion is a highly effective operation in FSH dystrophy (Fig. 16.3). However, it is also quite an ordeal for the patient as it involves not only the operation itself but 3 months in a cast or brace, and stress fractures of the ribs may occur during the rehabilitation phase. It says a lot for the operation that despite this, patients will usually request that the second side is done.

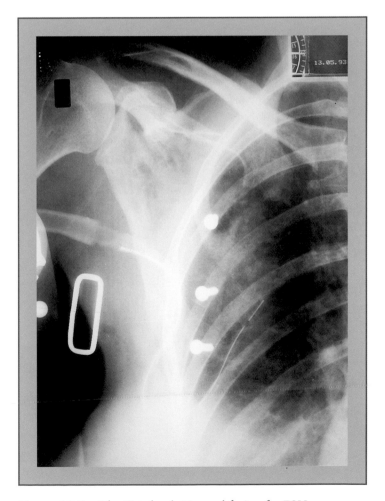

Figure 16.3 – *The Copeland–Howard fusion for FSH.*

Pseudowinging

No discussion of winging is complete without speaking of pseudowinging. Pseudowinging may be caused by pain or a space-occupying lesion lying between the scapula and the ribs.

Pseudowinging from pain is commonly seen in impingement and rotator-cuff tears as the patient brings the arm down from full elevation. In order to limit the impingement pain, the patient will lock the glenohumeral joint, and wing the scapula through the painful arc of movement. Once the arm has come down to 40° of elevation the patient will unlock the glenohumeral joint and the scapula will come back to its normal position. This is a trick-movement that patients learn to avoid pain.

The commonest space-occupying lesion between the scapula and chest wall is an osteochondroma of the scapula (Fig. 16.4). This may be an isolated lesion but is more commonly found in diaphyseal aclasia.

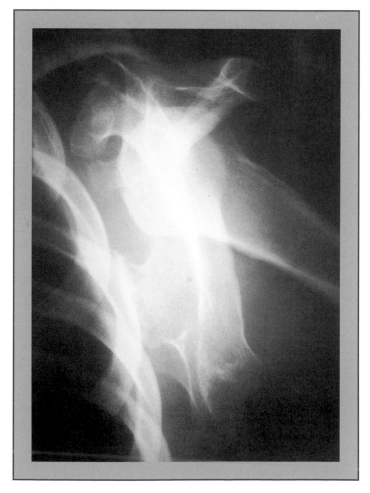

Figure 16.4 – *Osteochondromata of the scapula causing pseudowinging.*

Thoracic outlet syndrome

Thoracic outlet syndrome is a rare disease that stretches the diagnostic talents of vascular surgeons, neurosurgeons, thoracic surgeons, orthopaedic surgeons, neurologists and psychologists, because its symptoms may be vague and span the territory of all these specialists.

The thoracic outlet can be likened to a three-sided pyramid (Fig. 16.5). The actual outlet lies within the triangular floor of this pyramid. The medial half of the floor is the first rib and the outer half is the outlet itself. The triangular floor thus has three sides: the posterior side, the medial side, and the hypotenuse, which is the clavicle. The posterior wall of this pyramid is the scalenus medius and trapezius. The medial wall is the neck; this wall can be split into thirds, the posterior third being the lateral masses of the vertebra, the middle third is the carotid artery, and the anterior third is the internal jugular. Each of the three contents of the thoracic outlet (the subclavian vein, artery, and the brachial plexus) is donated from its third of the medial wall. So far this is very simple, a three-sided pyramid, arising from a three-sided triangular base and containing three structures. This simple pyramid is partitioned by scalenus anterior; this strap-like sheet of muscle partitions the brachial plexus from the carotid sheath and runs down to insert right into the mid-point of the triangular base on to the first rib at the scalene tubercle. The subclavian artery arises from the innominate artery or aorta in front of scalenus anterior and passes under it so that it emerges behind scalenus anterior with the plexus. The phrenic nerve passes down on the front of scalenus anterior.

This outlet can be narrowed in a variety of ways. If we look at the base triangle, to start with, the medial border can be stenosed by a cervical rib or fibrous band. Poor posture can lead to the arm drooping and the outlet closing. Deformity of the clavicle such as callus, shortening or hypertrophic non-union will constrict the hypotenuse. If the scalenus anterior is hypertrophied, unusually inserted, or fibrous it can crowd the outlet further. Crowding of the outlet in any way will cause compression of the artery, vein, or brachial plexus. The plexus is the most vulnerable to such compression, and neurological symptoms are thus the commonest. The lower roots of the brachial plexus — C8 and T1 — are the most vulnerable which leads to the peculiar radiation of neurological symptoms in TOS. The

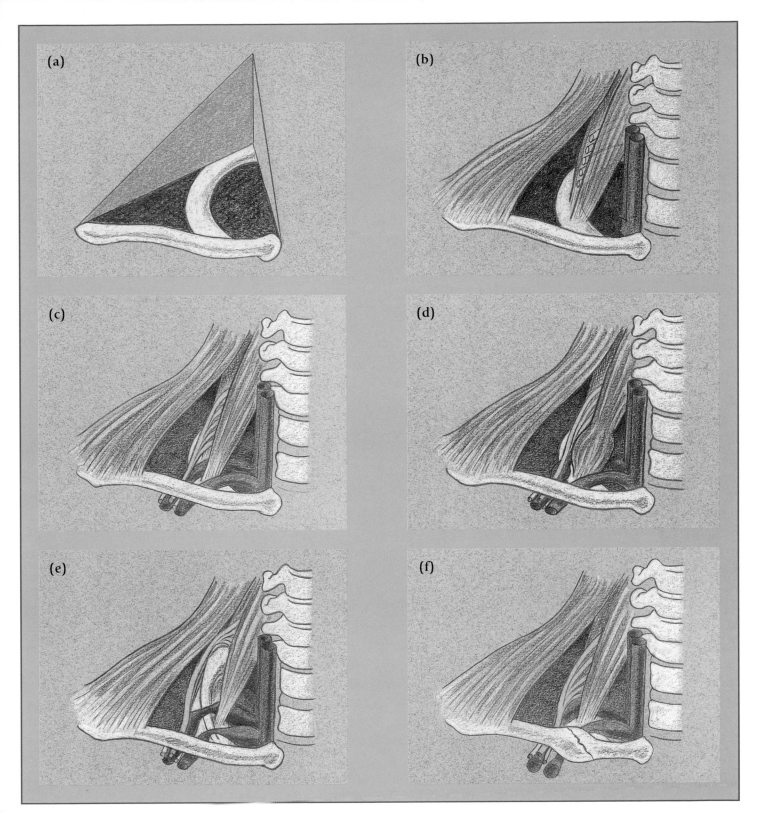

Figure 16.5 – *The thoracic outlet is like a three-sided pyramid (a). It is divided by scalenus anterior (b). It contains three structures: the subclavian vein, subclavian artery and brachial plexus (c). This outlet can be narrowed by (d) hypertrophy or a band in scalenus anterior, (e) a cervical rib or band or (f) malunion or callus from a fracture of the clavicle.*

radiation of the pain goes to the ulnar side of the wrist and the chest wall. True shoulder pain, on the other hand, always radiates to the radial side of the wrist. Alarm bells should ring if your patient describes pain in the ulnar nerve distribution or to the axilla and chest wall. The pain is made worse by carrying or lifting, and is severe when lying on that side at night.

Rarer is the upper plexus form of TOS which may present with shoulder pain radiating to the scapula and occiput, with distal radiation in the C5/C6 distribution. Headache and facial pain are common in this variety of TOS.

The sympathetic nerves also pass within the brachial plexus and they may be compressed causing a neuralgic-type pain (cold water running down the arm), and may cause skin colour changes with a cool, sweaty, dusky hand. These vasomotor changes are similar to Raynaud's disease.

Thirty percent of patients may have objective sensory loss, but muscle wasting is very rare occurring in less than 10% of cases.

There are three grades of vascular change in TOS. The first is diminished flow leading to exercise intolerance, particularly pain on overhead activity, and is the basis of Roos' test. The second is organic vascular change such as absent pulses, and thrombi thrown off the subclavian stenosis, or poststenotic dilatation; however, this is very rare, occuring in less than 10% of cases and usually presenting directly to the vascular surgeon. The third vascular manifestation is the sympathetic effect, which is very common. Venous compression is rare.

The diagnosis of TOS is made more difficult because the symptoms are hard for the patient to describe. The diagnosis is often confused with those homeopathic non-diagnoses beloved by orthopaedic physicians and fringe practitioners — fibromyalgia, shoulder girdle syndrome, postural pain, conversion syndrome and emotional disorders. This may lead to a chicken and egg situation for the patient is fobbed off for so long that they become depressed and emotionally unstable and the true diagnosis gets buried further.

There are three objective tests which should be used on all patients thought to have TOS. These are Roos' test, the military brace test and Adson's test.

Roos' test

This is the best objective test for TOS. The test is carried out by abducting both arms and shoulders to 90° and getting the patient to open and close the hands slowly but forceably for a period of 3 minutes. The test is sometimes called the overhead exercise test, and most patients with TOS will not be able to perform the test for anything like 3 minutes on the affected side. Roos' test is positive in 96% of cases proven at operation (Thompson, 1996).

The military brace test

This is also called the costoclavicular test. The patient stands with the hands comfortably to his sides. The surgeon then places a stethoscope over the supraclavicular fossa and feels the radial pulse with the other hand. The patient is asked to forceably brace the shoulders backwards, and downwards, as though a soldier on parade. The test is positive if the pulse fades, or a bruit appears.

Adson's test

Although this test was one of the first for TOS, it is not as accurate as Roos' test or the 'military brace test'. Adson called this his 'vascular test'. The patient sits comfortably, with the surgeon palpating the radial pulse. The patient is then asked to take a deep breath, as in a valsalva manoeuvre, and to turn the neck to the affected side with the chin thrust upwards. The test is postive if the pulse fades.

Auscultation over the subclavian artery may reveal a bruit. Tenderness to palpation over the brachial plexus may be found and a positive Tinel sign. Occasionally, intrinsic muscle wasting may be present. Grip strength may be reduced and two-point discrimination impaired in the ulnar nerve distribution.

The diagnosis of TOS is really a clinical one, there are very few investigations which may help to confirm the diagnosis. Arteriography will confirm subclavian compression or poststenotic dilatation. Arteriography has been superseded by duplex ultrasonography which may show a reduced flow in the axillary artery or even obstruction. Duplex ultrasound may show turbulence or velocity shifts in the subclavian artery (Fig. 16.6). The subclavian vein can also be examined by ultrasound and may show stenosis at the site of compression by the first rib. However, two-position venography remains the gold standard. Duplex ultrasound can be repeated pre- and postoperatively. Duplex scanning is positive in 93% of patients proven at surgery to have TOS (Thompson, 1996). The use of electrodiagnostic tests remains controversial.

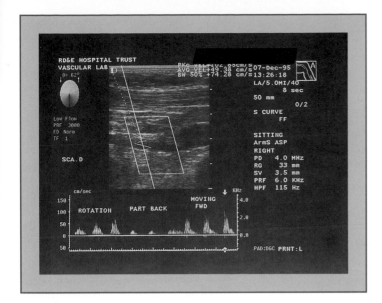

Figure 16.6 – *Duplex ultrasound investigation in TOS. Diminution of the pulse wave form can be seen as the trace at the bottom of the picture as the patient raises and then lowers the arm.*

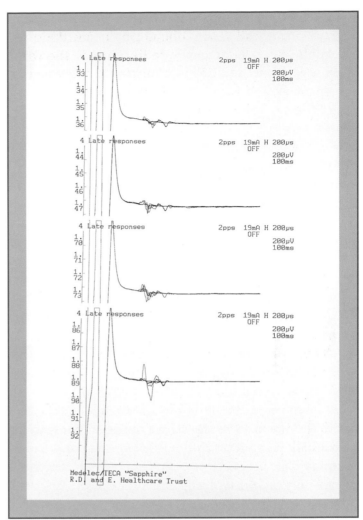

Figure 16.7 – *Abnormal reflex F-wave in TOS.*

The first use of neurophysiological testing is to exclude a more peripheral site of compression of the ulnar nerve. Abnormal reflex F-wave conduction and decreased sensory action potentials in the medial cutaneous nerve of the forearm may clinch the diagnosis (Fig. 16.7).

Treatment of TOS is initially always conservative. Postural retraining and physiotherapy, using exercises to strengthen the trapezius and levator scapulae are recommended. In patients who fail to improve with conservative therapy, consideration should be given to surgical decompression. Decompression may be either through the anterior approach, or more commonly today, using the transaxillary excision of the first rib.

A detailed description of these operations is beyond the limits of this chapter. In brief the anterior approach utilizes a half necklace incision. Platysma is divided and undermined to expose the posterior triangle of the neck. The clavicular head of sternomastoid is mobilized from the clavicle and the omohyoid is divided on stay-stitches. The fat pad is the mobilized, dividing the transverse cervical artery and suprascapular artery, in order to expose scalenus anterior. The phrenic nerve is exposed on the anterior border of scalenus anterior and is protected throughout. Scalenus anterior is then resected from the scalene tubercle, and if a cervical rib is present this is excised. This operation has gone out of favour since the results of transaxillary first-rib excision have shown better results.

In transaxillary excision of the first rib the assistant holds the arm abducted in a 'wrist lock', and a transverse incision is made over the third rib. The chest wall is followed up to the first rib taking great care not to damage the intercostobrachial nerves and the long thoracic nerve. Once the first rib is exposed it is resected taking great care not to damage the T1 root, subclavian artery or the more friable vein. At the end of the procedure, saline is introduced into the resulting cavity in order to check that there is no pneumothorax, which is common because the apex of the lung is just medial to the rib.

Brachial plexus injury

The surgical care of brachial plexus injury is one of the most specialized and demanding areas of orthopaedic surgery. For this reason most orthopaedic surgeons will assess the patient, stabilize them and then refer on, as soon as possible, to a regional specialist centre that deals with these patients. At the specialist centre the brachial plexus will be explored in a situation that allows microsurgical repair and grafting of the plexus (plexoplexal transfer), as well as nerve transfer (extraplexal transfer), for instance spinal accessory to suprascapular, and intercostal to musculocutaneous nerve, with interposed cable grafting from cervical sensory rami or lateral cutaneous nerve of the forearm. It is estimated that there are 350 supraclavicular brachial plexus injuries each year in the UK and 150 severe infraclavicular injuries. Even in highly specialized centres the number of explorations will be small, for instance Millesi performed 40 transfers in 10 years and Narakas (1987) 108 in 15 years.

Assessment of brachial plexus injury is dependent upon a good working knowledge of the anatomy of the region. The method of injury is important. Low-energy injury is seen in sportsmen and leads to the 'burner' or 'stinger' — a mild plexus injury seen in American football tackles. 'Burners' and 'stingers' usually have an excellent prognosis for early and complete recovery. At the other end of the scale is the high speed, high energy, motor cycle injury where a multiply injured motorcyclist arrives in the emergency room with life-threatening chest and head injuries. In this situation a high level of suspicion is required because the patient is often comatose from their head injury. Asymmetric loss of arm movement, swelling and bruising in the posterior triangle, and fractured transverse processes of the first and second ribs should alert the surgeon to the possibility of a brachial plexus injury. A Horner's syndrome suggests avulsion of the T1 root, and sometimes the C8 root. Fluoroscopic visualization of the diaphragm using an image intensifier may show a hemidiaphragmatic paralysis, which implies a supraganglionic lesion of C4 and C5. In this situation, resuscitation according to advanced trauma life support (ATLS) principles takes precedence over assessment of the plexus, but the surgeon should be just as alert for a plexus injury as he is for a cervical spine injury.

In the conscious patient, with an isolated brachial plexus lesion, manual muscle testing should build a picture of the level of the lesion. Total paralysis of the limb including serratus anterior with a persistent Horner's syndrome, accompanied by an insensate arm (with the exception of the epaulette region C4, and the lateral axilla supplied by the intercostobrachial nerve T2) implies root avulsion from C5 to T1. Paralysis of the shoulder and elbow with sensory loss in the radial border of the arm and the thumb and index finger imply a C5, C6 root injury, whilst paralysis of the hand with insensibility of the ring and little fingers and the ulnar border of the forearm implies a C8,T1 lesion. However, if serratus is intact, but the supraspinatus and infraspinatus are paralysed, this implies a lesion beyond the foraminal exits but proximal to Erb's point. Sensory examination should be performed for light touch and pin prick. If there is a significant neurological injury there are usually vasomotor changes because the sympathetic nerves accompany the ramifications of the brachial plexus, and will share their fate. Seventy-five percent of lesions are supraclavicular and only 25% retroclavicular or infraclavicular. The more distal the injury the better the prognosis following surgical reconstruction. Every patient should have plain radiographs of the cervical spine and shoulder girdle. If a vascular injury is suspected then immediate aortic arch arteriography should be performed. Immediate emergency surgery is mandatory if there is concomitant nerve and vascular injury. Precise diagnosis of the level of injury is now performed by early surgical exploration of the brachial plexus. In this context early means within 48 hours. The histamine test is no longer used. Further investigations such as computerized tomography (CT), magnetic resonance imaging (MRI) or electrodiagnosis should be performed at the regional centre.

Birch (1995) has summarized the results of nerve repair and transfer. He states that:

(a) Repair of ruptures in the posterior triangle gives worthwhile shoulder and elbow function in two-thirds of cases.
(b) Nerve transfer has improved the outlook for shoulder and elbow function in preganglionic injuries to C5, C6 and C7.
(c) In complete lesions, a combination of conventional grafting with nerve transfer gives a chance of some

modest return of hand function in children and young adults.

(d) Re-innervation of the limb secures significant pain-relief in many patients.

(e) Delay in repair is harmful. The earlier the repair the better. After 6 months failure is the rule.

(f) Results of primary grafting of nerves at the same time as urgent vascular repair are better than when nerve repair is delayed.

(g) A closely monitored programme of rehabilitation is essential.

Late reconstruction

The results of muscle transfers and arthrodeses are much poorer than the results of early nerve repair and grafting.

Arthrodesis of the shoulder may be indicated in the patient who has elbow flexion, a useful hand, and in whom there is some scapular control (trapezius and serratus anterior power MRC4+), but where the rotator cuff and deltoid are paralysed, and where re-innervation of these muscles is impossible or has failed. The aim of shoulder arthrodesis is to allow the hand to reach the mouth (Fig. 16.8).

External rotation osteotomy of the humerus is sometimes indicated in patients who have active elbow flexion, but a severe internal rotation contracture of the shoulder.

Latissimus dorsi transfer may be of some use in patients who have a powerful latissimus, but have lost suprascapular nerve function. It is based upon the operation of L'Episcopo for obstetric brachial plexus palsy. Unfortunately, this operation is nowhere near as good in adults, as it is in young children.

Obstetric brachial plexus palsy

There appear to be two major factors associated with obstetric brachial plexus palsy (OBPP) — overweight cephalic presentations with shoulder dystocia, and the underweight breech presentation. Narakas (1987) has classified OBPP into four groups and this classification is now widely used.

Group 1 (C5 and C6)

The shoulder and the flexors of the elbow are paralysed. The arm lies in the classic Erb Duchenne posture. Approximately 90% of babies make a full and spontaneous recovery of shoulder and elbow function. The hand is normal throughout.

Group 2 (C5, C6 and C7)

This is a more serious injury. There is paralysis of the shoulder, elbow flexion and wrist extension, and elbow extension. There is spontaneous recovery to 75% at the wrist and elbow, but only to 50% in the shoulder.

Group 3 (C5 to T1)

This is a severe injury. Paralysis of the whole arm is complete. Only one-third of babies will see spontaneous recovery in the limb, the shoulder having the worst prognosis.

Group 4 (C5 to T1 with Horner's syndrome)

All the spinal nerves have a preganglionic injury. This is a devastating injury from which there is never any recovery.

A full discussion of the management of babies with OBPP is beyond the remit of this text. In simple terms the baby should be examined by an experienced orthopaedic surgeon at the earliest opportunity. The smallest observation must be detailed, as it may drop the child from one group to another and make a great difference to the prognosis. Clearly a Horner's syndrome is of the most severe importance. The baby should have a radiograph of the shoulder and neck, because fracture of the clavicle may present as a pseudoparalysis, or may be associated with OBPP. The baby should be re-examined at 2 weeks, and then at monthly intervals. Babies in group 1 should show some recovery at 1 month and full recovery at around 5 months. The key

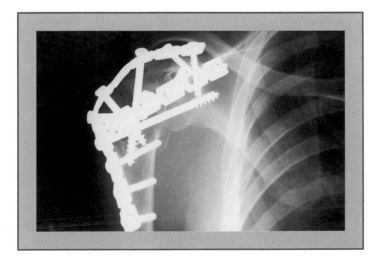

Figure 16.8 – *Arthrodesis of the shoulder. Two plates have been used as well as lag screws from the humerus to the acromion and glenoid.*

decision should be made at 3 months. If there is evidence of recovery of biceps function at this time then further conservative management is justified. However, if there is no recovery at the 3-month stage the baby should be referred to a major brachial plexus centre, as nerve grafting at this stage can improve the prognosis markedly. Half the children having grafting to C5, C6 will have an excellent to good recovery. If C7 is damaged and requires grafting, the excellent and good results drop to 25%.

Late surgery for OBPP should be undertaken in a strict order, firstly release of contractures, secondly correcting deformity and finally transferring muscles to regain power. Zancolli's modification of the L'Episcopo operation is the most widespread procedure to correct internal rotation at the shoulder. In this operation the latissimus dorsi is Z-plastied, and the distal part of the tendon is taken around the humerus and then sutured to the proximal part of the Z-plastied tendon, changing latissimus from an internal rotator to an external rotator. Pectoralis is transferred up to the distal end of subscapularis.

A derotation osteotomy of the humerus can be very helpful in the face of an internal rotation contracture, especially if there are significant changes to the bony architecture of the glenohumeral joint.

Suprascapular nerve-entrapment syndrome

This is a rare condition and consequently diagnosis may initially be difficult. The course of the suprascapular nerve is shown in Figure 16.9. In the early stages the patient presents with impingement-like shoulder pain. The pain is true shoulder pain, worse at night, and often increased on reaching and lifting. Radiographs are normal. The surgeon may be alerted to the diagnosis because the patient is not relieved of their pain by the impingement-test of Xylocaine injected into the subacromial bursa.

The differential diagnosis is helped by the rapid and severe wasting of the infraspinatus, which is noted at 8–12 weeks after the onset of pain. The differential diagnosis now becomes cuff tear or suprascapular nerve-entrapment syndrome, because there is marked wasting, weakness and true shoulder pain. However, the patient is usually much younger than the normally encountered cuff-tear patient aged late 50s to 70 years. Additionally, there is rarely a history of injury, there is no tenderness

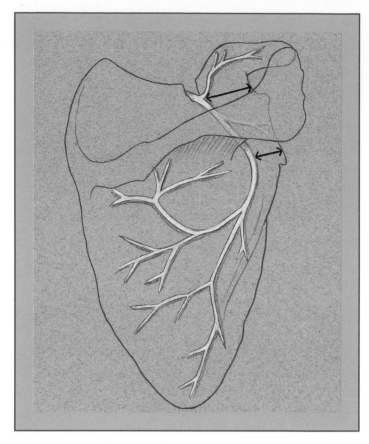

Figure 16.9 – *The course of the suprascapular nerve.*

over the supraspinatus insertion, no sulcus and eminence, no crepitus on elevation, and no easing of pain and motion on stooping. One variant of suprascapular nerve-entrapment syndrome is backpackers shoulder. This is thought to be caused by pressure from the shoulder straps of a backpack upon the suprascapular nerve.

In this situation an MRI is the investigation of choice because it will reveal two things. First it will reveal that there is no cuff tear, and second it may show a ganglion, at the spinoglenoid notch, compressing the suprascapular nerve (Fig. 16.10). However, a ganglion is unusual, normally the nerve is compressed in the suprascapular notch.

Neurophysiological studies confirm the diagnosis because they show that the infraspinatus is partially or totally denervated, and that there is a slow latency from Erb's point to infraspinatus. As soon as the diagnosis is confirmed the patient should undergo surgical decompression. There is no place for conservative treatment (Post, 1995) because the results of surgery are excellent and the incidence of complications miniscule.

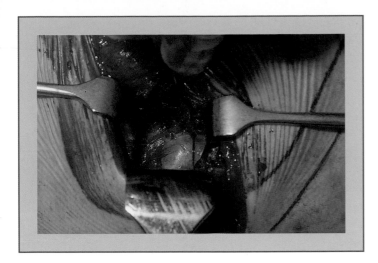

Figure 16.10 – *Surgery of spinoglenoid ganglion compressing the suprascapular nerve.*

The patient is placed in the lateral decubitus position. Surgery is best undertaken through a skin-crease incision over the top of the shoulder, and slightly medial to the normal Matsen deltoid-on approach. Although surgery can be undertaken using a trapezius split, access is poor and the author prefers to take the trapezius down from the clavicle, acromioclavicular joint, acromion and spine of the scapula, and then to re-attach it through drill holes at the close of the procedure. This gives an excellent approach to the supraspinatus fossa. The fat pad over the supraspinatus is divided and often contains a sizeable branch from the suprascapular artery. Supraspinatus is then retracted backwards to expose the floor of the suprascapular fossa. The suprascapular artery is found coursing over the suprascapular ligament, with the nerve below the ligament. Occasionally, the ligament may be ossified, in which case the nerve will be found emerging from a bony foramen in the scapula. The ligament is excised, and the notch is expanded and opened up using Cloward's spinal rongeurs.

In the case of a ganglion compressing the nerve at the spinoglenoid notch, a posterior approach is made, as for recurrent posterior dislocation. A skin-crease incision is made and the deltoid is split. The ganglion is usually quite obvious at this point, but sometimes the infraspinatus will need to be tenotomized on stay-sutures to expose the ganglion properly. Usually the ganglion will peel out like a grapeskin. Pain relief is felt almost immediately. The sling should be worn for 2 weeks. The degree of restitution of muscle bulk depends upon the delay to surgery. If surgery is performed early the muscle bulk will return to normal,

but if diagnosis is late (as often happens due to the rarity of this condition) then the muscle will not regain its normal bulk or strength.

Syringomyelia

This is a bizarre condition which often presents at the shoulder clinic. Remember the old aphorism 'If it's bizarre, do a WR' — WR standing for Wasserman reaction. Syphilitic Charcot joints are extremely rare these days, so consider all other forms of neuropathic or Charcot joints, and in particular diabetes and syringomyelia. As with all forms of neuropathic joint, these start painless, but become painful in the later stages and can be markedly destructive.

The patient presents with a painful shoulder. The radiograph shows a severely damaged glenohumeral articulation (Fig. 16.11). The head of the humerus and the glenoid are often resorbed; the joint-space is enlarged and contains loose fragments of bone. The rotator cuff may be destroyed with upward subluxation of the humeral stump,

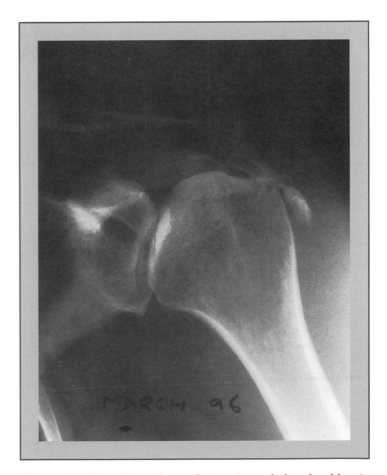

Figure 16.11 – *Gross bony destruction of the shoulder in syringomyelia.*

and the acromion may then become resorbed. The differential diagnosis is cuff-tear arthropathy, Milwaukee shoulder, or sepsis. However, the patient is usually three decades too young for the former two diagnoses, and infection can be ruled out with a normal white cell count, erythrocyte sedimentation rate (ESR), C-reactive protein (CRP) and synovial fluid culture. Men are more commonly affected than women, and the onset of the disease is usually between 20–40 years. The condition is almost exclusively found in the upper limbs, and is usually unilateral. Hence, the shoulder is the commonest joint to be affected by syringomyelia, and the elbow the second.

Careful neurological examination may reveal neurological loss in the arm, characteristically a loss of pain and temperature sensitivity, with preservation of fine touch and joint position sense. This is termed syringomyelic dissociation. Beware, these findings may be quite difficult to pick up.

The diagnosis is established by MRI scan of the cervical spine. The syrinx can be clearly seen on MRI, and its segmental extent can be measured (Fig. 16.12).

Treatment is controversial. Syringomyelia is a contraindication for shoulder replacement and yet the author knows several well known shoulder surgeons who admit to having performed a shoulder replacement in the early stages of syringomyelia, with short-term success. Time alone will show whether these patients' shoulder replacements will fail early.

The alternative treatment option, indeed the only option in the late stages when the cuff and acromion are destroyed, is shoulder fusion. Once again, the literature states that fusion is less successful in the patient with syringomyelia than in the normal situation. However, this may apply to old-fashioned methods of fusion. Certainly double plate fusion appears quite secure even in syringomyelia.

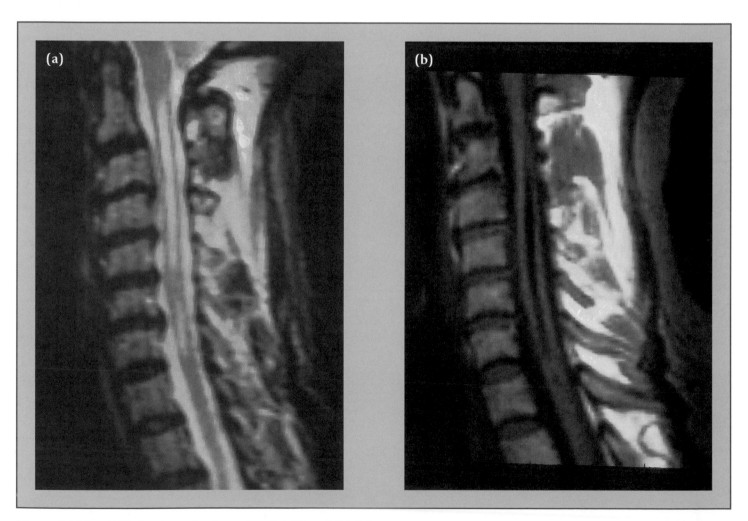

Figure 16.12 – *MRI showing extensive syrinx. (a) T1 and (b) T2 sequences.*

Dystonia

When we talk of the bizarre surely there can be nothing as bizarre, to the humble orthopaedic surgeon, as dystonia. The dividing line between dystonia and hysteria is narrow indeed. The patient will present with a bizarre posture of either the neck (torticollis) or of the shoulder. It is obvious that the shoulder is being held in an abnormal position by abnormal muscle tone. Examination under anaesthetic demonstrates an entirely normal shoulder joint. Upon induction of anaesthesia the offending muscle relaxes, posture returns to normal, and there is a full and free range of scapular and glenohumeral joint movement. As the anaesthetic wears off, the abnormal muscle spasm immediately returns. In the young patient with shoulder dystonia there may often be a psychological reason for this abnormal posture.

Treatment relies on attempting to define the secondary gain that the patient perceives they will get from the treatment of their condition, psychological support (from a psychologist and not from the orthopaedic surgeon) and the passage of time. Injection with botulinum toxin is of no help in this condition.

Stroke shoulder

Fortunately this condition is rare, now that stroke rehabilitation is mandatory in all major hospitals. Stroke shoulder is the painful stiff shoulder following a cerebrovascular episode. The shoulder is contracted and painful. Proper physiotherapy and rehabilitation of the stroke-patient involves passive mobilization of all affected joints, initially by the therapist, then by family, and finally by the patient themselves.

It is rare indeed for the patient nowadays to require surgical intervention. In the past when stroke shoulders were neglected, surgical release of pectoralis major and the subscapularis was occasionally needed followed by physiotherapy to maintain movement.

Axillary nerve palsy

The axillary nerve arises from the posterior cord of the brachial plexus, the rest of the cord passing on as the radial nerve. The nerve enters the quadralateral space with the posterior circumflex artery and a vein, both of

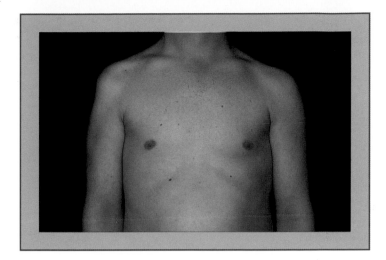

Figure 16.13 – *Deltoid-wasting in axillary nerve palsy of the right shoulder.*

which lie anterior to the nerve, and act as landmarks for the location of the nerve at this point. The neurovascular bundle emerges from the quadralateral space posteriorly between teres minor and teres major. Here it divides into a superficial and deep branch. The superficial branch supplies teres minor and the skin of the chevron area of the arm. The deep branch passes with the posterior circumflex artery and vein on the deep surface of the deltoid, which it supplies (Fig 16.13). The nerve is most often damaged by dislocations of the shoulder and by fracture dislocations. Birch (1995) recommends that if recovery has not occurred within 3 months that the nerve should be explored. If a neuroma in continuity or a division of the nerve is found, then it should be resected and cable grafted. Such an exploration should be performed by a specialist peripheral nerve surgeon.

Summary

Neurological presentations are the intellectual 'icing on the cake' for the shoulder surgeon. Some lesions such as FSH dystrophy are easily spotted others such as TOS are particularly difficult to diagnose. Diagnosis depends upon taking a careful history and conducting an obsessive neurological examination which is aided by a variety of investigations, in particular neurophysiological testing. Many neurological conditions around the shoulder are amenable to surgical correction, indeed many can only be successfully treated by surgery.

References

Chapter 1: The art of diagnosis

Emery RJ, Mullaji AB. Glenohumeral joint instability in normal adolescents. *J Bone Joint Surg* 1991; **73**B: 406–8.

Gerber C, Ganz R. Clinical assessment of instability of the shoulder with special reference to the anterior and posterior drawer tests. *J Bone Joint Surg* 1984; **66**B: 551–6.

Neer CS, Foster CR. Inferior capsular shift for involuntary inferior and multidirectional instability of the shoulder. *J Bone Joint Surg* 1980; **62**A: 897–908.

Richards RR, An K-N, Bigliani LU *et al*. A standardised method for the assessment of shoulder function. *J Shoulder Elbow Surg* 1994; **3**: 347–52.

Wiley AM. Arthroscopic appearance of frozen shoulder. *Arthroscopy* 1991; **7**(2): 138–43.

Chapter 3: Profit and loss: an account of the present state of shoulder arthroscopy

Andersen NH, Johannsen HV, Sheppen O, Sojbojerg JO. Frozen shoulder. Arthroscopy and manipulation in general anesthesia, followed by early passive mobilization (Danish). *Ugeskrift for Laeger* 1996; **158**(2): 147–50.

Berg EE, Oglesby JW. Loosening of a biodegradable shoulder staple. *J Shoulder Elbow Surg* 1996; **5**(1): 76–8.

Bigliani LU, Nicholson GP, Flatow EL. Arthroscopic resection of the distal clavicle. *Orthop Clin North Am* 1993; **24**(1): 133–41.

Brenneke SL, Morgan CJ. Evaluation of ultrasonography a a diagnostic technique in the assessment of rotator cuff tendon tears. *Am J Sports Med* 1992; **20**(3): 287–9.

Caspari RB, Geissler WB. Arthroscopic manifestations of shoulder subluxation and dislocation. *Clin Orthop* 1993; **291**: 54–66.

Caspari RB, Savoie FH. Arthroscopic reconstruction of the shoulder: The Bankart repair (suture technique). In: McGinty JB, Caspari RB, Jackson RW, Poehling GG (eds) *Operative Arthroscopy*, 2nd edn. Philadelphia: Lippincott–Raven Publishers, 1996; 695–708.

Chandnani VP, Yeager TD, DeBerardino T *et al*. Clenoid labral tears: Prospective evaluation with MRI imaging, MR arthrography, and CT arthrography. *Am J of Roentgenol* 1993; **161**(6): 1229–35.

Cofield RH. Arthroscopy of the shoulder. *Mayo Clinic Proceedings* 1983; **58**(8): 501–8.

Cordasco FA, Steinmann S, Flatow EL, Bigliani LU. Arthroscopic treatment of glenoid labral tears. *Am J Sports Med* 1993; **21**(3): 425–30.

Covall DJ, Fowble CD. Arthroscopic treatment of synovial chondromatosis of the shoulder and biceps tendon sheath. *Arthroscopy* 1993; **9**(5): 602–4.

D'Angelo GL, Ogilvie-Harris DJ. Septic arthritis following arthroscopy with cost-benefit analysis of antibiotic prophylaxis. *Arthroscopy* 1988; **4**(1): 10–14.

Detrisac DA, Johnson LL. Arthroscopic shoulder capsulorrhaphy using metal staples. *Orthop Clin North Am* 1993; **24**(1): 71–88.

Ellman H. Arthroscopic subacromial decompression. *Arthroscopy* 1987; **3**: 173–81.

Ellman H, Gartsman GM. Miscellaneous intra-articular conditions. In: *Arthroscopic Shoulder Surgery and Related Procedures*. Philadelphia: Lea and Febiger, 1993; 333–42.

Esch JC, Arthroscopic subacromial decompression and postoperative management. *Orthop Clin North Am* 1993; **24**(1): 161–71.

Farin PU, Jaroma H. Digital subtraction shoulder arthrography in determining site and size of rotator cuff tear. *Invest Radiol* 1995; **30**(9): 544–7.

Field LD, Savoie FH III. Arthroscopic suture repair of superior labral detachment lesions of the shoulder. *Am J Sports Med* 1993; **21**: 783–90.

Gartsman GM, Combs AH, Davis PF, Tullos HS. Arthroscopic acromioclavicular joint resection. An anatomical study. *Am J Sports Med* 1991; **19**(1): 2–5.

Flatow EL, Cordasco RA, Bigliani LU. Arthroscopic resection of the outer end of the clavicle from a superior approach: a critical, quantitative, radiographic assessment of bone removal. *Arthroscopy* 1992; **8**: 55–64.

Glousman RE. Instability versus impingement syndrome in the throwing athlete. *Orthop Clin North Am* 1993; **24**(1): 89–99.

Green A. Arthroscopic treatment of impingement syndrome. *Orthop Clin North Am* 1995; **26**(4): 631–41.

Gross RM, Fitzgibbons TC. Should Arthroscopy: A modified approach. *Arthroscopy* 1985; **1**: 156–9.

Hardy P, Thabit G III, Fanton GS *et al*. Arthroscopic management of recurrent anterior shoulder dislocation by combining a labrum suture with antero-inferior holmium: YAG laser capsular shrinkage (German). *Orthopade* 1996; **25**(1): 91–3.

Hinterman B, Gachter A. Arthroscopic findings after shoulder dislocation. *Am J Sports Med* 1995; **23**(5): 545–51.

Hoffmann F, Reif G. Arthroscopic shoulder stabilization using Mitek anchors. *Knee Surg Sports Traumatol Arthrosc* 1995; **3**(1): 50–4.

Imhoff A, Lederman T. Arthroscopic subacromial decompression with and without the Holmium: YAG-laser. A prospective comparative study. *Arthroscopy* 1995: **11**(5): 549–56.

Jobe FW, Kvitne RS. Shoulder pain in the overhand or throwing athlete: The relationship of anterior instability and rotator cuff impingement. *Orthop Rev* 1989; **18**: 963.

Johnson LL. The shoulder joint: An arthroscopist's perspective of anatomy and pathology. *Clin Orthop* 1987; **223**: 113–25.

Kaneko K, De Mouy EH, Brunet ME. Massive rotator cuff tears. Screening by routine radiographs. *Clinical Imaging* 1995; **19**(1): 8–11.

Karzel RP, Snyder SJ. Glenoid labrum tears: The role of arthroscopy. In: Parisien JS (ed) *Current Techniques in Arthroscopy*. Philadelphia: Current Medicine 1994; 65–74.

Klein AH, France JC, Mutschler TA, Fu FH. Measurement of brachial plexus strain in arthroscopy of the shoulder. *Arthroscopy* 1987; **3**(1): 45–52.

Kneisl JS, Sweeney HJ, Paige ML. Correlation of pathology observed in double contrast arthrotomography of the shoulder. *Arthroscopy* 1988; **4**(1): 21–4.

Lee HC, Dewan N, Crosby L. Subcutaneous emphysema, pneumomediastinum, and potentially life-threatening tension pneumothorax. Pulmonary complications from arthroscopic shoulder decompression. *Chest* 1992; **101**(5): 1265–7.

Markel MD, Hayashi K, Thabit G III, Thielke RJ. Changes in articular capsular tissue using holmium: YAG laser at non-ablative energy densities. Potential application in non-ablative stabilization procedures (German). *Orthopaedics* 1996; **25**(1): 37–41.

Martin DR, Garth WP Jr. Results of arthroscopic debridement of glenoid labral tears. *Am J Sports Med* 1995; **23**(4): 447–51.

Matthews LS, LaBudde JK. Arthroscopic treatment of synovial diseases of the shoulder. *Orthop Clin North Am* 1993; **24**(1): 101–11.

Matthews LS, Scerpella TA. Arthroscopic management of inflammatory arthritis and synovitis. In: McGinty JB, Caspari RB, Jackson RW, Poehling GG (eds) *Operative Arthroscopy*, 2nd edn. Philadelphia: Lippincott–Raven Publishers, 1996; 801–12.

McGinty JB. Arthroscopic removal of loose bodies. *Orthop Clin North Am* 1982; **13**(2): 313–28.

Neer CS. Anterior acromioplasty for the chronic impingement syndrome in the shoulder. *J Bone Joint Surg* 1972; **54A**: 41–50.

Nevasier TJ. Arthroscopy of the shoulder. *Orthop Clin North Am* 1987; **18**(3): 361–72.

Ogilvie-Harris DJ. Arthroscopy and arthroscopic surgery of the shoulder. *Semin Orthop Surg* 1987; **2**(4): 246–58.

Ogilvie-Harris DJ, Biggs DJ, Fitsialos DP, MacKay M. The resistant frozen shoulder. Manipulation versus arthroscopic release. *Clin Orthop* 1995; **319**: 238–48.

Ogilvie-Harris DJ, Boynton E. Arthroscopic acromioplasty: Extravasation of fluid into the deltoid muscle. *Arthroscopy* 1990; **6**(1): 52–4.

Ogilvie-Harris DJ, D'Angelo G. Arthroscopic surgery of the shoulder. *Sports Med* 1990; **9**(2): 120–8.

Ogilvie-Harris DJ, Demaziere A. Arthroscopic debridement versus open repair for rotator cuff tears. A prospective cohort study. *J Bone Joint Surg* 1993; **75**B(3): 416–20.

Ogilvie-Harris DJ, Demaziere A, Fitsialos D, Stevens JK. Arthroscopic acromioplasty. The superiority of the paterior portal over the latertal portal. *Orthop Clin North Am* 1993; **24**(1): 153–9.

Ogilvie-Harris EJ, Wiley AM. Arthroscopic surgery of the shoulder: A general appraisal. *J Bone Joint Surg* 1986; **68**B(2): 201–7.

Olsewski JM, Depew AD. Arthroscopic subacromial decompression and rotator cuff debridement for stage II and stage III impingement. *Arthroscopy* 1994; **10**(1): 61–8.

Palmer WE, Brown JH, Rosenthal DI. Rotator cuff: Evaluation with fat-suppressed MR arthrography. *Radiology* 1994; **188**(3): 683–7.

Parisien JS, Shaffer B. Arthroscopic managment of pyarthrosis. *Clin Orthop Related Res* 1992; **275**: 243–7.

Paulos LE. *Arthroscopic shoulder decompression: Technique and preliminary results*. Presented at the North American Arthroscopic Annual Meeting, Boston, April, 1985.

Pitman MI, Nainzadeh N, Ergas E, Springer S. The use of somatosensory evoked potentials for detection of neuropraxia during shoulder arthroscopy. *Arthroscopy* 1988; **4**(4): 250–5.

Pollock RG, Duralde XA, Flatow EL, Bigliani LU. The use of arthroscopy in the treatment of resistant frozen shoulder. *Clin Orthop* 1994; **304**: 30–6.

Reinus WR, Shady KL, Mirowitz SA, Totty WG. MR diagnosis of rotator cuff tears of the shoulder. Value of using T2-weighted fat-saturated images. *Am J Roentgeol* 1995; **164**(6): 1451–5.

Roye RP, Grana WA, Yates CK. Arthroscopic subacromial decompression: Two to seven-year follow-up. *Arthroscopy* 1995; **11**(3): 301–6.

Sachs RA, Stone ML, Devine S. Open vs. arthroscopic acromioplasty: A prospective randomized study. *Arthroscopy* 1994; **10**(3): 248–54.

Segmuller HE, Taylor DE, Hogan CS, Saies AD, Hayes MG. Arthroscopic treatment of adhesive capsulitis. *J Shoulder and Elbow Surg* 1995; **4**(6): 403–8.

Skyhar MJ, Altchek DW, Warren WF, Wickiewicz TL, O'Brien SJ. Shoulder arthroscopy with the patient in the beach-chair position. *Arthroscopy* 1988; **4**(4): 256–9.

Small NC. Complications in arthroscopy: The knee and other joints. Committee on Complications of the Arthroscopy Association of North America. *Arthroscopy* 1986; **2**(4): 256–8.

Small NC. Complications in arthroscopic surgery performed by experienced arthroscopists. *Arthroscopy* 1988; **4**(3): 215–21.

Snyder SJ, Karzel RP, Del Pizzo W, Ferkel RD, Friedman MJ. SLAP lesions of the shoulder. *Arthroscopy* 1990; **6**(4): 247–79.

Snyder SJ, Banas MP, Karzel RP. The arthroscopic Mumford procedure: An analysis of results. *Arthroscopy* 1995; **11**(2): 157–64.

Snyder SJ, Banas MP, Belzer JP. Arthroscopic evaluation and treatment of injuries to the superior glenoid labrum. *Instructional Course Lectures* 1996; **45**: 65–70.

Suder PA, Frich LH, Hougaard K, Lundorf E, Wulff Jakobsen B. Magnetic resonance imaging evaluation of capsulolabral tears after traumatic primary anterior should dislocation. A prospective comparison with arthroscopy of 25 cases. *J Shoulder and Elbow Surg* 1995; **4**(6): 419–28.

Wall MS, Warren RF. Complications of shoulder instability surgery. *Clin Sports Med* 1995; **14**(4): 973–1000.

Takenaka F, Fukatsu A, Matsuo S *et al*. Surgical treatment of hemodialysis-related shoulder arthropathy. *Clin Nephrol* 1992; **38**(4): 224–30.

Uitvlugt G, Detrisac DA, Johnson LL, Austin MD, Johnson C. Arthroscopic observations before and after manipulation of frozen shoulder. *Arthroscopy* 1993; **9**(2): 181–5.

Van Holsbeeck E, DeRycke J, Declerq G *et al*. Subacromial impingement: Open versus arthroscopic decompression. *Arthroscopy* 1992; **8**(2): 173–8.

Van Holsbeeck MT, Kolowich P, Eyler WR *et al*. US depiction of partial-thickness tear of the rotator cuff. *Radiology* 1995; **197**(2): 443–6.

Warner JJ, Miller MD, Marks P, Fu FH. Arthroscopic Bankart repair with the Suretac device. Part I: Clinical observations: *Arthroscopy* 1995; **11**(1): 2–13.

Warren RF, Moorman CT, Speer KP. Arthroscopic shoulder stablization using bioabsorbable tack. In: Parisien JS (ed) *Current Techniques in Arthroscopy*. Philadephia: Current Medicine, 1996; 125–33.

Wiley AM. Arthroscopic appearance of frozen shoulder. *Arthroscopy* 1991; **7**(2): 138–43.

Wolf EM. *Arthroscopic management of shoulder instabilities*. Presented at Speciality Day, American Academy of Orthopaedic Surgeons, Las Vegas, February, 1989.

Wolf EM. Arthroscopic capsulolabral repair using suture anchors. *Orthop Clin North Am* 1993; **24**(1): 59–69.

Wolf EM, Cheng JC, Dickson K. Humeral avulsion of glenohumeral ligaments as a cause of anterior shoulder instability. *Arthroscopy* 1995; **11**(5): 600–7.

Yamaguchi K, Flatlow EL. Arthroscopic evaluation and treatment of the rotator cuff. *Orthop Clin North Am* 1995; **26**(4): 643–59.

Yoneda M, Hirooka A, Saito S *et al*. Arthroscopic stapling for detached superior glenoid labrum. *J Bone Joint Surg* 1991; **73**B: 746–50.

Youssef JA, Carr CF, Walther CE, Murphy JM. Arthroscopic Bankart suture repair for recurrent traumatic unidirectional anterior shoulder dislocations. *Arthroscopy* 1995; **11**(5): 561–3.

Zvijac JE, Levy HJ, Lemak LJ. Arthroscopic subacromial decompression in the treatment of full thickness rotator cuff tears: A 3- to 6-year follow-up. *Arthroscopy* 1994; **10**(5): 518–23.

Chapter 4: Impingement: needle, scope or scalpel?

Armstrong JR. Excision of the acromion in the treatment of the supraspinatus syndrome. *J Bone Joint Surg* 1949; **31**B: 436–42.

Banas MP, Miller RJ, Totterman S. Relationship between the lateral acromial angle and rotator cuff disease. *J Shoulder Elbow Surgery* 1995; **4**: 454–61.

Bigliani LH, Morrison DS, Apri EW. The morphology of the acromion and relationshp to rotator cuff tears. *Orthop Trans* 1986; **10**: 228.

Brox JI, Staff PH, Ljunggren AE, Brevik JI. Arthroscopic surgery compared with supervised exercises in patients with rotator cuff disease. *Br Med J* 1993; **307**: 899–903.

Bunker TD, Wallace WA (ed) *Shoulder Arthroscopy*. London: Dunitz 1991.

Craig EV (ed). *Master Tecniques in Orthopaedic Surgery; The Shoulder*. New York; Raven Press, 1995.

Daluga DJ, Dobozi W. The influence of distal clavicle resection and rotator cuff repair on the effectiveness of anterior acromioplasty. *Clin Orthop* 1989; **247**: 117–23.

DePalma AF. Surgery of the shoulder (2nd edn.) Philadelphia: JB Lippincott, 1973.

Dines OM, Warren RE, Inglis AE *et al*. The coracoid impingement syndrome. Presented at the *Second Open Meeting of the ASES*, New Orleans, February 1986.

Edelson JG, Taitz C. Anatomy of the coracoacromial arch. *J Bone Joint Surg* 1992; **74**B: 589–94.

Edelson JG, Zuckerman J, Hershovitz I. Os Acromiale: Anatomy and surgical implications. *J Bone Joint Surg* 1993; **75**B: 551–5.

Gerber C, Terrier F, Ganz R. The role of the coracoid process in the chronic impingement syndrome. *J Bone Joint Surgery* 1985; **67**B: 703–8.

Golser K, Sperner G, Hauser C *et al*. Sensory innervation of the should joint. *J Shoulder Elbow Surg* 1995; **4**(Suppl.): S34.

Grant JCB. *Grant's Atlas of Anatomy* (6th edn.) Baltimore: Williams & Wilkins, 1972.

Holt ME, Allibone RO. Anatomic variants of the coraco-acromial ligament. *J Shoulder Elbow Surg* 1995; **4**: 370–5.

Ide K, Shirai MD, Ito H, Sibasaki T, Takayama A. The neurohistological study in the subacromial bursa. *J Shoulder Elbow Surg* 1994; **3**(Suppl.): S60.

Jobe FW, Jobe CM. Painful athletic injuries of the shoulder. *Clin Orthop and Related Research* 1982; **173**: 117.

Johnson LL. Uses and abuses of arthroscopy. *J Bone Joint Surg* 1983; **65**A:

McLaughlin HL. Lesions of the musculotendinous cuff of the shoulder. *J Bone Joint Surg* 1944; **26**: 31–51.

Meyer AW. The minute anatomy of attritional lesions. *J Bone Joint Surg* 1931; **13**A: 341.

Miniaci A, Dowdy PA, Willits KR, Vellet AD. Magnetic resonance imaging evaluation of the rotator cuff tendons in the asymptomatic shoulder. *Am J Sports Med* 1995; **23**(2): 142–5.

Morrison D, Bigliani LU. The clinical significance of variations in acromial morphology. *Orthop Trans* 1987; **11**: 234.

Neer CS. Anterior acromioplasty for the chronic impingement syndrome in the shoulder. *J Bone Joint Surg* 1972; **54**A: 41.

Neer CS. Impingement lesions. *Clin Orthop and Related Research* 1983; **173**: 70–8.

Neviaser TJ, Neviaser RJ, Neviaser JS, Neviaser JS. The four in one arthroplasty for the painful arc syndrome. *Clin Orthop* 1982; **163**: 107–12.

Ogilvie-Harris DJ, Demazaire A. Arthroscopic debridement versus open repair for rotator cuff tears. *J Bone Joint Surg* 1993; **75**B: 416–20.

Petersson CJ, Gentz CF. Ruptures of the supraspinatus tendon. *Clin Orthop* 1983; **174**: 143–8.

Reinus WR, Shady KL, Mirowitz SA, Totty WG. Magnetic resonance imaging in the evaluation of rotator cuff tears. *Am J Roentgenol* 1995; **164**(6): 1451–5.

Rockwood CA, Lyons FR. Shoulder impingement syndrome: Diagnosis, radiographic evaluation, and treatment with a modified Neer acromioplasty. *J Bone Joint Surg* 1993; **75**A: 409.

Uhtoff HK, Sarkar K. Surgical repair of rotator cuff ruptures. *J Bone Joint Surg* 1991; **73**B: 399–401.

Smith Petersen MN, Aufranc OE, Larson CB. Useful surgical procedures for rheumatoid arthritis involving joints of the upper extremity. *Arch Surg* 1943; **46**: 764–70.

Stuart MJ, Azevedo AJ, Cofield RH. Anterior acromioplasty for the treatment of the shoulder impingement syndrome. *Clin Orthop* 1990; **260**: 195–200.

Tivoinen DA, Tuite MJ, Orwin JF. Acromial structure and tears of the rotator cuff. *J Shoulder Elbow Surg* 1995; **4**: 376–83.

Thorling J, Bjerneld H, Hallin G, Hovelius L, Hagg O. Acromioplasty for impingement syndrome. *Acta Orthop Scand* 1985; **56**: 147–8.

Walch G, Boileau P, Noel E, Donnell ST. Impingement of the deep surface of the supraspinatus tendon on the posterosuperior glenoid rim. *J Shoulder Elbow Surg* 1992; **1**: 238–45.

Withrington RH, Girgis FL, Seifert MH. A placebo controlled trial of steroid injections in the treatment of supraspinatus tendonitis. *Scand J Rheumatol* 1985; **14**: 76–8.

Chapter 5: The management of rotator-cuff tears

Andrews JR, Broussard TS, Carson WG. Arthroscopy of the shoulder in the management of partial tears of the rotator cuff. *Arthroscopy* 1985; **1**: 117–22.

Bateman JE. *The Shoulder and Neck*. Philadelphia; WB Saunders, 1972.

Bigliani LU, Cordasco FA, McIlveen SJ, Musso ES. Operative treatment of failed repairs of the rotator cuff. *J Bone Joint Surg* 1992; **74**A: 1505.

Brooks CH, Revell WJ, Heatley RW. A quantitative histological study of the vascularity of the rotator cuff tendon. *J Bone Joint Surg* 1992; **74**B: 151–3.

Burkhart SS. Reconciling the paradox of rotator cuff repair versus debridement. *Arthroscopy* 1994; **10**(1): 4–19.

Bunker TD, Anthony PP. The pathology of frozen shoulder; A Dupuytren's like disease. *J Bone Joint Surg* 1995; **77**B: 677–83.

Bunker TD, Wallace WA. Shoulder Arthroscopy. London: Dunitz, 1991.

Clark JM, Harryman DT. Tendons, ligaments and capsule of the rotator cuff. *J Bone Joint Surg* 1992; **74**A: 713–25.

Codman EA. The Shoulder. Rupture of the supraspinatus tendon and other lesions in or about the subacromial bursa. Boston: Thomas Todd, 1934.

Colachis SC, Strohm BR. Effect of suprascapular and axillary nerve blocks on muscle force in the upper extremity. *Arch Phys Med Rehab* 1971; **50**: 22–9.

Cooper DE, O'Brien SJ, Arnoczky SP, Warren RF. The structure and function of the coracohumeral ligament. *J Shoulder Elbow Surg* 1993; **2**: 70–7.

Edelson JG, Taitz C, Grisham A. The coracohumeral ligament. *J Bone Joint Surg* 1991; **73**B: 150–3.

Ellman H, Kay SP, Wirth M. Arthroscopic treatment of full thickness tears of the rotator cuff. *Arthroscopy* 1993; **9**: 195–200.

Gerber C, Vinh TS, Hertel R, Hess CW. Latissimus dorsi transfer for the treatment of massive tears of the rotator cuff. *Clin Orthop* 1988; **232**: 51–61.

Gohlke F, Essikrug B, Schmitz F. The pattern of the collagen fibre bundles of the capsule of the glenohumeral joint. *J Shoulder Elbow Surg* 1994; **3**: 111–28.

Harryman DT, Sidles JA, Harris SL, Matsen FA. The role of the rotator interval capsule. *J Bone Joint Surg* 1992; **74**A: 53–65.

Hinton MA, Parker AW, Drez D, Altcheck D. An anatomic study of the subscapularis tendon and myotendinous junction. *J Shoulder Elbow Surg* 1994; **3**: 224–9.

Howell SM, Imobersteg AM, Seger DH, Marone PJ. Clarification of the role of the supraspinatus muscle in shoulder function. *J Bone Joint Surg* 1986; **68**A: 398–404.

Karas SE, Giachello TL. Subscapularis transfer for reconstruction of massive tears of the rotator cuff. *J Bone Joint Surg* 1996; **78**A: 239.

Keating JF, Waterworth P, Shaw Dunn J, Crossan J. The relative strengths of the rotator cuff muscles. A cadaver study. *J Bone Joint Surg* 1993; **75**B: 137–40.

Lazarus MD, Chansky HA, Misra S, Williams GR, Ianotti JP. Comparison of open and arthroscopic subacromial decompression. *J Shoulder Elbow Surg* 1994; **3**: 1–11.

Lohr JF, Uhtoff HK. The microvascular pattern of the supraspinatus tendon. *Clin Orthop* 1989; **254**: 35–8.

Lyons AR, Tomlinson JE. Clinical diagnosis of tears of the rotator cuff. *J Bone Joint Surg* 1992; **74**B: 414–15.

McLaughlin HL. Asherman EF. Lesions of the musculotendinous cuff of the shoulder. *J Bone Joint Surg* 1951; **33**A: 76–86.

Moseley HF, Goldie I. The arterial pattern of the rotator cuff of the shoulder. *J Bone Joint Surg* 1963; **45**B: 780.

Nakajima T, Rokuuma N, Hamada K, Tomatsu T, Fukuda H. Histological and biomechanical characteristics of the supraspinatus tendon. *J Shoulder Elbow Surg* 1994; **3**: 79–87.

Neer CS, Saterlee CC, Dalsey RM, Flatow EL. The anatomy and potential effects of contracture of the coracohumeral ligament. *Clin Orthop* 1992; **280**: 182–5.

Nobuhara K, Ikeda H. Rotator interval lesions. *Clin Orthop* 1987; **223**: 44–50.

Norwood LA, Barrack R, Jacobsen KE. Clinical presentation of complete tears of the rotator cuff. *J Bone Joint Surg* 1986; **71**A: 499.

Ozaki J, Fujimoto S, Nakagawa Y, Masuhara K, Tamai S. Tears of the rotator cuff of the shoulder associated with pathological changes in the acromion. *J Bone Joint Surg* 1988; **70**A: 1224.

Pettersson G. Rupture of the tendon aponeurosis of the shoulder joint in anterior inferior dislocation. *Acta Chir Scand* 1942; **77**(suppl.): 1–184.

Post M, Silver R, Singh M. Rotator cuff tear. Diagnosis and treatment. *Clin Orthop* 1983; **173**: 78–91.

Rathbun JB, MacNab I. The microvascular pattern of the rotator cuff. *J Bone Joint Surg* 1970; **52**B: 540.

Rothman RH, Parke WW. The vascular anatomy of the rotator cuff. *Clin Orthop* 1965; **41**: 176–86.

Savoie FH, Field LD, Jenkins RN. Cost analysis of successful rotator cuff repair surgery. *Arthroscopy* 1995; **11**(6): 672–6.

Stableforth 1995 (Personal communication).

Sward L, Hughes JS, Amis A, Wallace WA. The strength of surgical repairs of the rotator cuff. *J Bone Joint Surg* 1992; **74**B: 585.

Swiantkowski M, Iannotti JP, Esterhaj JL et al. *Intraoperative Assessment of Rotator Cuff Vascularity Using Laser Doppler Flowmetry*. Presented at the 56th Annual Meeting of the AAOS, Las Vegas, Feb 10, 1989.

Turkel SJ, Panio MW, Marshall JL et al. Stabilizing mechanisms preventing anterior dislocation of the glenohumeral joint. *J Bone Joint Surg* 1981; **63**A: 1208–17.

Uhtoff HK, Loehr J, Sarkar K. *The pathogenesis of rotator cuff tears*. In: Proceedings of the Third International Shoulder Conference. Japan, Fukuora: 1986.

Van Linge B, Mulder JD. Function of the supraspinatus muscle; An experimental study in man. *J Bone Joint Surg* 1963; **45**B: 750–4.

Zuckerman JD, Leblanc JM, Choueka J, Kummer F. The effect of arm position and capsular relaease on rotator cuff repair. A biomechanical study. *J Bone Joint Surg* 1991; **73**B: 402–5.

Chapter 6: The young sportsman with traumatic recurrent dislocation

Baker CL, Uribe JW, Whitman. Arthroscopic evaluation of acute initial anterior shoulder disloction. *Am J Sports Med* 1990; **18**: 25–8.

Barber FA. Strength of sutures and suture anchors: State of the art. Presented at the American Academy of Orthopaedic Surgery Specialty Day, 1995.

Bayley 1990 (see Mok *et al.*)

Broca A, Hartman H. Contribution a l'etude des luxations de l'epaule. *Bull et memoirs Soc Anat Paris* 1890; **4**: 312–36.

Ellman H, Gartsman G. *Arthroscopic Shoulder Surgery and Related Procedures*. Philadelphia: Lea and Febiger, 1993.

Emery RJ, Mullaji AB. Glenohueral joint instability in normal adolescents. *J Bone Joint Surg* 1991; **73**B: 406–8.

Gerber C, Ganz R. Clinical assessment of instability of the shoulder with special reference to anterior and posterior drawer tests. *J Bone Joint Surg* 1984; **66**B: 551–6.

Glousman R, Jobe F, Tibone J, Moynes D, Antonelli, Perry J. Dynamic electromyographic analysis of the throwing shoulder with glenohumeral instability. *J Bone Joint Surg* 1988; **70**A: 220.

Hovelius L. Anterior dislocation of the shoulder in teenagers and young adults. Five year prognosis. *J Bone Joint Surg* 1987; **69**A: 393–9.

Itoi E, Keuchle DK, Newman SR, Morrey BF, An K-N. Stablising function of the biceps in stable and unstable shoulders. *J Bone Joint Surg* 1993; **75**B: 546–50.

Jakobsen BW, Sjobjerg JO. *Primary Repair After Traumatic Anterior Dislocation of the Shoulder Joint*. Presented at the European Shoulder and Elbow Surgeons Meeting, Nottingham, 1996.

Kumar VP, Balasubramaniam P. The role of atmospheric pressure in stabilising the shoulder. An experimental study. *J Bone Joint Surg* 1985; **67**B: 719–21.

Kronberg M, Brostrom L-A, Soderlund V. Retroversion of the humeral head in the normal shoulder and its relationships to the normal range of motion. *Clin Orthop* 1990; **253**: 113–17.

Lephart SM, Warner JP, Borsa PA, Fu F. Proprioception of the shoulder joint in healthy, unstable, and surgically repaired shoulders. *J Shoulder Elbow Surg* 1994; **3**: 371–80.

McAulife TB, Pangayatselvan T, Bayley JIL. Failed surgery for anterior recurrent anterior dislocation of the shoulder. *J Bone Joint Surg* 1984; **70**B: 798–801.

Mok DW, Fogg AJ, Hokan R, Bayley JIL. The diagnostic value of arthroscopy in glenohumeral instability. *J Bone Joint Surg* 1990; **72**B: 698–700.

Neer CS, Foster CR. Inferior capsular shift for involuntary inferior and multidirectional instability of the shoulder. *J Bone Joint Surg* 1980; **62**A: 1208–17.

O'Driscoll S, Evans D. Contralateral shoulder instability following anterior repair. *J Bone Joint Surg* 1991; **73**B: 941–6.

Perthes G. Uber operationen bei: Habitueller schulterluxation. *Deutsch Ztschr Chir* 1906; **85**: 199–227.

Ribbans WJ, Mitchell R, Taylor GJ. Computed arthrotomography of primary anterior dislocation of the shoulder. *J Bone Joint Surg* 1990; **72**B: 181–5.

Solomonow LJ, Guanche C, Wink C et al. Mechanoreceptors and the reflex arc in the feline shoulder. *J Shoulder Elbow Surg* 1996; **5**: 139–46.

Turkel SJ, Panio MW, Marshall JL et al. Stabilizing mechanisms preventing anterior dislocation of the glenohumeral joint. *J Bone Joint Surg* 1981; **63**A: 1208–17.

Uhtoff HK, Picopo M. Anterior capsular redundancy of the shoulder: Congenital or traumatic? An embryological study. *J Bone Joint Surg* 1985; **67**B: 363–6.

Walch G, Nove-Josserand L, Levigne C, Renaud E. Tears of the supraspinatus tendon associated with hidden lesions of the rotator interval. *J Shoulder Elbow Surg* 1994; **3**: 353–60.

Chapter 7: The teenager with atraumatic shoulder instability

Beighton P, Soloman L, Soskolne CL. Articular mobility in an African population. *Ann Rheum Dis* 1973; **32**: 413–18.

Bigliani LU, Pollock RG, McIlveen SJ, Endrizzi DP, Flatow EL. Shift of the posteroinferior aspect of the capsule for recurrent posterior glenohumeral instability. *J Bone Joint Surg* (Am) 1995; **77**A: 1011–20.

Boyd HB, Sisk TD. Recurrent posterior dislocation of the shoulder. *J Bone Joint Surg* (Am) 1972; **54**A: 779–86.

Burkhead WZ, Rockwood Jr. CA. Treatment of instability of the shoulder with an exercise program. *J Bone Joint Surg* (Am) 1992; **74**A: 890–6.

Carter C, Wilkinson J. Persistent joint laxity and congenital dislocation of the hip. *J Bone Joint Surg* (Br) 1964; **46**B: 40–5.

Cooper RA, Brems JJ. The inferior capsular-shift procedure for multidirectional instability of the shoulder. *J Bone Joint Surg* (Am) 1992; **74**A: 1516–21.

Duncan R, Savoie III FH. Arthroscopic inferior capsular shift for multidirectional instability of the shoulder: A preliminary report. *Arthroscopy* 1993; **9**: 24–7.

Emery RJH, Mullaji AB. Glenohumeral joint instability in normal adolescents. Incidence and significance. *J Bone Joint Surg* (Br) 1991; **73**B: 406–8.

Kronberg M, Broström LA, Németh G. Differences in shoulder muscle activity between patients with generalised joint laxity and normal controls. *Clin Orthop* 1991; **269**: 181–92.

Lephart SM, Warner JJP, Borsa PA, Fu FH. Proprioception of the shoulder joint in healthy, unstable, and surgically repaired shoulders. *J Shoulder Elbow Surg* 1994; **3**: 371–80.

Mallon WJ, Speer KP. Multidirectional instability: Current concepts. *J Shoulder Elbow Surg* 1995; 4: 54–64.

Maruyama K, Sano S, Saito K, Yamaguchi Y. Trauma-instability-voluntarism classificaction for glenohumeral instability. *J Shoulder Elbow Surg* 1995; 4: 194–8.

Matsen III FA, Thomas SC, Rockwood Jr. CA. Glenohumeral instability. In: Rockwood Jr. CA, Matsen III FA (eds) *The Shoulder*. v. 1. Philadelphia: W.B. Saunders Company, 1990; 526–622.

Morrey BF, An K-N. Biomechanics of the shoulder. In: Rockwood CA Jr., Matsen FA III (eds.) *The Shoulder*. Philadelphia: W.B. Saunders Company, 1990; 208–45.

Neer II CS, Foster CR. Inferior capsular shift for involuntary inferior and multidirectional instability of the shoulder. A preliminary report. *J Bone Joint Surg* (Am) 1980; **62**A: 897–908.

Rowe CR. Prognosis in dislocations of the shoulder. *J Bone Joint Surg*; 1956; **38**A: 957–77.

Rowe CR, Pierce DS, Clark JG. Voluntary dislocation of the shoulder. A preliminary report on a clinical, electromyographic, and psychiatric study of twenty-six patients. *J Bone Joint Surg* (Am) 1973; **55**A: 445–60.

Scott Jr. DJ. Treatment of recurrent posterior dislocations of the shoulder by glenoplasty. Report of three cases. *J Bone Joint Surg* (Am) 1967; **49**A: 471–6.

Silliman JF, Hawkins RJ. Classification and physical diagnosis of instability of the shoulder. *Clin Orthop* 1993; **291**: 7–19.

Tsutsui H, Yamamoto R, Kuroki Y et al. Biochemical study on collagen from the loose shoulder joint capsules. In: Post M, Morrey BF, Hawkins RJ (eds.) *Surgery of the Shoulder*, St. Louis: Mosby, 1991; 108–11.

Wallace WA. Recurrent instability of the shoulder and its management. In: Kelly IG (ed.) *The Practice of Shoulder Surgery*. Oxford: Butterworth Heinemann 1993; 163–79.

Weber BG, Simpson LA, Hardegger F. Rotational humeral osteotomy for recurrent anterior dislocation of the shoulder associated with a large Hill–Sachs lesions. *J Bone Joint Surg* (Am) 1984; **66**A: 1443–50.

Chapter 8: Frozen shoulder

Baird KS, Crossan JF, Ralston SH. Abnormal growth factor and cytokine expression in Dupuytren's contracture. *J Clin Pathol* 1993; **46**: 425–8.

Bayley JIL. Arthroscopy of frozen shoulder. (Personal communication) 1994.

Boardman ND, Debski RE, Warner JP, Taskiran E, Maddox L, Imhoff AB, Fu FH, Woo SL-Y. Tensile properties of the superior glenohumeral and coracohumeral ligaments. *J Shoulder Elbow Surg* 1996; **5**: 249–54.

Bonnici AV, Birjandi F, Spencer JI, Fox SP, Berry AC. Chromosomal abnormalities in Dupuytren's contracture and carpal tunnel syndrome. *J Hand Surg* 1992; **17**B: 349–55.

Bridgeman JF. Periarthritis of the shoulder and diabetes mellitus. *Ann Rheum Dis* 1972; **31**: 69–71.

Bunker TD. Time for a new name for frozen shoulder. *Br Med J* 1985; **290**: 1233–4.

Bunker TD, Anthony PP. The pathology of frozen shoulder. *J Bone Joint Surg* 1995; **77**B: 677–83.

Bunker TD, Esler CNA. Frozen shoulder and lipids. *J Bone Joint Surg* 1995; **77**B: 684–6.

Bunker TD, Lagae K, DeFerm A. Arthroscopy and Manipulation in Frozen Shoulder. *J Bone Joint Surg* 1994; **76**B(suppl.): 53.

Charnley JC. Periarthritis of the shoulder. *Postgrad Med J* 1959; 384–8.

Codman EA. *Tedinitis of the short rotators*. In: *Ruptures of the Supraspinatus Tendon and Other Lesions in or About the Subacromial Bursa*. Boston: Thomas Todd and Co, 1934.

Cooper De, O'Brien SJ, Arnoczky SP, Warren RF. The structure and function of the coracohumeral ligament. *J Shoulder Elbow Surg* 1993; **2**: 70–7.

DePalma AF. Loss of Scapulohumeral Motion (frozen shoulder). *Ann Surg* 1953; **135**(2): 194–204.

Duplay ES. De la periarthrote scapulohumerale. *Arch Gen Med* 1872; **20**: 513–42.

Duralde XA, Jelsma RD, Pollock RG, Bigliani LU. Arthroscopic treatment of resistant frozen shoulder. *Arthroscopy* 1993; **9**(3): 345.

Edelson JG, Taitz G, Grishkan A. The coracohumeral ligament. anatomy of a substantial but neglected structure. *J Bone Joint Surg* 1991; **73**B: 150–3.

Emig EW, Schweizer ME, Karasick D, Lubowitz J. Adhesive capsulitis of the shoulder: MR diagnosis. *Am J Radiol* 1995; **164**: 1457–9.

Enziger FM, Weiss SW. Soft Tissue tumours 1988 (2nd edn). St Louis: Mosby.

Esch JC. Athroscopic treatment of resistant primary frozen shoulder. *J Shoulder Elbow Surg* 1994; **3**(1)(suppl.): S71.

Fazzi UG. Dupuytren's disease: The use of corticosteroids. *J R Coll Surg Edinb* 1995; **40**: 76.

Fisher L, Kurtz A, Shipley M. Association between cheiro-arthropathy and frozen shoulder in patients with insulin dependent diabetes mellitus. *Br J Rheum* 1986; **25**: 141–6.

Gagey O, Bonfait H, Gillot C, Hureau J, Mazas F. Anatomic basis of ligamentous control of elevation of the shoulder. *Surg Radiol Anat* 1987; **9**: 19–26.

Ha'Eri GB, Maitland A. Arthroscopic findings in frozen shoulder. *J Rheumatol* 1981; **8**(1): 149–52.

Havel RJ. Disorders of lipid metabolism. In: Beeson PB, McDermott W, Wyngaarden JB (eds.) *Cecil's textbook of medicine*, 15th edn. Philadelphia: W.B. Saunders, 1979; 2002–11.

Hannafin JA, DiCarol EF, Wickiewicz TL. Adhesive Capsulitis: Capsular Fibroplasia of the Shoulder Joint. *J Shoulder Elbow Surg* 1994; **3**(1) (suppl.): S5.

Harryman DT, Sidles JA, Harris SL, Matsen FA. The role of the rotator interval capsule. *J Bone Joint Surg* 1992; **74**A: 53–65.

Janda DH, Hawkins RJ. Shoulder manipulation in patients with adhesive capsulitis and diabetes mellitus. *J Elbow Shoulder Surg* 1993; **2**: 36–8.

Kay NRM, Slater DN. Fibromatosis and Dupuytren's Disease. *Lancet* 1981; **2**(8241): 303.

Lequesne M, Dang N, Banassonn M, Mery C. Increased association of diabetes mellitus with capsulitis of the shoulder and shoulder hand syndrome. *Scand J Rheumatol* 1977; **6**: 53–6.

Lundberg BJ. The frozen shoulder. *Acta Orthop Scand* 1969; **119**: 1–59.

Meulengracht E, Schwartz M. Course and prognosis of periarthritis scapulohumerale. *Acta Med Scand* 1952; **143**: 350–60.

McLaughlin HL. The frozen shoulder. *Bull Hosp J Disease* 951; **20**: 126–31.

Midorikawa K, Hara, Shibata, Izaki, Ogata. Manipulation of frozen shoulder: Application of arthroscopic surgery. *J Shoulder Elbow Surg* 1994; **3**(suppl.): S42.

Neer CS, Saterlee CC, Dalsey RM, Flatow EL. The anatomy and potential effects of contracture of the coracohumeral ligament. *Clin Orthop* 1992; **280**: 182–5.

Neviaser JS. Adhesive Capsulitis of the Shoulder. *J Bone Joint Surg* 1945; **27**: 211–21.

Neviaser JS. Arthrography of the shoulder. Springfield III: Charles C Thomas, 1975; 60–6.

Nobuhara K, Ikeda H. Rotator interval lesions. *Clin Orthop* 1987; **223**: 44–50.

Ozaki J, Nakagawa Y, Sakurai G, Tamai S. Recalcitrant chronic adhesive capsulitis of the shoulder. *J Bone Joint Surg* 1989; **71A**: 1511–15.

Ogilvie-Harris DJ, Wiley AM. Arthroscopic surgery of the shoulder. *J Bone Joint Surg* 1986; **68**: 201–7.

Pal B, Anderson J, Dick WC, Griffiths ID. Limitation of joint mobility and shoulder capsulitis in insulin and non-insulin dependent diabetes mellitus. *Br J Rheumatol* 1986; **25**: 147.

Quigley TB. Checkrein shoulder, a type of frozen shoulder. *Surg Clin North Am* 1969; **43**: 1715–20.

Reeves B. The natural history of frozen shoulder. *Scand J Rheumatol* 1975; **4**: 193–6.

Sanderson PL, Morris MA, Stanley JK, Fahmy NRM. Lipids and Dupuytren's disease. *J Bone Joint Surg* 1992; **74B**: 923–7.

Schaer H. Die ätiologie der periarthritis humeroscapularis. *Ergebn Chir Orthop* 1936; **29**: 11.

Segmuller HE, Taylor DE, Hogan CS, Saies AD, Hayes MG. Arthroscopic treatment of adhesive capsulitis. *J Shoulder Elbow Surg* 1995; **4**: 403–8.

Sergovich FR, Botz JS, MacFarlane RM. Nonrandom cytogenetic abnormalities in Dupuytren's disease. *New England J Med* 1983; **308**: 162–3.

Schaffer B, Tibone JE, Kerlan RK. Frozen shoulder: A long term follow up. *J Bone Joint Surg* 1992; **74A**: 738–46.

Simonds FA. Shoulder pain: With particular reference to the frozen shoulder. *J Bone Joint Surg* 1949; **31**(B): 426–32.

Uitvligt G, Detrisac DA, Johnson LL, Austin MD, Johnson C. Arthroscopic observations before and after manipulation of frozen shoulder. *Arthroscopy* 1993; **9**(2): 181–5.

Wiley AM. Arthroscopic appearance of frozen shoulder. *Arthroscopy* 1991; **7**(2): 138–43.

Wright V, Haq AM. Periarthritis of the shoulder II. *Ann Rheum Dis* 1976(a); **35**: 220–6.

Wright V, Haq AM. Periarthritis of the shoulder I. *Ann Rheum Dis* 1976(b); **35**: 213–19.

Wurster Hill DH, Brown F, Park JP, Gibson SH. Cytogenetic studies in Dupuytren's contracture. *Am J Human Gen* 1988; **43**: 285–92.

Zuckerman JD, Cuomo F, Rokito S. Definition and classification of frozen shoulder. *J Shoulder Elbow Surg* 1994; **3**(1) (suppl.): S5.

Chapter 9: Stepping stones towards the ideal shoulder replacement

Boilleau P, Walch G. Morphological study of the humeral proximal epiphysis. *J Bone Joint Surg* 1992; **74B**: 14.

Brems J. The glenoid component in total shoulder arthroplasty. *J Shoulder Elbow Surg* 1993; **2**: 47–54.

Bunker TD, Feldman AY. Rotational dissociation of the glenoid component of a shoulder prosthesis. *J Shoulder Elbow Surg* (In press) 1997.

Collins D, Tencer A, Sidles J, Matsen FA. Edge displacement and deformation of glenoid components in response to eccentric loading. *J Bone Joint Surg* 1992; **74A**: 501–7.

Harryman DT, Sidles JA, Clark JM *et al.* Translation of the humeral head on the glenoid with passive glenohumeral motion. *J Bone Joint Surg* 1990; **72**: 1334–43

Harryman DT, Sidles JA, Harris SL, Lippitt SB, Matsen FA. The effect of articular conformity and the size of the humeral head component on laxity and motion after glenohumeral arthroplasty. *J Bone Joint Surg* 1995; **77A**: 555–63.

Hovelius L, Augistini BG, Fredin H *et al.* Primary anterior dislocation of the shoulder in young patients. *J Bone Joint Surg* 1996; **78A**: 1677–84.

Ianotti JP, Gabriel JP, Schneck SL, Evans BG, Misra S. The normal glenohumeral relationships. *J Bone Joint Surg* 1992; **74A**: 491–500.

Jonsson U, Halvorsen D, Abbaszadegan H, Revay S, Salmonsson B. *Better Function One Year After Randomisation to Shoulder Arthroplasty with a Glenoid Component than Without. 9th Congress of the European Society for Surgery of the Shoulder and Elbow.* 19–21 September 1996, Nottingham UK.

Neer CS. Articular replacement of the humeral head. *J Bone Joint Surg* 1955; **37**: 215–28.

Neer CS, Morrison DS. Glenoid bone grafting in total shoulder arthroplasty. *J Bone Joint Surg* 1988; **70**: 1154–62

Norris TR, Iannotti JP. *A Prospective Outcome Study Comparing Humeral Head Replacement with Total Shoulder Replacement. 9th Congress of the European Society for Surgery of the Shoulder and Elbow.* 19–21 September 1996, Nottingham UK.

Roberts S, Foley AP, Swallow H, Wallace WA, Coughland DP. The geometry of the humeral head. *J Bone Joint Surg* 1991; **73B**: 647–50.

Wallace WA, Neumann L, Frostick SP, Kiss J. *Classifying Re-operations After Shoulder Arthroplasty. 9th Congress of the European Society for Surgery of the Shoulder and Elbow.* 19–21 September 1996, Nottingham UK.

Wirth MA, Rockwood CA. Current concepts review. Complications of total shoulder replacement arthroplasty. *J Bone Joint Surg* 1996; **78A**: 603.

Chapter 10: The acromioclavicular joint

Alman FL Jr. Fractures and ligamentous injuries of the clavicle and its articulation. *J Bone Joint Surg* (Am) 1967; 49A: 774–84.

Bannister GC, Wallace WA, Stableforth PC, Hutson MA. The management of acute acromio-clavicular dislocation. *J Bone Joint Surg* (Br) 1989; 71B: 848–50.

Bosworth BM. Acromioclavicular separation. *Surg Gyn Obstet* 1941; 73: 866–71.

Ciullo JV. Endoscopic resection of the A/C Joint: Seven years experience. *6th Int Congress on Surgery of the Shoulder*: Helsinki, June 1995.

Dawe CJ. Acromioclavicular joint injuries. *J Bone Joint Surg* (Br) 1980; 62B: 269.

Dias JJ, Steingold RF, Richardson RA, Tesfayohannes B, Gregg PJ. The conservative treatment of acromioclavicular dislocation. *J Bone Joint Surg* (Br) 1987; 69B: 719–22.

Flatow EL. Arthroscopic treatment of acromioclavicular disorders. In: Vastamäki M, Jalovaara P (eds.) *Surgery of the Shoulder*. Amsterdam: Elsevier, 1995.

Fukuda K, Craig EV, Kai-Nan AN, Cofield RH, Chao YS. Biomechanical study of the ligamentous system of the acromioclavicular joint. *J Bone Joint Surg* (Am) 1986; 68A: 434–40.

Glick JM, Milburn LJ, Haggerty JF, Nishimoto D. Dislocated acromioclavicular joint: Follow-up study of 35 unreduced acromioclavicular dislocations. *Am J Sport Med* 1977; 5: 264–70.

Groh GI, Badwey TM, Rockwood CA. Treatment of cysts of the acromioclavicular joint with shoulder hemiarthroplasty. *J Bone Joint Surg* (Am) 1993; 75A: 1790–4.

Imatani RJ, Hanlon JJ, Cady GW. Acute, complete acromioclavicular separation. *J Bone Joint Surg* (Am) 1975; 57A: 328–32.

Larsen E, Bjerg-Nielsen A, Christensen P. Conservative or surgical treatment of acromioclavicular dislocation. *J Bone Joint Surg* (Am) 1986; 68A: 552–5.

Lizaur A, Marco L, Cebrian R. Acute dislocation of the acromio-clavicular joint. *J Bone Joint Surg* (Br) 1984; 76B: 602–6.

Neviaser JS. Acromioclavicular dislocation treated by transference of the coraco-acromial ligament. *Clin Orthop* 1968; 58: 57–68.

Paavolainen P, Bjorkenheim J-M, Paukku P, Slatis P. Surgical treatment of acromioclavicular dislocation: A review of 39 patients. *Injury* 1983; 14: 415–20.

Phemister DB. The treatment of the acromioclavicular joint by open reduction and threaded-wire fixation. *J Bone Joint Surg* (Am) 1942; 24: 166–8.

Rawes ML, Dias JJ. Long-term results of conservative treatment for acromioclavicular dislocation. *J Bone Joint Surg* (Br) 1996; 78B: 410–12.

Rowe CR. *The Shoulder*. New York: Churchill Livingstone, 1988.

Takagishi K, Yonemoto K, Tsukamoto Y, Itoman M, Yamamoto M. A cautionary note to treatment of complete acromioclavicular separation using artificial materials. *Orthop Int* 1996; 4(5): 343–7.

Tossy JD, Mead NC, Sigmond HM. Acromioclavicular separations: Useful and practical classification for treatment. *Clin Orthop* 1963; 28: 111–19.

Urist MR. Complete dislocations of the cromioclavicular joint. *J Bone Joint Surg* 1946; 28: 813–37.

Weaver JK, Dunn HK. Treatment of acromioclavicular injuries, especially complete acromioclavicular separation. *J Bone Joint Surg* (Am) 1972; 54A: 1187–94.

Warren-Smith CD, Pailthorpe CA, Ward MW. The Weaver–Dunn procedure for the late repair of acromioclavicular dislocation. *J Bone Joint Surg* (Br) 1994; 76B (Supp. I): 39.

Warren-Smith CD, Ward MW. Operation for acromioclavicular dislocation. *J Bone Joint Surg* (Br) 1987; 69B: 715–18.

Chapter 11: The patient with swelling at the sternoclavicular joint

Acus RW, Bell RH, Fisher DL. Proximal clavicle excision: An analysis of results. *J Shoulder Elbow Surg* 1995; 4(3): 182–7.

Beckman T. A case of simultaneous luxation of both ends of the clavicle. *Acta Chir Scand* 1924; 56: 156–63.

Brower AC, Sweet DE, Keats TE. Condensing osteitis of the clavicle: A new entity. *Am J Roentgenol* 1974; 121: 17–21.

Brown JE. Anterior sternoclavicular dislocation. A method of repair. *Am J Orth* 1961; 184–9.

Buckerfield CT, Castle ME. Acute restrosternal dislocation of the clavicle. *J Bone Joint Surg* (Am) 1984; 66A: 379–85.

Chigira M, Maehara S, Nagase M, Ogimi T, Udagawa E. Sternoclavicular hyperostosis. *J Bone Joint Surg* (Am) 1986; 68A: 103–12.

Clark RL, Milgram JW, Yawn DH. Fatal aortic tamponade due to a Kirschner wire migrating from the right sternoclavicular joint. *South Med J* 1974; 67: 316–18.

Daus GP, Drez D, Newton BB, Kober R. Migration of a Kirschner wire from the sternum to the right ventricle. *Am J Sport Med* 1993; 21(2): 321–2.

Denham RH, Dingley AF. Epiphyseal separation of the medial end of the clavicle. *J Bone Joint Surg* (Am) 1967; 49A: 1179–83.

Eskola A, Vainionpää S, Vastamäki M, Slätis P, Rokkanen P. Operation for old sternoclavicular dislocation. *J Bone Joint Surg* (Br) 1989; 71B: 63–5.

Jackson Burrows H. Tenodesis of subclavius in the treatment of recurrent dislocation of the sternoclavicular joint. *J Bone Joint Surg* (Br) 1951; 33B: 240–3.

Kruger GD, Rock MG, Munro TG. Condensing osteitis of the clavicle. *J Bone Joint Surg* (Am) 1987; 69A: 550–7.

Langen. *Virchow's Arch Path Anat.* 1934; 293: 381.

Lewonowski K, Bassett GS. Complete posterior sternoclavicular epiphyseal separation. *Clin Orthop* 1992; 281: 84–8.

Lowman CL. Operative correction of old sternoclavicular dislocation. *J Bone Joint Surg* 1928; 10: 740–1.

Nettles JL, Lindscheid RL. Sternoclavicular dislocations. *J Trauma* 1968; 8(2): 158–64.

Milch H. The Rhomboid Liagament in surgery of the sternoclavicular joint. *J Int Coll Surg* 1952; XVIII(1): 41–51.

Omer GE. Osteotomy of the clavicle in surgical reduction of anterior sternoclavicular dislocation. *J Trauma* 1967; 7(4): 584–90.

Rowe CR. *The Shoulder*. New York: Churchill Livingstone, 1988.

Sanders JO, Lyons FA, Rockwood CA. Management of dislocations of both ends of the clavicle. *J Bone Joint Surg* (Am) 1990; **72**A: 399–402.

Smolle-Juettner FM, Hofer PH, Pinter H, Friehs G, Szyskowitz R. Intracardiac malpositioning of a sternoclavicular fixation wire. *J Orth Trauma* 1992; **6**(1): 102–5.

Treble NJ. Normal variations in radiographs of the clavicle: Brief report. *J Bone Joint Surg* (Br) 1988; **70**B: 490.

Wood VE. The results of total claviculectomy. *Clin Orthop* 1986; **207**: 186–90.

Worman LW, Leagus C. Intrathoracic injury following retrosternal dislocation of the clavicle. *J Trauma* 1967; **7**: 416.

Yasuda MD, Tamura K, Fujiwara M. Tuberculous arthritis of the sternoclavicular joint. *J Bone Joint Surg* (Am) 1995; **77**A: 136–9.

Chapter 12: Management strategies for two- and three-part proximal humeral fractures

Bernstein J, Adler LM, Blank JE *et al*. Evaulation of the Neer system of classification of proximal humeral fractures with computerized tomographic scans and plain radiographs. *J Bone Joint Surg* 1996; **78**(A) 9: 1371–5.

Bigliani LU. Fractures of the shoulder. Part I: Fractures of the proximal hemerus. In: Bucholz RW (eds.) *Fractures in Adults*. Rockwood CA: Green DP, 1991; 881–2.

Brien H, Noftall F, MacMaster S, Cummings T, Rockwood P. Neer's classification system: a critical appraisal. *J Trauma* 1995; **38**(2): 257–60.

Buhr AJ, Cooke AM. Fracture patterns. *Lancet* 1959; 531–6.

Clifford PC. Fractures of the neck of the humerus: a review of the late results. *Injury* 1981; **12**: 91–5.

Constant CR, Murley AHG. A clinical method of functonal assessment of the shoulder. *Clin Orth and Related Research* 1985; **214**: 160–4.

Cornell CN, Levine D, Pagnani MJ. Internal fixation of proximal humerus fractures using the screw-tension band technique. *J Orthop Trauma* 1994; **8**(1): 23–7.

De Laat EAT, Visser DPJ, Coene LNJEM, Pahlplatz PVM, Tavy DLJ. Nerve lesions in primary shoulder dislocations and humeral neck fractures. *J Bone Joint Surg* 1994; **76**B: 381–3.

Esser RD. Treatment of three- and four-part fractures of the proximal humerus with a modified cloverleaf plate. *J Orthop Trauma* 1994; **8**(1): 15–22.

Flatow EL, Cuomo F, Maday MG *et al*. Open reduction and internal fixation of two-part displaced fractures of the greater tuberosity of the proximal part of the humerus. *J Bone Joint Surg* 1991; **73**A(8): 1213–18.

Hawkins RJ, Bell RH, Gurr K. The three-part fracture of the proximal part of the humerus. *J Bone Joint Surg* 1986; **68**A, 9: 1410–14.

Hawkins RJ, Kiefer GN. Internal fixation techniques for proximal humeral fractures. *Clinical Orthop and Related Research* 1987; **223**: 77–85.

Hawkins RJ. Displaced proximal humeral fractures. *Orthopaedics* 1993; **16**(1): 49–54.

Jaberg H, Warner JJP, Jakob RP. Percutaneous stabilization of unstable fractures of the humerus. *J Bone Joint Surg* 1992; **74**(A) 4; 508–15.

Jupiter JB, Mullaji AB. Blade plate fixation of proximal humeral non-unions. *Injury* 1994; **25**(5): 301–3.

Kocialkowski A, Wallace WA. Closed percutaneous K-wire stabilization for displaced fractures of the surgical neck of the humerus. *Injury* 1990; **21**: 209–12.

Kristiansen B. Treatment of displaced fractures of the proximal humerus: Transcutaneous reduction and Hoffmann's external fixation. *Injury* 1989; **20**: 195–9.

Kristiansen B, Christensen SW. Proximal humeral fractures. Late results in relation to classification and treatment. *Act Orthop Scand* 1987; **58**: 124–7.

Lee CK, Hansen HR. Post-traumatic avascular necrosis of the humeral head in desplaced proximal humeral fractures. *J Trauma* 1981; **21**(9): 788–91.

Leyshon RL. Closed treatment of fractures of the proximal humerus. *Acta Orthop Scand* 1984; **55**: 48–51.

Lind T, Krøner K, Jensen J. The epidemiology of fractures of the proximal humerus. *Arch Orthop Trauma Surg* 1989; **108**: 285–7.

Mills HJ, Horne G. Fractures of the proximal humerus in adults. *J Trauma* 1985; **25**: 801–5.

Mouradian WH. Displaced proximal humeral fractures. *Clin Orthop and Related Research* 1986; **212**: 209–18.

Nayak NK, Schickendantz MS, Regan WD, Hawkins RJ. Operative treatment of nonunion of surgical neck fractures of the humerus. *Clin Orthop and Related Research* 1994; **313**: 200–5.

Neer CS. Displaced proximal humeral fractures. Part I. Classification and evaluation. *J Bone Joint Surg* 1970(a); **52**A: 1077–89.

Neer CS. Displaced proximal humeral fractures. Part II. Treatment of three-part and four-part displacement. *J Bone Joint Surg* 1970(b); **52**A: 1090–103.

Neer CS. Fractures and dislocations of the shoulder. In: Rockwood CA, Green DP (eds.) *Fractures in Adults*. Philadelphia: JB Lippincott 1984(c); 675–721.

Rasmussen S, Hvass I, Dalsgaard BS, Holstad E. Displaced proximal humeral fractures: results of conservative treatment. *Injury* 1992; **23**(1): 41–3.

Robinson CM, Christie J. The two-part proximal humeral fracture: A review of operative treatment using two techniques. *Injury* 1993; **24**(2): 123–5.

Sidor ML, Zuckerman JD, Lyon T *et al*. The neer classification system for proximal humeral fractures. *J Bone Joint Surg* 1993; 75A **12**: 1745–50.

Siebenrock KA, Gerber C. The reproducibility of classifcation of fractures of the proximal end of the humerus. *J Bone Joint Surg* 1993; 75A **12**: 1751–5.

Stableforth PG. Four-part fractures of the neck of the humerus. *J Bone Joint Surg* 1984; **66**B: 104–8.

Szyszkowitz R, Seggl W, Schleifer P, Cundy PJ. Proximal humeral fractures. Management techniques and expected results. *Clin Orthop and Related Research* 1993; **292**: 13–25.

Young TB, Wallace WA. Conservative treatment of fractures and fracture-dislocations of the upper end of the humerus. *J Bone Joint Surg* 1985; **67**B (3): 373–7.

Weseley MS, Barenfeld PA, Eisenstein AL. Rush pin intramedullary fixation for fractures of the proximal humerus. *J Trauma* 1977; **17**(1): 29–37.

Zifko B, Poigenfürst J, Pezzei C, Stockley I. Flexible intramedullary pins in the treatment of unstable proximal humeral fractures. *Injury* 1991; **22**(1): 60–2.

Chapter 13: The four-part fracture: rebuild or replace?

Compito CA, Self EB, Bigliani LU. Arthroplasty and acute shoulder trauma. *Clin Orthop* 1994; **307**: 27–36.

Darder A, Darder A Jr., Sanchis V, Gastaldi E, Gomar F. Four-part displaced proximal humeral fractures: Operative treatment using Kirschner wires and tension band. *J Orthop Trauma* 1993; **7**(6): 497–505.

Esser RD. Treatment of three- and four-part fractures of the proximal humerus with a modified cloverleaf plate. *J Orthop Trauma* 1994; **8**(1): 15–22.

Goldman RT, Koval KJ, Cuomo F, Gallagher MA, Zuckerman JD. Functional outcome after humeral head replacement for acute three- and four-part proximal humeral fractures. *J Shoulder Elbow Surg* 1995; **4**(2): 81–6.

Hawkins RJ, Switlyk P. Acute prosthetic replacement for severe fractures of the proximal humerus. *Clinical Orthop and Related Research* 1991; **289**: 156–60.

Jakob RP, Miniaci A, Anson PS *et al*. Four-part valgus impacted fractures of the proximal humerus. *J Bone Joint Surg* 1991; **73**B: 295–8.

Kofoed H. Revascularisation of the humeral head. *Clin Orthop* 1983; **179**: 175–8.

Kraulis J, Hunter G. The results of prosthetic replacement in fracture-dislocations of the upper end of the humerus. *Injury* 1977; **8**: 129–31.

Lee CK, Hansen HR. Post-traumatic avascular necrosis of the humeral head in displaced proximal humeral fractures. *J Trauma* 1981; **21**(9): 788–91.

Leyshon RL. Closed treatment of fractures of the proximal humerus. *Acta Orthop Scand* 1984; **55**: 48–51.

Mouradian WH. Displaced proximal humeral fractures. *Clin Orthop and Related Research* 1986; **212**: 209–18.

Neer CS. Displaced proximal humeral fractures. Part I. Classification and evaluation. *J Bone Joint Surg* 1970(a); **52**A: 1077–89.

Neer CS. Displaced proximal humeral fractures. Part 2. Treatment of three-part and four-part displacement. *J Bone Joint Surg* 1970(b); **52**A: 1090–103.

Rasmussen S. Displaced proximal humeral fractures: Results of conservative treatment. *Injury* 1992; **23**(1): 41–3.

Resch H, Beck E, Bayley I. Reconstruction of the valgus-impacted humeral head fracture. *J Shoulder Elbow Surg* 1995; **42**: 73–80.

Rietveld ABM, Daanen HA, Rozing PM, Obermann WR. The lever arm in glenohumeral abduction after hemiarthroplasty. *J Bone Joint Surg* 1988; **70**B 4: 561–5.

Schai P, Imhoff A, Preiss S. Comminuted humeral head fractures. A multicenter analysis. *J Shoulder Elbow Surg* 1995; **4**(5): 319–30.

Stableforth PG. Four-part fractures of the neck of the humerus. *J Bone Joint Surg* 1984; **66**B: 104–8.

Sturzenegger M, Fornaro E, Jakob RP. Results of surgical treatment of multifragmented fractures of the humeral head. *Arch Orthop Trauma Surg* 1982; **100**: 249–59.

Szyszkowitz R, Seggl W, Schleifer P, Cundy PJ. Proximal humeral fractures. Management techniques and expected results. *Clin Orthop and Related Research* 1993; **292**: 13–25.

Tanner MW, Cofield RH. Prosthetic arthroplasty for fractures and fracture dislocations of the proximal humerus. *Clin Orthop and Related Research* 1983; **179**: 116–29.

Chapter 14: Fractures of the clavicle

Allman FL. Fractures and ligamentous injuries of the clavicle and its articulations. *J Bone Joint Surg* 1967; **49**A: 774–84.

Anderson K, Østergaard Jensen P, Lauritzen J. Treatment of clavicular fractures. *Acta Orthop Scand* 1987; **57**: 71–4.

Ballmer FT, Gerber C. Coraco-clavicular screw fixation for unstable fractures of the distal clavicle. *J Bone Joint Surg* 1991; **73**B: 291–4.

Bartosh RA, Dugdale TW, Nielsen R. Isolated musculo-cutaneous nerve injury complicating closed fracture of the clavicle. *Am J Sports Med* 1992; **20**(3): 356–9.

Boehme D, Curtis RJ, DeHaan JT *et al*. Non-union of fractures of the mid-shaft of the clavicle. *J Bone Joint Surg* 1991; **73**A (8): 1219–25.

Capicotto PN, Heiple KG, Wilbur JH. Midshaft clavicle nonunions treated with intramedullary steinman pin fixation and onlay bone graft. *J Orthop Trauma* 1994; **8**(2): 88–93.

Edwards DJ, Kavanagh TG, Flannery Mc. Fractures of the distal clavicle: A case for fixation. *Injury* 1992; **23**(1): 44–6.

Eskola A, Vainiopää S, Myllynen P, Pätiälä H, Rokkanen P. Surgery for ununited clavicular fracture. *Acta Orthop Scand* 1986; **57**: 366–7.

Fagg PS. The shoulder. In: Foy MA, Fagg PS (eds.) *Medicolegal Reporting in Orthopaedic Trauma*. Churchill Livingstone, 1990; **42**.

Gerber C, Schneeberger AG, Vinh T-S. The arterial vascularization of the humeral head. An anatomical study. *J Bones Joint Surg* 1990; **72**(10): 1486–94.

Howard FM, Shafer SJ. Injuries to the clavicle with neurovascular complications. *J Bone Joint Surg* 1965; **47**A (7): 1335–46.

Jupiter JB, Leffert RD. *J Bone Joint Surg* 1987; **69**A (5): 753–60.

Kona J, Bosse M, Staeheli JW, Rosseau RL. Type II distal clavicle fractures: A retrospective review of surgical treatment. *J Orthop Trauma* 1990; **4**(2): 115–20.

Manske DJ, Szabo RM. The operative treatment of mid-shaft clavicular non-unions. *J Bone Joint Surg* 1985; **67**A (9): 1367–71.

Marsh HO, Hazarian E. Pseudarthrosis of the Clavicle. *J Bone Joint Surg Proceedings* 1970; **52**B: 793.

Middleton SB, Foley SJ, Foy MA. Partial excision of the clavicle for nonunion in national hunt jockey. *J Bone Joint Surg* 1995; **77**B: 778–80.

Miller DS, Boswick JA. Lesions of the brachial plexus associated with fractures of the clavicle. *Clin Orthop and Related Research* 1969; **64**: 144–7.

Mullaji AB, Jupiter JB. Low-contact dynamic compression plating of the clavicle. *Injury* 1994; **25**(1): 41–5.

Neer CS. Fractures of the distal third of the clavicle. *Clin Orthop and Related Research* 1968; **58**: 43–50.

Neer CS. Fractures and dislocations of the shoulder. In: Rockwood CA, Green DP (eds.) *Fractures in Adults*. JB Lippincott Publishers, Philadelphia, 1984; 675–721.

Neviaser RJ. Injuries to the clavicle and acromioclavicular joint. *Orthop Clin North Am* 1987; **18**(3): 433–8.

Nordqvist A, Petersson C. The incidence of fractures of the clavicle. *Clin Orthop and Related Research* 1994; **300**: 127–32.

Nordqvist A, Petersson C, Redlund-Johnell I. The natural course of lateral clavicle fracture. *Acta Orthop Scand* 1993; **64**(1): 87–91.

Poigenfürst J, Rappold G, Fischer W. Plating of fresh clavicular fractures: results of 122 operations 1992; **23**(4): 237–41.

Post M. Current concepts in the treatment of fractures of the clavicle. *Clin Orthop and Related Research* 1988; **245**: 89–101.

Schuind F, Pay-Pay E, Andrianne Y *et al*. External fixation of the clavicle for fracture of non-union in adults. *J Bone Joint Surg* 1988; **70**A (5): 692–5.

Schwarz N, Höcker K. Osteosynthesis of irreducible fractures of the clavicle with 2.7 mm ASIF plates 1992; **33**(2): 179–83.

Stanley D, Trowbridge EA, Norris SH. The mechanism of clavicular fracture. *J Bone Joint Surg* 1988; **70**B (3): 461–4.

Stanley D, Norris SH. Recovery following fractures of the clavicle treated conservatively. *Injury* 1988; **19**: 162–4.

Tse DH, Slabaugh PB, Carlson PA. Injury to the axillary artery by a closed fracture of the clavicle. A case report. *J Bone Joint Surg* 1980; **62**A (8): 1372–4.

Ideberg R. Fractures of the scapula involving the glenoid fossa. In: Bateman JE, Welsh RP (eds.) *Surgery of the Shoulder*. Philadelphia: BC Decker, 1984; 63–6.

Kavanagh BF, Bradway JK, Cofield RH. Open reduction and internal fixation of displaced intra-articular fractures of the glenoid fossa. *J Bone Joint Surg* 1993; **75**A(4): 479–84.

Kuhn JE, Blasier RB, Carpenter JE. Fractures of the acormion: A proposed classification system. *J Orthop Trauma* 1994; **8**(1): 6–13.

Leung KS, Lam TP, Poon KM. Operative treatment of displaced intra-articular glenoid fractures. *Injury* 1993; **24**(5): 324–8.

Leung KS, Lam TP. Open reduction and internal fixation of ipsilateral fractures of the scapular neck and clavicle. *J Bone Joint Surg* 1993; **75**A (7): 1015–18.

Müller ME, Allgöwer M, Schneider R, Willenegger H. *Manual of Internal Fixation*. 3rd edition. Springer-Verlag, 1991.

Nordqvist A, Petersson C. Fracture of the body, neck, or spine of the scapula. *Clin Orthop and Related Research* 1992; **283**: 139–44.

Ogawa K, Yoshida A, Takahashi M, Ui M. Fractures of the coracoid process. *J Bone Joint Surg* 1997; **79**B (1): 17–19.

Oni OOA, Hoskinson J. The 'stove-in shoulder': Results of treatment by early mobilization. *Injury* 1992; **23**(7): 444–6.

Robinson CM, Court-Brown CM. Non-union of the scapula spine fracture treated by bone graft and plate fixation. *Injury* 1993; **24**(6): 428–9.

Wallace WA. The shoulder. In: Colton CL, Hall AJ (eds.) *Atlas of Orthopaedic Surgical Approaches*. 1991; **9**: 134–46.

Chapter 15: The fractured scapula

Ada JR, Miller ME. Scapular fractures. Analysis of 113 cases. *Clin Orthop and Related Research* 1991; **269**: 174–80.

Armstrong CP, Van der Spuy. The fractured scapula: Importance and management based on a series of 62 patients. *Injury* 1984; **15**: 324–9.

Aulicino PL, Reinert C, Kornberg M, Williamson S. Displaced intra-articular glenoid fractures treated by open reduction and internal fixation. *J Trauma* 1986; **26**(12): 1137–41.

Bauer G, Fleischmann W, Dußler E. Displaced scapular fractures: Indication and long-term results of open reduction and internal fixation. *Arch Orthop Trauma Surg* 1995; **114**: 214–19.

Eyres KS, Brooks A, Stanley D. Fractures of the coracoid process. *J Bone Joint Surg* 1995; **77**B (3): 425–8.

Goss TP. Fractures of the glenoid cavity. *J Bone Joint Surg* 1992; **74**A (2): 299–305.

Hall RJ, Calvert PT. Stress fracture of the acromion: An unusual mechanism and review of the literature. *J Bone Joint Surg* 1994; **77**B (1): 153–4.

Hardegger FH, Simpson LA, Weber BG. The operative treatment of scapular fractures. *J Bone Joint Surg* 1984; **66**A–B (5): 725–9.

Hersovici D, Sanders R, DiPasquale T, Gregory P. Injuries of the shoulder girdle. *Clin Orthop and Related Research* 1992; **318**: 54–60.

Ho KMT, Schranz PJ, Wallace WA. 'Stress' fracture of the scapula. *Injury* 1993; **24**(7): 498.

Chapter 16: Paralysis and dystrophy around the shoulder

Bigliani LU, Perez Sanz JR, Wolfe IN. Treatment of trapezius palsy. *J Bone Joint Surg* 1985; **67**A: 871–7.

Birch R. Nerves of the thoracoscapular and glenohumeral joints. In: Copland S (ed.) *Operative Shoulder Surgery*. New York: Churchill Livingston 1995.

Flowers MJ, Cowling P. Brachial neuritis after human parvovirus B19 infection. *J Shoulder Elbow Surg* 1993; **2**: 321–3.

Frostick S. Compression of the long thoracic nerve. 9th Congress of the European Society for Surgery of the Shoulder and Elbow. Nottingham (UK), 19–21 September, 1996.

Kaupilla LI. The long thoracic nerve: possible mechanisms of injury based on an autopsy study. *J Shoulder Elbow Surg* 1993; **2**: 244–8.

Manning P, Frostick SP, Wallace WA. *Winging of the Scapula, a Fresh Look at the Long Thoracic Nerve. 9th Congress of the European Society for Shoulder and Elbow Surgery*, 19–21 September 1996, Nottingham UK.

Narakas AO. Obstetrical brachial plexus injuries. In: Lamb DW (ed.) *The Paralysed Hand*. Edinburgh: Churchill Livingstone 1987.

Post M. Pectoralis major transfer for winging of the scapula. *J Shoulder Elbow Surgery* 1995(a); **4**: 1–9.

Post M. Operative repair of suprascapular nerve entrapment. In: Craig EV (ed.) Master Techniques in Orthopaedic Surgery: *The Shoulder*. New York: Raven Press Ltd 1995.

Spillane JD. Localised neuritis of the shoulder girdle. *Lancet* 1943; **ii**: 532–5.

Thompson J. Thoracic outlet syndromes. *Br J Surg* 1996; **83**: 435–6.

Vastamaki M, Kaupilla LI. Aetiological factors in isolated paralysis of the serratus anterior muscle. *J Shoulder Elbow Surg* 1993; **2**: 240–3.

Index

A